RECONCILABLE DIFFERENCES

RECONCILABLE
DIFFERENCES

Andrew Christensen, PhD
and
Neil S. Jacobson, PhD

THE GUILFORD PRESS
New York   London

© 2000 The Guilford Press
A Division of Guilford Publications, Inc.
72 Spring Street, New York, NY 10012
http://www.guilford.com

Printed in the United States of America

This book is printed on acid-free paper.

Last digit is print number: 9 8 7 6 5 4 3 2

Library of Congress Cataloging-in-Publication Data

Christensen, Andrew.
    Reconcilable differences / by Andrew Christensen and
  Neil Jacobson.
       p.   cm.
    Includes bibliographical references and index.
    ISBN 1-57230-261-5 (hardcover)
    1. Conflict management. 2. Couples. 3. Man–woman
  relationships. 4. Interpersonal communication.
  5. Interpersonal relations.   I. Jacobson, Neil S.
  II. Title.
  HM1126.C48   1999
  303.6 9—dc21   99-41183
                                                       CIP

During the production phase of this book, Neil S. Jacobson died suddenly and unexpectedly. His death is an incalculable loss to his family and friends and to the three fields in which he was a leading scholar and researcher: marital therapy, domestic violence, and depression.

As his close collaborator and friend for years, I will miss him terribly. This book is dedicated to his honor and memory.

—A. C.

Contents

PART II. From Argument to Acceptance

PART III. Deliberate Change through Acceptance

PART IV. When Acceptance Is Not Enough

Acknowledgments

*T*here are those who influenced my ideas, those who helped me articulate them in this book, those who helped me implement these ideas with couples, and those who helped me live the reality of these ideas. All deserve acknowledgment.

Clearly my coauthor, Neil Jacobson, has had the foremost influence on my ideas about couple therapy. Through years of productive discussion, joint writing projects, and joint supervision of our clinicians, we have developed and refined our approach to couple therapy. We each might have been able to develop this approach alone, but not nearly as well and not nearly as enjoyably. Aside from Neil, other important influences on my thinking were Robert Weiss, a father of behavioral couple therapy and my first marital therapy supervisor; Gayla Margolin, with whom I conducted my first clinical study of marital therapy; Harold Kelley, an influential social psychologist; and Dan Wile, whose clinical writings, though coming from a dramatically different theoretical perspective, directly influenced my own work with couples. And finally, the couples with whom I worked, either directly in my private practice or indirectly by watching hours of their therapy sessions on videotape, were a continued challenge to my thinking and a repeated reminder that the dirty and tender reality of conflict and love is always more complicated than our theories envision.

My editor at The Guilford Press, Christine Benton, was an enormous help in translating my ideas into ink. She understood what I was trying to say about acceptance in relationships, and she kept the rudder of this book clearly on that course. She helped me say what I wanted to say—which is all that anyone can ask of an editor. I also want to thank Melissa Fu and Betty Horng for their secretarial assistance with this book. They cheerfully worked on the manuscript as it went through its various drafts.

The therapists on our project, in both Los Angeles and Seattle, brought the ideas of our treatment approach to bear on the lives of our struggling couples. Alfredo Crespo, Shelly Harrell, Megan Sullaway, and Anthony Zamudio, in Los Angeles, and Peter Fehrenbach, Carol Henry, Christopher Martel, and Debra Wilk, in Seattle, are talented therapists who have the special skill of attending to the research demands of our project without letting it interfere with the clinical needs of each case. The graduate student coordinators, Kathleen Eldridge at UCLA and Sara Berns at the University of Washington, are remarkably able administrators of the day-to-day operations of the research project. They helped the project get up and going and now make sure that it runs smoothly and happily. I also want to thank my other graduate students at UCLA, Brian Doss, Amanda Jensen, and Janice Jones, who skillfully recruit, screen, and assess couples. These graduate students at UCLA and the University of Washington not only make the project run, they have contributed conceptually and clinically to it. Finally, Betty Horng's efficiency and care have ensured a smoothly running project.

And finally, I want to thank those who have helped me live my ideas of conflict, acceptance, and intimacy in a true learning laboratory of love, our home: my wife, Louise; my daughter, Lisa; and my son, Sean.

ANDREW CHRISTENSEN

Just as my coauthor, Andy Christensen, has acknowledged me, I want to acknowledge him, first and foremost. Since 1991, when our collaboration began, Andy has been a friend and an ideal collaborator. To loosely paraphrase Humphrey Bogart in *Casablanca,* this was the start of a beautiful collaboration/friendship. Although I had been actively engaged in couple therapy research since 1972, the post-Christensen era definitely represents the most rewarding nine years of that history. Andy and I worked together so well because we shared a deep conviction that couple therapy could be more than it had been up until that time. Andy understands the workings of intimate relationships as no other collaborator of mine ever has, and his clinical acumen is matched with the highest level of integrity as well as scientific rigor. In the creation of this new form of couple therapy, I feel like I have found my true soul mate.

The insights of other couple therapists have also been instrumental to the development of our approach. Dan Wile and Susan Johnson deserve special mention. I have also benefited from an unusually competent group of graduate students: Stacey Prince and James Cordova were involved in our initial pilot study, which showed the promise of this approach; more recently, Sara Berns, Jennifer Wheeler, and Dave Atkins have made important contributions at both the clinical and the conceptual levels. In particular, Sara Berns has shown great dedication and clinical skill in her coordination of our current study; her scientific leadership has resulted in one of the smoothest run studies I have ever been associated with. In Seattle, I have also been fortunate to be associated with an outstanding group of research therapists: Christopher Martell, Debra Wilk, Carol Henry, and Peter Fehrenbach. Peter has also played an invaluable role as a clinical supervisor. Finally, I want to acknowledge the contribution of my extraordinarily skilled administrative assistant, Catherine Holmes, who has a unique combination of qualities without which our work would have been much more difficult; her high level of administrative skills and her interpersonal qualities, which include a keen intelligence, wit, and people skills, helped us get through hard times.

This book and the project as a whole have been a labor of love. Everyone mentioned here was indispensable to its success.

NEIL S. JACOBSON

Preface

No matter how much we have in common with the one we love, each of us remains a unique human being. And no matter how much we love each other, the differences between us will eventually cause conflict. We feel hurt or ignored, resentful or angry, and our arguments often make the problem worse. Something's got to give, and we usually nominate our partner.

Sound familiar? If so, you're not alone. Trying to get your partner to change when strife seems to be pulling your relationship apart is human nature. It's easy to understand your own point of view; it's much harder to see where the one you love is coming from. That your relationship would improve drastically if only he or she would see things your way and make a few little alterations in behavior seems like an obvious conclusion.

As you undoubtedly know, however, trying to change another person, even one motivated by love and loyalty toward you, is a tall order. Eliciting change from your spouse without demonstrating acceptance of his or her unique position is difficult, often impossible, as we have learned through over two decades of clinical practice and research in the field of couple therapy.

When we met twenty-three years ago, we were both proponents of the behavioral approach to couple therapy in which we had been trained. This type of therapy teaches couples communication and problem-solving skills so that partners can make positive changes in their behavior toward each other. In studies conducted in North America, Germany, Australia, and elsewhere, the behavioral approach has proved superior in helping couples improve their degree of satisfaction and reduce the conflict in their relationship compared to getting no treatment at all. The efficacy of the behavioral approach is also supported by more research than any other therapy for couples. Neil became a leading exponent of this type of couple therapy and produced some of the best research studies showing its effectiveness. However, his studies and those of others showed the limitations of this approach: a good third of couples did not respond to the treatment, and even among those who did respond positively, a substantial number relapsed in the years following treatment. From a scientific standpoint, the best available wasn't that good.

In 1991, when Neil invited me to speak at the University of Washington, we discovered that we had, separately and simultaneously, started to experiment with a different approach to couples in conflict. Though they were not identical, our interventions had one thing in common: the promotion of acceptance over change. We had developed ways in which partners could experience and accept the normal vulnerabilities that we all have and the very natural incompatibilities that crop up between two unique individuals. With this acceptance, something paradoxical often occurred: many of the needs and demands for change evaporated, and each partner became more amenable to making the changes that were truly important to the other.

We decided to combine forces in developing our new treatment and in seeking a grant that would allow us to test its effectiveness. In 1993 we obtained a three-year grant from the National Institute of Mental Health to conduct a small pilot study comparing our treatment against traditional behavioral couple therapy. As part of our pilot study, we trained five therapists in our new approach, which we called integrative couple therapy, as well as in the traditional behavioral approach. Twenty-one distressed couples were randomly assigned to one of the two approaches and received up to twenty-six sessions of therapy. Based on extensive evaluations of these couples prior to treatment, immediately after treatment, and at follow-up periods, the couples in our integrative treatment performed substantially better than those in the traditional treatment, even though they, as expected, also showed improvement.

Encouraged by these results, we knew that only a larger study with a more diverse sample of couples and more extensive evaluation and follow-up would prove that our treatment was superior to behavioral couple therapy. In 1997 we received funding from the National Institute of Mental Health for a five-year study of 180 couples, which to our knowledge will be the largest and most extensive evaluation of couple therapy conducted to date. All couples who receive our integrative couple therapy get this book as a companion manual to their treatment. Although it does not come with one of the therapists we have trained, we believe that couples can use this book to lessen conflict and increase intimacy in their relationships on their own.

Our study is focused exclusively on married couples, albeit a diverse sample of married couples, and so this book is written with spouses in mind. But we have also used this approach successfully with unmarried couples. Indeed, we believe that as long as both partners are committed to the relationship, the same principles apply. The universal themes of conflict and closeness that enter all romantic relationships make this book widely relevant whether you are married or living together; heterosexual, gay, or lesbian partners. Because of its underlying principle of acceptance, couples from different ethnicities and backgrounds should find it adaptable to their needs.

If there is one thing we have discovered in our years of work with couples, it is that advice is easy to give, hard to take, and even harder to implement. Although this book is aimed at ushering you both toward an understanding of how couples interact, what causes conflict, and how you might lessen yours, it purposely avoids "sounds-good," "one-size-fits-all" advice. Instead, we guide you toward an understanding of your own unique relationship and suggest ways to foster acceptance. To bring our points home, we have filled the pages with illustrations of couples facing problems a lot like yours. As the primary author of this book, I have generated these examples from my own practice, my supervision of couple therapy, and my personal experience, but each is a constructed amalgam so as to protect the confidentiality of any real couple.

Because conflict is a window on the vulnerabilities and sensitivities of warring partners, it offers the promise of greater connection as well as the threat of alienation. We believe that by understanding your conflicts and emotionally accepting your positions in the conflict, the two of you can achieve genuine intimacy. You can, in the end, reconcile the differences that keep you apart.

ANDREW CHRISTENSEN

RECONCILABLE DIFFERENCES

CHAPTER 1

Three Sides
to Every Story

DEBRA'S STORY

How long can you be married to a stranger? Looks like I may be about to set a record of some kind.

After eight years of marriage and almost two years of courtship before that—ten years of being together—I still can't communicate with Frank. The problem is, he doesn't listen to me. He never shares his feelings with me, just turns off, withdraws. I hardly ever can figure out what's going on with him.

It's gotten to the point where I feel closer to Joan, a woman I've been working with for just a year, than I do to Frank. At least I never have to wonder what she's thinking or feeling—she lets me know. A coffee break with her is always stimulating because we have so much to say and so little time to say it. We're so tuned in to each other, we even finish each other's sentences sometimes.

It's completely different with Frank. We are intimate in some ways, of course. I know his body very well, from years of stroking and exploring. And from his grunts and moans, I've figured out his sexual preferences pretty well. I could write a book about his personal habits: the obsessive way he flosses his teeth, the careful way he blow-dries his hair to cover his bald spot, the meticulous way he lines up his clothes in the closet.

But I sure don't know what he's thinking and feeling most of the time. He gets this look that's part tired, part concerned, part preoccupied. But when I ask him if anything's wrong, he says "No." When I ask him what he's feeling, he says, "Tired." When I ask him what he's thinking about, he says, "Work." If I ask him *what* about work, he says, "Just some problems." All his answers seem perfunctory and dutiful, like he doesn't want to tell me but has to. He might as well say it right out: "I don't want to talk about this anymore." He'd rather watch a stupid sitcom on TV than connect with his own wife.

Sometimes I wonder if he even *has* any feelings other than tiredness. (Is that really a feeling?) He just plods through life, always taking care of business, preoccupied with getting his work done but never showing much excitement or pain. He says his style shows how emotionally stable he is. I say it just shows he's passive and bored.

In many ways I'm just the opposite: I have a lot of ups and downs. But most of the time I'm energetic, optimistic, spontaneous. Of course I get upset, angry, and frustrated sometimes. He says this range of feeling shows I'm emotionally immature, that "I have a lot of growing up to do." I think it just shows I'm human.

I do share most of my thoughts and feelings with him: my problems at work, my reactions to my friends, my emotional highs and lows. His response to all this? A sort of bland tolerance most of the time—sometimes interested, sometimes not, sometimes just going along out of habit, sometimes. . . . I really don't know. How can I, when he doesn't tell me what's going on with him? So I just ramble on, feeling more and more like I'm talking to myself. The chatterbox wife with the bored husband.

It wasn't like this at first. He was never very open, but he enjoyed listening to me. And he would tell me things about himself. In the beginning, even though the communication between us was never balanced, it was at least mutual. I thought he'd eventually get more comfortable with me and confide in me more, but he actually confides less now than when we first met!

His lack of communication bothers me most when we disagree about something. I want to discuss our differences and try to work out a solution. I expect conflict in a close relationship; I'm not threatened by it; and I want to deal with it openly. But Frank won't even discuss it. At the first sign of tension, he runs. He offers some feeble platitude like "Things will work themselves out."

I think the root of our problem is Frank's sensitivity to criticism and anger. He can't stand any suggestion that he might have done something wrong, especially if I show that I'm angry about it. What does he think a close relationship is, some continuous recording of soft Muzak? He's not perfect, I'm not perfect—we're different people with different needs. So of course we're going to get angry sometimes. That doesn't mean we don't love each other. Yet whenever I get critical or angry, he acts as if I've violated some sacred law of nature. And then he gets even more critical and angry at me (for being critical and angry at him) than I was with him in the first place.

I remember one incident that kind of sums up the way I see Frank. We went out to dinner with a couple who had just moved to town. The husband was a friend of one of Frank's college roommates, and the evening started out great. They were a charming couple, and since we'd never met and they were new in town, we had a lot to talk about. As the evening wore on, I became more and more aware of how wonderful their life was. They seemed genuinely in love with one another, even though they had been married longer than we have. No matter how much the man talked to us, he always kept in contact with his wife: touching her, or making eye contact with her, or including her in the conversation. And he used "we" a lot to refer to them. Watching them made me realize how little Frank and I touch, how rarely we look at each other, and how separately we participate in a conversation. We hardly ever mention "we" or "us." I wanted to put my hand on Frank's knee or hold his hand, just to have the look of two couples. But I was afraid Frank wouldn't respond or, worse, give me that look that says "Not now!" Sometimes I think he is embarrassed to be with me.

Anyway, I admit it. I was envious of this other couple. And to make matters worse, they had *money*. Of course, they were much too polite to mention it, but as they casually referred to the private schools their kids went to and the vacations that they took, I realized that they were not struggling to get by. After dinner, we went back to their place, and their house was incredible—not ostentatious, but tasteful, classy, and expensive, with some beautiful antique furniture and some oriental rugs that I was tempted to steal. We once looked for a house in their neighborhood, but we couldn't afford even the least expensive ones.

They seemed to have it all: loving family, beautiful home, leisure, luxury. What a contrast to Frank and me: struggling along, both working full-time jobs, trying to save money, sometimes barely managing to pay the bills. I wouldn't mind that so much, if only we worked at it *together*. But we're so distant. Even though we have similar goals in mind, it doesn't feel like we're on the same team.

When we got home, I started expressing those feelings. I wanted to reevaluate our life—as a way of getting closer. I don't like the materialistic side of myself; envying other people's wealth makes me feel shallow. I thought maybe we needed to adjust our priorities, not struggle so much for the almighty dollar. Maybe we couldn't be as wealthy as these people, but there was no reason we couldn't have the closeness and warmth they had.

As usual, Frank didn't want to talk about it. When he said he was tired and wanted to go to bed, I got angry. It was Friday night, and neither of us had to get up early the next day; the only thing keeping us from being together was his stubbornness. It made me mad. I was fed up with giving in to his need for sleep whenever I brought up an issue to discuss. I thought, Why can't he stay awake just for me sometimes?

I wouldn't let him sleep. When he turned off the lights, I turned them back on. When he rolled over to go to sleep, I kept talking. When he put a pillow over his head, I talked louder. He told me I was a baby. I told him he was insensitive. It escalated from there and got ugly. No violence but lots of words. He finally went to the guest bedroom, locked the door from the inside, and went to sleep.

The next morning we were both worn out and distant. He criticized me for being so irrational. Which was probably true. I do get irrational when I get desperate. But I think he uses that accusation as a way of justifying himself. It's sort of like "If you're irrational, then I can dismiss all your complaints and I am blameless." But I didn't make much of a protest. I just thought, What's the use?

FRANK'S STORY

Debra never seems to be satisfied. I'm never doing enough, never giving enough, never loving enough, never sharing enough. You name it, I don't do enough of it. There's a line from an old song that goes "Too much is not enough." That's Debra.

Or to put it another way, I sometimes think of the old Dylan song, "Too Much of Nothing." Debra sometimes acts like everything I do to please her amounts to nothing. I get no credit for what I do for her.

Sometimes she gets me believing I really am a bad husband. I start feeling as though I've let her down, disappointed her, not met my obligations as a loving, supportive husband. But then I give myself a dose of reality. What have I done that's wrong? I'm an okay human being. People usually like me, respect me. I hold down a responsible job. I don't cheat on her or lie to her. I'm not a drunk or a gambler. I'm moderately attractive, and I'm a sensitive lover. I even make her laugh a lot. Yet I don't get an ounce of appreciation from her—just complaints that I'm not doing enough.

I think she must be insecure. She wants constant reassurance. I told her once in desperation, "Look. I love you. Until further notice to the contrary, you can assume that I still love you. I promise to inform you of any change in the status of these feelings. You don't need to keep checking in." Maybe she's bored with her life. She's always looking for high drama and excitement in the relationship. It's really a soap-opera view of love, where everything has to be heavy and emotional. But I want our relationship to be a place where I can retreat from the stresses and demands of my life, not one more addition to them.

She's always asking me how I'm feeling. The truth is, sometimes I'm not feeling a damn thing. She seems to assume that my emotions are always bubbling and that I'm just stingy in refusing to share my inner life with her. But that's not the way it is. Often I'm exhausted from work and just want to vegetate. I'll flip on the TV, plop down on the sofa, suck on a beer, and "veg out." It doesn't matter what program is on—give me a good sitcom over PBS any day. Heck, I even like the commercials. I'm like a sponge, just soaking up sensations from the tube. I'm not there for intellectual stimulation or social chitchat. Maybe one of these days I'll start growing vines from my ears, as Debra suggests. But to me it's relaxing. Now I ask you: Is what I'm doing morally wrong? Is it constitutionally forbidden? Is it a positive sign of decadence? To hear Debra, you'd certainly think so.

Don't get me wrong. I'm not always exhausted or stressed out. In fact, I think I pace myself rather well—especially compared to Debra. I organize my life so I'm prepared for the demands and stresses that go with my job and my home life. I'm not thrown by events the way Debra is. Her feelings are like a roller coaster: sometimes up, sometimes down. I can't live that way. A nice steady cruising speed is more my style.

But I don't put Debra down for being the way she is. I'm basically a tolerant person. People, including spouses, come in all shapes and sizes. They aren't tailored to fit your particular needs. So I don't take offense at little annoyances; I don't feel compelled to talk about every difference or dislike; I don't feel every potential area of disagreement has to be explored in detail. I just let things ride.

When I show that kind of tolerance, I expect my partner to do the same for me. When she doesn't, I get furious. When Debra picks at me about every detail that doesn't fit with her idea of what's right, I do react strongly. My cool disappears, and I explode.

Debra accuses me of being an emotional pack rat, of storing bad feelings until an opportune time, but that's not true. I don't go around dwelling on whatever injustices or irritations I've had to put up with. I don't hoard them in secret until I can reveal them in some dramatic display. But when I'm criticized for some small thing, I suddenly remember what I've suffered without a word, and I get furious at the injustice of it.

I can handle most of my problems myself. I don't lay them on other people, and I don't hold others responsible for solving my problems. Debra can't seem to understand that there are certain things that I can only work through alone.

I remember driving home with Debra after a night out with a couple we had just met. The husband was a friend of my college roommate, Willie. They were an attractive, impressive couple. He had come to town to manage one of our commercial banks; she had joined one of our family law firms. I was surprised that old goofball Willie, whom I had always thought of as sort of shallow, had such interesting and classy friends.

On the way home I was wondering what kind of impression I'd made on them. I was tired that evening and not at my best. Sometimes I can be clever and funny in a small group, but not that night. Maybe I was trying too hard. Sometimes I have high standards for myself and get down on myself when I can't come up to them. But this other couple wasn't particularly clever either. Maybe we were all sizing each other up, like on a first date. I never much liked first dates, always wanted to get past them to the comfortable stage.

Debra interrupted my ruminations with a seemingly innocent question: "Did you notice how much in tune those two were with each other?" Now I know what's behind that kind of question—or at least where that kind of question will lead. It always leads right back to us, specifically to me. Eventually the point becomes "We aren't in tune with each other," which is code for "You're not in tune with me."

I dread these conversations that chew over what's wrong with us as a couple, because the real question, which goes unstated in the civil conversations, but gets stated bluntly in the uncivil ones, is "What's wrong with Frank?" So I sidestepped the issue on this occasion by answering that they were a nice couple.

But Debra pushed it. She insisted on evaluating them in comparison to us. They had money and intimacy. We had neither. Maybe we couldn't be wealthy, but we could at least be intimate. Why couldn't we be intimate? Meaning: Why couldn't *I* be intimate? I tried to lighten up the conversation, suggesting that maybe we lacked an intimacy gene. She was not amused.

When we got home, I tried to defuse the tension by saying I was tired and suggesting that we go to bed. I *was* tired, and the last thing I wanted was one of these conversations. But Debra was relentless. She argued that there was no reason we couldn't stay up and discuss this. She often acts like my fatigue is just an excuse.

I proceeded with my bedtime routine, giving her the most minimal of responses. If she won't respect my feelings, why should I respect hers? She talked at me while I put on my pajamas and brushed my teeth; she wouldn't even let me alone in the bathroom. When I finally got into bed and turned off the light, she turned it back on. I rolled over to go to sleep, but she kept talking. You'd think she'd have gotten the message when I put the pillow over my head—but no, she pulled it off. At that point I lost it. I told her she was a baby, a crazy person—I don't remember everything I said. Finally, in desperation, I went to the guest bedroom and locked it from the inside. I was too upset to go to sleep right away, and I didn't sleep well at all.

In the morning, I was still angry at her. I told her she was irrational. For once, she didn't have much to say. The truth is, we were both exhausted.

AN OUTSIDER'S STORY

The differences that Frank and Debra find so upsetting in each other were there from the beginning. Debra was emotional and moody. She formed close ties to others and got emotional support and stimulation from these relationships. Her style was to speak her mind and be open about her feelings.

Frank, on the other hand, was shy and private. An only child, he had grown up an outsider, with few friends. To this day, he didn't like to socialize much and often felt uncomfortable in the presence of others. He sought security, not so much in the company of others, but in a stable, organized, rational life. You could always depend on Frank. His checkbook was always balanced, literally and figuratively. His life was a lesson in the avoidance of excess.

Frank and Debra had much in common: similar backgrounds, almost identical values, and some common interests in sports. They found each other physically attractive, and even the differences between them were a source of attraction. Frank's calm manner was a nice balance for Debra's moodiness, while her comfort in social situations allowed him to be private but still take part in the conversation. Frank's penchant for organization helped Debra lead a less frenetic pace, while her optimism and enthusiasm added energy to his plodding style.

Ideally, these differences would have brought them to a happy medium. Frank might have learned to be more open about how he felt, while Debra might have become more comfortable with privacy and time alone. He might have developed a more zestful, spontaneous approach to life, while she might have learned to pace herself. He might have become more comfortable in social situations, while she might have learned to value the peace and quiet of solitude.

Because the contrasts between them at first seemed appealing, Frank and Debra appreciated them and were open to mutual influence and change early in their relationship. However, in time, their own needs and the inability of the other to satisfy them made those already existing differences larger. Frank's need for time alone conflicted with Debra's need for time together. The more he sought independence, the more she pressed for closeness. The more emotional she became, the more he "turned off." Before long, she began to see his shyness as inadequacy, his careful, deliberate style as boring, and his reluctance to communicate as lack of love. He began to see her emotionality as immaturity, her energetic tempo as exhausting, and her desire for closeness as weakness.

Their differences then became a source of argument, featuring criticism, defensiveness, withdrawal, and counterattack. Given her greater comfort with communication, especially negative communication, Debra was more likely to start a conversation about their differences by expressing her needs or feelings. But Frank felt criticized by her statements—partly because they often *were* critical and partly because he was already sensitive to criticism and had become more so during the course of his relationship with Debra.

For example, Debra's comments about the other couple on the way home from their evening out seemed to Frank a statement about him—one carrying the strong implication that he wasn't as "in tune" with Debra as their new male friend was with his wife. It's hardly surprising that Frank took the comment as a criticism, since she has criticized him many times for not being sensitive to her. Debra has often complained, with some justification, that Frank is not attentive and involved enough with her. So, although her remark about the other couple was heard by Frank as a criticism, criticism was not what she had intended. In fact, her feeling at the time was more envy of their friends than concern with her husband or herself. However, their past conflicts over intimacy and being "in tune" with each other, plus Frank's acquired sensitivity to Debra's criticism, led him to take her comment personally.

Because Frank feared an ugly argument with Debra, he sidestepped her comment. Sometimes diversions like this work for Frank because they bypass the conversation and avert an argument. However, sometimes—as on this occasion—his tactics frustrate Debra and contribute to the very conflict he is trying to prevent. The more he withdraws, the angrier she gets. What little conversation they have consists of mutual attacks and defensive maneuvers. So destructive does their behavior become that they fail to recognize the feelings they have in common. On this particular evening, for example, they were both envious of their new friends.

As Debra and Frank's problems have accumulated, each has developed a theory of how the other's difficulties are damaging the relationship. They each think the other is at fault, and thus they both selectively remember parts of their life, focusing on those parts that support their own points of view. For example, Debra thinks Frank is socially awkward and afraid of intimacy. He has few friends, and no close friends. When she tries to talk to him about their own lack of closeness—such as after the night out with their new acquaintances—he avoids the discussion. This avoidance, in Debra's view, proves that his fear of intimacy, even with his own wife, is the source of their problems.

In contrast, Frank believes Debra's insecurity is the source of their problems. He uses the same incident, but interpreted differently, to support his point of view. As he sees it, Debra got upset that night merely because their friends made more money and were more affectionate in public than he and Debra. Frank thinks they have problems because Debra cannot accept herself and others (even her own husband) for what they are.

As they each carry around these theories about the other, they become entrenched in their positions and blinded to the various ways one *could* look at their problems. Debra ignores any evidence of Frank's social competence, such as his sense of humor, his kindness and consideration toward others, or his passionate lovemaking. Yet these positive qualities were reasons why Debra was attracted to Frank. In parallel fashion, Frank overlooks obvious signs of Debra's psychological security, such as her persistence and optimism in the face of disappointment. Each expects the other to be inadequate, acts as if he or she is, and in so doing promotes the very characteristic that is so disliked. Debra, assuming Frank won't participate much in social encounters, provides little opportunity or incentive for him to speak and thus contributes to his shyness and social withdrawal. Frank, assuming Debra will get upset at any bad news, doesn't tell her things that he thinks will bother her. When she eventually finds out, she gets more upset than she would have if he had told her in the first place. Plus now she is angry with him for concealing information from her.

Every couple starts out, like Frank and Debra, with a number of differences between them—differences that may nourish the relationship or damage it. When the differences cause problems, as they have for Debra and Frank, couples may argue. Each partner alternates between criticizing the other for being different and defending against the other's criticisms. Or, instead of outright argument, they may withdraw from each other, expressing their dissatisfaction through avoidance. Rather than solving the problems or minimizing the differences, these destructive cycles can maintain and even exaggerate the very differences that caused the problems in the first place. The end product of this vicious cycle is that the differences often seem irreconcilable.

THE PURPOSE OF THIS BOOK

In the last ten years, we have developed a new approach to couple therapy, called integrative couple therapy, and done research on it. We have written several scientific papers and one book describing our approach and the data we have collected that shows its effectiveness. Currently, we are in the middle of an extensive, five-year research study, funded by the National Institute of Mental Health, to conduct the largest and most comprehensive evaluation of couple therapy ever, including an evaluation of integrative couple therapy. This book is also about our approach to couple therapy, but it is written for you: ordinary people who are struggling with conflict in your own relationships. *Reconcilable Differences* is designed to be used by you whether you are in therapy to improve your relationship or going it alone.

The purpose of this book is to help you understand the conflicts you have with your partner and then to transform those conflicts into greater peace and intimacy. When you get embroiled in conflict with your partner, you both may blame the trouble on faults in the other. You each try to correct these faults by changing the other. But the other resists change, and so you get locked in a struggle that tears away at your good feelings for each other. Each of you can feel stuck, not knowing how to cope with unwelcome differences in the other and resorting to blame, criticism, defensiveness, and withdrawal. These ways of coping serve only to hurt each other's feelings. Bruised and injured by your attempts to resolve your differences, you may feel that the chasm has become impossible to breach.

In this book we will show you a way out of this impasse: by accepting your partner. The natural inclination is to try to change your partner, but efforts directed solely at such change often make the conflict worse. When you genuinely accept your partner, you may achieve peace from the conflict and, paradoxically, change from your partner. Your partner probably wants to make you happy. When you are able to accept each other's experience, and often the behavior that results from that experience, you both may make spontaneous changes to accommodate to the other. Acceptance offers a route for you both to move toward a happier and closer union.

How can you achieve genuine acceptance? And how can acceptance transform conflicts into intimacy? Although they are painful, conflicts offer a window into the emotions of both of you: your disappointments, hopes, strengths, and weaknesses. If you can look at these conflicts not with the goal of blaming and fault finding but with the goal of understanding the strong emotions that drive each of you, you can learn more about yourself and your partner individually as well as how you interact. This understanding allows you to appreciate each other more completely and more honestly and can inspire compassion for each other's position. Through this understanding you also may gain some perspective that will lessen your conflicts, perhaps even enabling you to laugh at them at times. Understanding and compassion for each other and greater perspective on your conflicts may then lead you to an acceptance of each other's feelings and behavior, which in turn breaks your vicious cycles of argument, disagreement, and withdrawal—or at least allows you to recover from those cycles more quickly. At the very least, the process of analyzing and discussing your differences and conflicts in an atmosphere of acceptance will promote greater tolerance between you; in the best case, it can enhance the intimacy between you. Conflict offers not only the threat of alienation but also the possibility of intimacy.

Change is the brother of acceptance, but it is the younger brother. When acceptance comes first, it paves the way for change. When you and your partner experience greater acceptance from each other, your resistance to change often dissolves. You may be more open to adapting to each other and accommodating in ways that reduce conflict. You may be able to communicate more clearly and negotiate and problem-solve more effectively since you are no longer adversaries. In this book we will also discuss strategies for promoting change in relationships once greater acceptance has been achieved.

Finally, we will discuss some special problems in relationships. When your partner has an individual psychological disorder, such as depression, the relationship itself is challenged. Maintaining a close relationship under these circumstances is especially difficult, but the relationship can be either a profound help or a serious deterrent to your partner who is struggling with a disorder. There can be even more serious challenges to relationships, such as when your partner deceives you with a secret affair or when your partner abuses you verbally or physically. Should you leave the relationship or stay? If you stay, how should you cope? How much can you and should you accept in these situations? What changes should you insist on? When should you seek professional help? We will discuss all these issues.

Our book is divided into four parts. The first, "The Anatomy of Arguments," dissects typical relationship conflicts so that you can better understand how a simple comment or gesture can explode into battle and how the war between you is likely to escalate over time. You will be given plenty of illustrations from other couples and will be asked to start looking at the specific trouble between you and your own partner. By the time you have finished reading Part I, you will have an essential foundation for using the rest of the book. Part II, "From Argument to Acceptance," shows the ways that you and your partner can foster acceptance of each other. Acceptance cannot be demanded or forced, yet it is anything but a passive state. It is crucial to establish some measure of acceptance if you hope to ease the conflict in your relationship and facilitate the changes in each other that are really important to you. In these chapters you will learn the important difference between acceptance and resignation and see how even small steps toward mutual acceptance and compassion can improve your relationship. Part III, "Deliberate Change through Acceptance," discusses ways in which you can pursue change directly, but in the context of acceptance. So often efforts to change merely lead to more of the same. To achieve genuine changes in your relationship, you may need to accept, at times, your own difficulties in implementing those changes and your partner's negative reactions to those changes. Finally,

Part IV, "When Acceptance Is Not Enough," looks at those cases when your partner presents special challenges because of his or her own disorder, such as depression, or when your partner mistreats you, such as by having an affair. This section also discusses professional help for individual and relationship problems.

Each chapter in the book relies heavily on examples from couples. To preserve confidentiality, these case examples are an amalgam of the hundreds of couples we have seen in therapy, of couples we have known socially, and even of our own relationships. These examples provide "living evidence" of how our ideas play out in real life. Each chapter ends with a short summary of the main ideas and an exercise that will bring the ideas of this chapter home to your own unique relationship.

The ideal way to read this book is jointly with your partner. After each of you reads the chapter, it is helpful to discuss the ideas and relate them to yourselves. The exercises can easily be turned into joint exercises. But a word of caution is in order: it will be easier to find your partner in these chapters than it will be to find yourself. To prevent the discussions from leading to blame ("You do exactly what they talk about in Chapter . . . "), it is always helpful to focus on applications to yourself rather than applications to your partner.

If your partner doesn't want to read this book, it can still be helpful for you to read it. If your partner does want to read the book, but discussions about the book lead to further arguments between you, each of you should read it alone and do the exercises alone. After you have completed the first section, you may want to try to discuss the book together again. At that point, you may find it possible to have an enlightening and helpful discussion of what you have learned.

RECAP

This chapter took a single conflict from a married couple and presented three sides to that conflict: the wife's view, the husband's view, and a more objective view that incorporated both spouses' positions. This three-sided view of conflict gives a taste of what is to come in Part I, where we explain conflict from the perspective of the participants as well as from a broader, more objective perspective.

This chapter also gave an overview of the focus of the book, with its emphasis on acceptance as a path toward resolving conflict, and an overview of the format of the book.

Exercise

Pick a recent argument between you and your partner. Write down three sides to that incident: first the story that you would tell, next the story that your partner would probably tell, and finally the story that an observer might tell. Compare the three stories. How are they different?

PART I

The Anatomy of an Argument

CHAPTER 2

"You're Wrong!"

RELATIONSHIP PROBLEMS

AS FAULTS

> How wonderful to have someone to blame! How
> wonderful to live with one's nemesis! You may be
> miserable, but you feel forever in the right. You
> may be fragmented, but you feel absolved of all the
> blame for it.
> —ERICA JONG,
> *How to Save Your Own Life* (1977)

What starts arguments? What are they about?

Don Peterson, a psychologist at Rutgers University, tried to answer those questions by asking a group of volunteer couples to record important daily marital events. Each couple got together every evening to determine the most important contact they had had with each other during that day. They then wrote separate, detailed accounts of that important contact. They explained what started the event, noted what each said and did, and described their respective thoughts and feelings about the event. Not surprisingly, many of the most important contacts were arguments. Peterson took all the reports of arguments and, using scientific methods, classified them in various ways. He found that there were four typical events that started arguments.

Not surprisingly, the most common trigger for argument was *criticism*. We all know that certain kinds of remarks, those intended to put our partners down, are likely to ignite a conflict. Carol, for example, who was sensitive about her forgetfulness, became only mildly defensive when her husband, Ron, pointed out that he'd found the door unlocked upon arriving home. When he referred to her as a "space cadet," however, she became enraged.

Ron's comment is an example of an obvious and intended criticism. But sometimes criticisms are unintentional. A wife may make what she views as a constructive suggestion or a passing observation, but her husband reacts with hurt feelings and feels either falsely maligned or blamed for something that isn't his fault. When Vivian said to Steve, "You sometimes have trouble dealing with the kids," she may have intended it merely as a statement of fact, given that a temper tantrum by their four-year-old had recently shattered the evening's domestic tranquillity. But to Steve her remark felt like an unjustified attack on him as a father. He believes that at times every parent, including his wife, has trouble handling the temper tantrums of young children. Why does she have to comment on it? What for her was simply an observation, for him was a hurtful criticism.

A second common trigger for argument was a *demand* that struck the recipient as unfair or illegitimate. Alicia asked Victor to stay home from his weekly card game with his friends because she was sick with the flu. She thought she would feel better if he stayed with her and took care of her. Victor, however, viewed her request as unreasonable: "I am not a doctor; I cannot help you. Furthermore, you are not that sick. Why should I give up something that's important to me just because you feel bad?" Similarly, Carol's request that Ron type up a report she needed seemed reasonable to her since she was already stressed out from trying to finish the report for tomorrow's deadline and still had to prepare some evaluations that were also due. But Ron did not see it her way: "You want me to be your secretary because you procrastinated as usual and created the mess that you're in. Why is it my job to bail you out?"

Conflicts were also triggered by what Peterson called "*cumulative annoyance.*" If Steve repeatedly forgets to put the dishes in the dishwasher, Vivian gets irritated, and they argue. If Carol is late now and then, Ron can tolerate it, but when she is constantly late, he gets angry. He wonders how she can be so inconsiderate, always keeping him waiting. Carol realizes that she is often late, but she also figures that she has never missed an important event or incurred the wrath of anyone other than Ron. Her coworkers treat her habitual tardiness as an endearing foible. Why can't he?

A final common trigger for conflict was a rebuff or a *rejection.* For example, Steve put his arms around Vivian as a gesture of affection, but when Vivian responded with "Not now," Steve got angry: "You say you want me to be affectionate with you, but then you brush me off!" "Yes, in general, I want you to be more affectionate," Vivian retorted, "but can't you accept that I am not always in the same mood as you?"

Ron felt rebuffed when he made a special effort to cook pasta primavera, Carol's favorite dish, and Carol said, "Thanks, but I have a bad stomachache. I think I'll just have some tea and get into bed." Ron wondered out loud, "How can you be so insensitive?" Carol responded defensively, "I just don't feel well, and I'm not hungry!" She couldn't understand why he had to make such a big deal out of her refusal to eat his meal.

In each of these cases an argument begins with the actions or inactions of one partner. In the case of a criticism, an unfair demand, and cumulative annoyance, one partner offends the other. In the case of rejection, it is a partner's failure to respond appropriately that leads to conflict.

In all of these cases a single act by one partner upsets the other and they argue. When such events occur repeatedly, however, each person gets more sensitive to the triggers, such that over time it takes less and less provocation to ignite an argument. Mary does not need to make a full-fledged critical comment about George's dealings with the kids to provoke a reaction from him. After years of enduring critical comments, George may interpret Mary's innocent request "Would you help Max with his homework?" as criticism because it suggests that he *should* have helped Max with his homework or that he *should* have noticed that Max needed help. If George reacts defensively to even these relatively benign comments, Mary may do her best to avoid anything that sounds blaming or accusatory. However, even Mary's carefully chosen words at a family outing at the beach, "Remember that Max can't swim well," may contain a hint of judgment (i.e., George won't be careful about watching Max in the water) that comes across to George as criticism.

Similarly, Anna does not need to attempt a passionate kiss with Greg to experience his rejection. After many rejections she rarely makes such obvious gestures to excite his passion. Now even his distracted look when he greets her or his apparent lack of interest when she talks about her day feels like rejection. By now, Greg may be aware of her sensitivity to rejection, so he may try to "psych himself up" to make an enthusiastic response. But she may see through these forced and insincere efforts and feel rejected anyway.

If you were watching these encounters, you might wonder why each person had such a strong reaction to such apparently unimportant actions. Why did Ron feel so rejected when Carol's illness made it impossible for her to eat the dinner he had cooked? Why was George so stung by Mary's minor criticism of how he handled the kids? Your confusion would be understandable because you are not privy to the inner experience of these couples, let alone privy to all the past incidents that led to that experience. You would be seeing only a small slice of a long, complicated, and painful history that explains these heightened sensitivities to seemingly innocent remarks.

"WHY IS THIS HAPPENING TO US?": THE SEARCH FOR AN EXPLANATION

When any important event occurs in our lives, we seek an explanation. If the event is painful and occurs repeatedly, such as an argument, our search takes on a sense of urgency. We need to understand the event to gain some control over it. If we can accurately determine the cause of the event, we may be able to alter its cause and thus avoid future pain. With some sense of crisis, then, we put on our trenchcoats and, like detectives, search for the culprit. Who perpetrated this crime?

There are two obvious suspects in any relationship conflict: you and your partner. Assuming the conflict did not include other people, you two are the agents in the argument. The culprit has to be one of you. But which one?

Psychologists have conducted extensive research on the kinds of explanations that people develop to make sense of the events in their lives. Perhaps not surprisingly, our analyses tend to differ depending on whether we are looking at ourselves or at others. When we explain our own actions in a conflict, we tend to look outside ourselves. The pressure of a deadline or the nasty comments of others made us do what we did. Our eyes and ears are directed at the outside world, so we are acutely aware of the external pressures that impinge on us and influence our behavior. But when we explain the actions of others, we generally look to factors within them, such as their personality traits. Because our eyes and ears are focused on them, we may be less aware of the factors in their own world that have influenced them. We see them—and them alone—as the cause of their own behavior. It's like the differences noted between biography and autobiography: in telling another's story, we tend to assign more responsibility for sins and errors to our subject than we do when we are our own subject.

These human tendencies are constantly at work in close relationships. If a husband and wife both agree that she should ask her boss for a raise but she insists that now is not the time, her husband may explain her reluctance as cowardice while she may blame her boss's mood—she knows when her boss is open to these requests. Similarly, if both husband and wife have agreed to limit their visits to his parents but he almost immediately accepts another invitation for dinner with them, she may explain his response as personal weakness while he may explain it as guided by his parents' feelings.

In the case of arguments, we are acutely aware of the hurtful actions or inactions of our partners but regard our own hurtful behavior as merely a reaction to our partners' misdeeds.

In the end, if you ask yourself why a painful argument occurred, you are likely to point an accusing finger at your partner. It's your partner who is culpable, and his or her own qualities caused the event. And as for you? No matter how unseemly your actions were, you were merely provoked.

YOUR PARTNER'S ROLE IN CONFLICT

"It's All Your Fault": Indictment and Conviction

> More trials and guilty verdicts take place in the heads of married couples than in courts of law.

As we think over our partners' actions, we often conduct a kind of legal inquiry in our heads. We hold a mental trial to evaluate their emotional crimes against us. While limited in its jurisdiction, this court deals with the largest and most profound of claims: high crimes of love and character.

Like everyone else, you undoubtedly have mentally reviewed evidence of your partner's misdeeds and analyzed what these misdeeds mean. Each wrongful action suggests your partner has some bad trait. He didn't listen to your point of view—maybe he is inconsiderate. She did what she wanted to do without taking you into account—maybe she is selfish. He criticized you for things he does too—maybe he is unfair. She angrily interrupted you and called you names—maybe she is hostile.

Your partner's wrongful acts may suggest the absence of positive traits rather than the presence of negative ones. If your partner ignores your feelings, maybe he doesn't care about you. If your partner forgets what you've told her, maybe she doesn't value your input. If your partner doesn't show affection to you, maybe he no longer loves you. If your partner seems uninterested in sex, maybe she has lost her attraction to you. If your partner doesn't spend much time with you, maybe he hasn't made you a priority in his life.

As you think over your partner's recent behavior toward you, you remember similar acts in the past. A recent bit of selfishness brings to mind a string of selfish actions. Recent clues that your partner doesn't really love you remind you of other such evidence. In your mind you review these pieces of evidence, both current and past. They are the exhibits you present in your mental court. They are the incriminating testimony about which your cerebral jury deliberates. A verdict of guilty seems certain.

But a verdict is only the first step toward achieving justice. Next we want our partners to confess their guilt. They need to admit that they are selfish or inconsiderate or lacking in respect and love. At the very least, they should apologize to us. More important, they need to change. They should work on their problem. They should make consistent efforts to be more giving, more considerate, and more loving.

"You're Sick": The Diagnosis

Those of us who are more psychologically inclined may search for explanations of our partners' behavior in their personality makeup. Rather than look for moral deficiency, we look for emotional impairment. Rather than holding a court hearing, we conduct a psychiatric examination. Rather than demanding indictment and conviction, we seek an accurate diagnosis.

Often such a diagnosis points to emotional problems. If your partner shows a need for reassurance, appreciation, and love that seems excessive, perhaps he doesn't really like himself and is therefore insecure about whether others love him. If she doesn't confide in you or doesn't shower you with affection, maybe she has a deep fear of intimacy with others. If he doesn't wish to socialize much with your family and friends, maybe he has a troubling lack of confidence in himself. If she is too critical of you, maybe it is because she doesn't accept herself and thus can't accept others.

Your diagnosis of your partner may suggest something even more serious than emotional problems: a specific mental disorder. If your partner is moody and irritable, you may conclude he is depressed. If her accusations concerning you seem wild and unfounded, you may diagnose her as paranoid. If his behavior during arguments seems irrational, you may call him crazy. It is their madness, not their badness, that causes our partners' hurtful behavior toward us.

In our effort to understand our partners' emotional difficulties or mental illness, we may search their past. We often discover clues in the behavior of our in-laws. His family always papers over their differences and never faces their conflicts directly, so no wonder he avoids conflict. Her father always babies her, so now she wants me to spoil her. His parents never forced him to be responsible, so he is irresponsible. Her mother is humorless and often depressed, so maybe that explains her bad moods.

After we have diagnosed our partners' maladies, we naturally want them to listen to our careful analysis of their problems and admit that we are right. Despite our lack of professional training, we genuinely believe that we understand what makes our partners tick. They should face up to their emotional limitations or their mental disorders by accepting our diagnoses.

Once they have openly and nondefensively acknowledged their problem, they will presumably want to improve themselves. We may suggest some self-help books that will buttress our keen insight into what is wrong with them. We may advise some real therapy for them and perhaps even for their parents and siblings. If needed, we could choose the appropriate therapist for them, and even provide necessary background to the therapist and a tentative diagnosis. Long-term, intensive psychotherapy would undoubtedly be the treatment of choice. However, the cost and length of that treatment may be prohibitive. Perhaps a high dose of Prozac, or another of those highly touted new psychiatric medications, could restore sanity!

"You're Not Good Enough": The Performance Evaluation

We may spare our partners the profound knowledge we have of their personalities and instead evaluate their performance as spouses, partners, parents, providers, or simply people. Rather than search for a diagnosis, we now look for potential inadequacy. Rather than examine for moral weakness, we scrutinize for incompetence. We judge our partners not on their morality or their mental health, but rather on their ability to be a good lover, spouse, or parent.

Our standards for satisfactory performance are gleaned from watching others. If your wife is not physically affectionate but you have seen other wives who shower their husbands with hugs and kisses, you may conclude that she does not know how to express her love properly. If your husband is upset when you go out with friends but you know husbands who encourage their wives to go out with their friends, then maybe your husband is too possessive. If your partner is too clingy and needy for you, maybe she hasn't developed the ability to be alone or to cultivate friends as others have. Conversely, if your partner doesn't spend enough time with you, maybe he hasn't truly realized that he is now married; his single life is over.

You may conclude that your partner is not mature enough for marriage. She is ill prepared for intimacy. He never learned to listen attentively, or provide support or love properly. Somehow she didn't get the training to be intimate or to tolerate separation, to be sexually open or to be patient sexually, to be ambitious on the job or to prioritize home life, to be open and honest in a close relationship, or to show judgment in what to say and when to say it, or to be spontaneous and free, or to be responsible and committed.

As in addressing judgments of moral inadequacy or diagnoses of mental problems, our partners' first step in correcting their failings is to admit that we are right. They are inadequate spouses. They should acknowledge their deficiencies. Once they do that, they can address their inadequacies in several ways. They can look to other couples for models of proper behavior. If we know other husbands, for example, who are not concerned when their wives go out weekly with their friends, then why should our husbands be concerned? If we have read how often most couples in America have sex, why can't our wives at least meet that standard? Even more important than looking to other couples, our partners can look to us. We, after all, are models of what a good spouse should be: we know how to prioritize our time; we aren't needy; we know how to be physically affectionate. We can lead them back to the Promised Land of a happy marriage—if only they would listen to us.

YOUR OWN ROLE IN CONFLICT

"Poor Me": Victims

Because we believe we are only reacting to our partners' provocations, we tend to cast ourselves in the role of victim and our partners in the role of villain. If gregarious Rodney spends lots of time visiting with other people at a party, leaving his shy wife Donna to fend for herself, she will likely be angry and feel like a victim of his actions. She may wonder whether he really cares about her or if he is just incredibly inconsiderate. If she voices her distress to Rodney on the way home from the party, he in turn may feel attacked. He may wonder about her insecurity or neediness. Will he always have to look out for her? All he did was have a good time at the party. He didn't get drunk or flirt with other women or act inappropriately. Why is he being attacked? He too may feel victimized.

"Maybe It Does Take Two": Coconspirators

Rodney and Donna illustrate one difficulty with villain–victim casting. If both of you insist you're the victim, you can't hope to take the first step toward resolving conflict. But there is another reason it's hard to maintain the view that you are both innocent victims. A verdict about your partner highlights his or her misdeeds, but it casts a troubling shadow on you as well. If your partner is selfish, inconsiderate, or unfair, why did you two get together? Did you exercise bad judgment? Were you fooled by the classic bait-and-switch trick, seeing your partner's true colors only after you were invested in the relationship? Were you fooled by superficial attractions? Did you encourage or fail to discourage your partner's flaws? Are you a coconspirator in your partner's crimes against you?

Your diagnoses and performance evaluations of your partner can also cast a suspicious light on you. Why did you choose such a damaged or incompetent person as a partner? Did you want or need such a flawed person? If your partner didn't have emotional problems or inadequacies when you two met, did you play some role in fostering these problems? If your partner did have these problems to begin with, why didn't you discern them? Did you contribute to his or her difficulties? Do you share some complicity in your partner's problems? Are you an "enabler," someone who does not have a particular problem but contributes to it in the other by "enabling" it to take place?

"What Does This Problem Say about Me?": Secret Villains

Occasionally many of us stop blaming our partners long enough to wonder whether the way they treat us implies that there really is something wrong with us. If your partner is critical of you, does that mean you are inadequate? If your partner is depressed, does that mean you have not been kind and loving? If she seems an emotional wreck, does that mean you have not been patient and supportive? If he is not attracted to you, does that mean you are unattractive? If she shows little interest in you, does that mean you are uninteresting? If he has so little love to give, does that mean you are unlovable? While you may ultimately discard these possibilities, it is difficult not to wonder about them. You may harbor a nagging fear that you, not your partner, is the real villain.

"LET ME EXPLAIN WHY WE HAVE SO MANY PROBLEMS": THE BATTLE OF ACCUSATIONS

It's only natural to want to share your conclusions once you have so carefully assessed your partner's misbehavior. If you don't tell your partner about the moral weaknesses or mental problems or inadequacies that you have discovered in him or her, how will your partner learn? Your partner will never be able to change unless someone who knows him or her well is honest enough to reveal these flaws. How your partner reacts to your frankness, however, depends on how and when you broach the subject. If you are bristling from a recent argument, you may tell your partner angrily, even vindictively. Your own distress propels your revelations. Your explanations, although voicing what you believe is true, sound like blame and accusation. Not surprisingly, your partner does not react well to these accusations, however truthful you think they are.

When you are not reacting to an immediate argument, you may try to tell your partner about your conclusions in a calmer, gentler, more respectful way. You may couch your verdict in compassion. You may use your best bedside manner. You may mix positive comments with negative ones in your evaluation.

Even with these extra efforts, you have probably found that your partner seldom reacts positively to your conclusions about his or her faults. Your judgments are not afforded the respect that your care in formulating them should warrant. Your partner may interrupt you. He or she may deny, wholesale, all of your conclusions. Your partner may vigorously defend himself or herself.

As distressing as these reactions may be, even more distressing are the accusations delivered in return. Your partner has gone through his own moral evaluation, diagnostic assessment, and performance evaluation *of you*. She has concluded that it is your faults, your emotional immaturity, and your inadequacy, much more than any of her own, that cause the unhappiness between you. Your partner matches your conclusions with conclusions of his or her own.

What can erupt next is a battle of explanations that quickly turns into a war of accusations. Many of us start out wanting to share our concerns sympathetically or kindly or respectfully, but our partners' reactions put us on the defensive. In the accusations and counteraccusations that follow, neither party would dare voice any fear of having played a role in the problem. To admit that we too may have been villains, or at least coconspirators, would make us too vulnerable.

To protect ourselves, then, any admissions we make are delivered in the service of an accusation. We may, for example, admit to having been blind to our partners' faults early on. We may admit to a lover's foolish optimism that the one we love would eventually change his or her personality. Admissions like these just emphasize the faults in our partners.

During the battle of accusations, we certainly don't feel much closeness and love for our partners. We may even feel active dislike for them. If the argument is particularly heated, we may admit to feelings and attitudes that were once there but are now, regrettably, absent. We may acknowledge "The old feelings just aren't there" or "I don't care that much anymore." The clear references to time ("old feelings" and "anymore") suggest that the feelings and attitudes were once there and that in *those* days appropriate behavior followed quite naturally. But to act in a loving manner given the present feelings would be a lie. And we will not lie. Statements of our integrity often accompany confessions of our lack of feelings: "I have to tell you the truth—I simply don't care anymore" or "I won't lie to you. The feelings just aren't there." The statements often suggest a pressure to engage in dishonesty, presumably to protect the partner in the short run, but a commendable resistance to that pressure for the sake of truth.

Thus, what starts out as an attempt to explain our views of our partner can easily degenerate into a battle of accusations, then into admissions that highlight the accusations, and finally into statements about not caring or not loving the other. These latter comments can be particularly injurious and threatening.

What gets lost in these discussions are the actions or inactions that initially triggered pain in us and led to our attempts at understanding. The fact that we feel so often rebuffed in our attempts to reach out to our partners may never get voiced. Instead, our accusations about their fear of intimacy and their counteraccusations about our insecurity may preclude any discussion of what it is that hurts us. If the conversation deteriorates to "admissions" that we no longer feel the way we used to or that they no longer love us, these discussions may create more pain and hurt than the pain and hurt that led to the discussion in the first place.

Raul and Adreanna often have conflicts over the care of their toddler, Joey. Adreanna is a dedicated, concerned mother who has read a lot about child health and development. She knows that her first responsibility as a mother is Joey's safety and health. Raul takes parenthood in general, and safety in particular, much more casually. He likes to say "Kids learn from their bruises." Given these different stances toward child care, it is not surprising that they have different opinions about how closely to watch Joey and about what kind of activities he should be allowed. In his frustration over Adreanna's views, Raul sometimes diagnoses her as irrational: "You are so neurotically worried about everything. You would raise him in an isolation chamber if you had your way." In her frustration with Raul, Adreanna judges him to be inadequate as a father and lacking in the moral values a parent should have: "You are so preoccupied with your own stuff, you hardly bother to pay attention to Joey. You don't care about his welfare. I'm just grateful he hasn't seriously hurt himself under your watch." With these exchanges of accusations, both will defend themselves and make countercharges. What won't get discussed or at least acknowledged is that Adreanna does really worry when Raul is in charge of Joey and that Raul feels bad about being under surveillance by Adreanna and not trusted by her. What also doesn't get discussed in these battles of accusation is the specific issue of concern that brought up the conflict to begin with: Should Joey be allowed to play in the backyard by himself, with a parent checking in occasionally, or should a parent be with him at all times? Can Joey climb the stairs by himself, or should someone be right behind him to help him? If the discussion deteriorates into "admissions" of lack of love or caring for the other, these comments may be more painful than the anxiety and distrust that started the discussion in the first place.

"YOU ALWAYS . . . ": BURYING THE KERNEL OF TRUTH

What makes one partner in a couple insist on his explanation of the problem and the other insist on hers? First of all, both of you know that there is some truth in your respective explanations. Each of you has witnessed your partner's behavior many times over and seen direct evidence of the characteristic you accuse the other of having. Second, your partner's stubborn resistance to acknowledging any validity in your assertion only makes you press on. How can your partner so willfully refuse to recognize an obvious truth!

Unless one of you is crazy—that is, clearly out of touch with reality—the accusations made by both of you have kernels of truth in them. But those kernels are exaggerated truths, distorted by the heat of the argument and the pressure of your partner's resistance. When you expand on a genuine characteristic, making it more dramatic and excessive than it really is, your partner naturally feels justified in denying the caricature you have drawn. For example, the wife who accuses her husband of overreacting may, in the heat of the argument, claim that he is *always* "out of control." He can vigorously defend such an extreme characterization of him and perhaps even turn the tables on her: "Just who's out of control? You're the one who's overreacting!"

Research in the social sciences provides some support for the truth in our accusations. Studies have shown that partners in bad marriages are more likely to be impulsive, while partners in happy marriages are more likely to be agreeable and conscientious. Even more compelling evidence shows that emotional difficulties are associated with relationship dissatisfaction. For example, neurotic tendencies, alcoholism, and depression are linked to relationship dissatisfaction. Finally, there is even evidence implicating inadequacy as a predictor of relationship problems. Spouses who are less skilled at communication and conflict resolution are more likely to be in dissatisfied relationships. Thus, the spouse who accuses the partner of being bad or mad or inadequate and implicates these qualities as contributing to the relationship problems may have a point.

But these accusations are off the mark in several ways. First, the research shows that traits such as impulsivity and depression only make a good marriage difficult, not impossible. Being agreeable and conscientious makes a good marriage more likely, but by no means guarantees it. Many couples are able to sustain a fulfilling relationship despite all sorts of personal inadequacies. Second, the accusation focuses only on the partner's negative characteristics and not on one's own. And as we have said, the accusation is likely to exaggerate the characteristic in the partner. Third, and most important, the accusation, defense, and counteraccusation—the battle of explanation between the partners—does nothing to improve or alter those characteristics under consideration, except perhaps to make them worse.

When all we do is accuse the one we love of misdeeds and character flaws, when we lay blame at every turn, we thwart the very goal we aspire to: change in our partners. Finding fault and exaggerating the human frailties we've identified in this person most dear to us only discourages cooperation and exhausts goodwill toward us. We rarely elicit change from someone else this way. We cannot force change through repeated, futile attacks. There must be a better way.

RECAP

Seen from our own perspective, arguments begin with actions or inactions by our partners that cause us pain. Criticism, unfair demands, cumulative annoyance, and rejection are the kinds of behaviors and responses that may trigger conflict. If these events happen only rarely, we can ignore them. When they happen repeatedly, we try to understand why they happen. We almost always begin our quest by focusing on the other person. What is it about our partners that leads to these painful actions? In our heads we may conduct a kind of legal inquiry into their transgressions and conclude that our partners have certain moral and character deficiencies: they are selfish, unfair, or inconsiderate. If we are more psychologically minded, we may conduct a diagnostic evaluation rather than a legal inquiry, concluding that the one we love has emotional problems such as immaturity, neurotic insecurity, or clinical depression. Or we may instead evaluate our partners' adequacy, determining that lack of training as a parent, lack of skill at communication, or inadequacy at expressing love is at the root of their hurtful behavior.

While we are engaging in this analysis of our partners, we may also wonder about our own contribution to the problems. We may feel like victims but wonder if we are possibly coconspirators. At the very least, we selected a partner with these faults. Might we have also permitted these faults or even fostered them? Could it be that inadequacies in us are also to blame? Although these possibilities may trouble us intermittently, typically we refocus on our partners' culpability rather than our own.

When we finish our analyses, we naturally want to share them, because we believe that informing our partners of their flaws is the best way to get them to work on changing them. But even when we believe we are acting out of constructive honesty and we present our conclusions tactfully, our partners are rarely receptive. Feeling blamed, they are likely to defend themselves and, even more upsetting, share their own conclusions about us. It is our faults, not theirs, that cause the problems. In the battle of explanations that follows, the only admissions that are made are ones that serve to highlight the accusations. Lost are discussions of the concrete events that initially triggered pain. If the battle of explanations is particularly heated, one or both partners may say things that are more painful than the original actions that led to the discussion in the first place. Even if there is some truth in our accusations, albeit exaggerated, that truth often gets lost in the din of battle. Conflict becomes entrenched, if not heightened, and we both dig in our heels and refuse to admit any need for self-change. Thus, actions made in an attempt to stimulate change end up preventing it.

Exercise

Think about the arguments you have with your partner. What is your usual first reaction when rehashing them?

- Do you focus immediately on your partner's role, your own role, or both? What do you do with the fears you have about your own role in conflict?
- When finding fault with your partner, do you usually focus on character issues (my partner is bad), mental problems (my partner is emotionally unstable or immature), or incompetence (my partner doesn't know how to be a good partner, spouse, parent, etc.)? Jot down the specific flaws that you're most likely to identify repeatedly.
- When your partner finds fault with you, what does he or she focus on? Write down the litany of complaints about you and your behavior that you usually hear from the one you love.
- What is the pairing between you two? Have you begun to assign certain caricaturist images to each other during conflict? For example, in an exchange of fault finding, does he see you as in some way emotionally unstable while you see him in some way as a bad person?
- What do you expect your partner to do about the flaws that you have identified? What do you think he or she expects you to do about the faults identified in you?

Keep your answers in a drawer where you can retrieve them for review later.

CHAPTER 3

"How Can You Be That Way?"

RELATIONSHIP PROBLEMS AS INCOMPATIBILITIES

> Marriage is the process of choosing the right
> woman with whom to be incompatible.
> —EVAN ESAR,
> *20,000 Quips and Quotes* (1968)

Soon after he reached his 81st birthday, my* father discovered he had colon cancer. The cancer was removed, but the surgeon reported that it had spread and would be terminal. His oncologist predicted that his remaining life would be measured in months. Fortunately, the surgery left him free from pain. During a visit to our home by my parents, I set up a video camera and interviewed first my father alone about his life and then my mother and father together about their almost forty-five years as a married couple. They talked openly about their life together and its many ups and downs. Toward the end of the interview, my father spontaneously observed: "I have often been amazed at how different we really are."

My mom and dad were at least as similar as most married couples. They both were Danish immigrants and shared their Danish-American heritage as well as values, such as education and hard work. Yet their

*As stated earlier, all personal and case examples are from Andrew Christensen.

individual personalities often pushed them in different directions. Mom was a doer; Dad was a dreamer. Mom was ambitious; Dad was laid back. Mom was a realist; Dad was an idealist. These differences fired their attraction as well as ignited their controversies with each other.

DIFFERENCES THAT MAKE A DIFFERENCE

> Differences—eternal differences, planted by God in a single family, so that there may always be color; sorrow perhaps, but color in the daily grey.
> —E. M. FORSTER

A major source of attraction between men and women is the differences between their bodies and the happy way in which these differences mesh. The French expression "Vive la différence" celebrates this.

It is not just physical differences that are a source of attraction and pleasure. Different ideas and opinions can enliven conversation between people. A couple may get together because of their spirited discussions about their differing views of politics or religion or philosophy. Different roles facilitate the accomplishment of necessary life tasks. Although traditional sex roles had many drawbacks, those roles did allow for a clear division of labor: he worked out in the world, she worked at home; he handled business issues, she handled childcare; he managed the upkeep of things outside the house, such as the yard and car, she took care of things inside the house, such as cooking and laundry.

Personality differences may also attract and interest us. June may find Mel's talkativeness appealing because it contrasts with her own reticence. If she were with someone as quiet as she is, little communication would occur. Allen may find Sue's energetic ambition helpful to him because it motivates him to get his own career going. Andrea may admire Daren's accomplishments in life and his sense of responsibility.

Differences that are initially appealing, however, may later show a darker side. The different views of religion that inspired such interesting conversations early on may cause serious problems when decisions must be made about children and their religious affiliation. Now something—or someone—has to give.

The roles that develop in a relationship can confine as well as facilitate tasks. They can also be alienating. If Bill is a house dad and Joanne is a working mom, they may find it difficult to share their worlds with each other because each develops little expertise in the other's domain.

Bill should develop broader interests, thinks Joanne. Joanne needs to step down off the fast track now and then, thinks Bill.

Finally, and perhaps most dramatically, personality characteristics that are attractive early in the relationship may become problematic later. Over time June may find Mel's talkativeness irritating; is he afraid of silence? Allen may feel pressure from Sue's energetic ambition; pushing herself is one thing, the way she pushes others has to stop. Andrea may come to feel that Daren is hyperresponsible; can't he ever "kick back" and just relax? As the accompanying "Cathy" cartoon illustrates, the same differences that attract can also repel.

Many differences, of course, were neither sources of attraction nor bones of contention. They were just part of the package of qualities that made up each person. But now they are a source of conflict. Blake did not feel strongly about Sondra's being less social than he, but this difference has since caused them many struggles. Initially Carrie was not particularly concerned that Parker was close to his controlling mother, but his attachment has since led to many arguments.

CATHY © 1997 Cathy Guisewite. Reprinted with permission of Universal Press Syndicate. All rights reserved.

No matter how widely we survey the range of possible mates through dating, no matter how carefully we select our potential partners through matchmaking services, singles parties, personal ads, or "fix-ups" via friends and family, the partners we select will be different from us, and often enough these differences will eventually cause us grief.

Ted Huston and Renate Houts, psychologists at the University of Texas, tried to mathematically determine the likelihood of similarities and differences between partners. They studied 168 couples and found that the likelihood that a man and a woman would match each other on the two separate dimensions of leisure interests and role preferences was only 33 percent. The estimated likelihood of matching on a hypothetical third dimension was about 17 percent. Matching on more than three dimensions was even less likely. On average, the couples in their study had dated only five different partners more than casually before marriage. This limited exposure, plus the low likelihood of finding a match on three or more dimensions, meant that spouses were incompatible in a variety of characteristics. Incompatibility was a mathematical certainty.

A cynic once remarked that "love is the delusion that one woman [or man] differs from the other." Perhaps the more common delusion of love is that our partners are more similar to us than they really are.

HOW OUR DIFFERENCES EVOLVE

> I will always cherish the initial misconceptions I had about you.
>
> —UNKNOWN

Early in our relationships, we may be shielded from differences that make us incompatible. Courtship practices maximize the opportunities for pleasure and minimize the chances for conflict. We dress up so that we look our best. We go out on dates, recreational events designed to please both of us. We are primed to try to impress and please the other. It is only as we begin to spend more time together, to experience each other in different, nonrecreational circumstances, and to meet each other's friends and families, that we are exposed to possible incompatibilities. Our moods are brought to light; our habits are revealed; our idiosyncrasies are bared. It is virtually certain that in some of these ways we will not fit well. When we find that the attractions are not strong enough or the incompatibilities are too great with a particular person, we end the relationship.

Fortunately, greater contact not only reveals more incompatibilities but also fosters greater closeness and attraction. We become more comfortable together and feel closer as we share more and more of our lives. Unanticipated areas of pleasure may turn up. We begin to find that life with a partner is a complex balance of positives and negatives. Eventually we make a commitment to someone when the attractions seem strong and the incompatibilities manageable.

Of course, we hope for a happy life together, but in love as in life, the only certainty is change. Attraction may fade or love may grow; manageable differences may mushroom into troublesome incompatibilities or big issues may shrink to minutiae. You may expect to spend a lot of time as a couple with your parents, while your husband thinks the occasional Sunday dinner with his in-laws is plenty. Over time your husband may become fonder of your parents and enjoy spending extra time with them, or you may find you need less contact, in which case the difference between you dissipates. But it's just as likely that you could both harden in your positions so that what was a minor problem at first becomes a major problem later.

Incompatibilities may change through individual experiences as well as through shared experiences. Kyle and Patrice were in perfect agreement on how much time they should spend together until Patrice got a job promotion. The challenge, excitement, and pressure of her new job made her spend more and more of her time working, and Kyle began to feel left out of her life.

Whether incompatibilities are present to begin with or develop over time, they cause difficulty for couples because they mean deprivation or pain for one or both. When Patrice spends less time with Kyle, he feels neglected and unloved. He worries about being a low priority in Patrice's life. However, if Patrice neglects her job responsibilities, she will feel anxious and worried.

If your husband wants less contact with your parents and you comply with his wishes, you may miss this contact and feel guilty about neglecting them. If your husband goes along with you, he may feel bored with your parents or, worse, resentful toward you because you pushed him into going. Incompatibilities have consequences for each partner.

THE LIGHT AND DARK SIDES
OF SIMILARITIES

Similarities are probably more important than differences in determining whom we choose as mates. Research indicates that people choose partners who are similar to themselves in age, background, and values. This is not surprising since our similarities give us common ground for conversation, for laughter, for the people we choose as friends, for activities, and for decision making. As a bonus, similarities beget similarities. Our common interests promote joint activities, which then further our common interests. If we both love politics, our discussion of politics and our attendance at political rallies are shared experiences that may increase our interest in politics. Likewise, if we play bridge together, we may become more skilled at being bridge partners and find more enjoyment and success in playing bridge.

Similarities may also cause conflict, however, although probably less so than differences. Partners who both believe they have impeccable taste and want to have the final word on decorating decisions may battle over what furniture to buy and what color carpet to order. Two people who are better talkers than listeners may battle over "airtime," each resenting that the other doesn't listen well. Besides inciting competition, similarities can create conflict when circumstances don't permit partners to express their similar interests. What happens when you both enjoy independent activity with friends, but someone has to stay home with the children? What if both of you are close to your parents and want to spend the Christmas holidays at their respective homes? Also, similarities can cause conflict by creating an imbalance in the relationship. Neither Nate nor Makiko, both spontaneous, live-for-the-moment kind of people, bothered to save any money, and when they found that they had nothing to show for their years of work and that home prices had appreciated beyond their ability to buy, they blamed each other: Makiko blamed Nate for not being more responsible; as the man, he should have taken charge of savings and financial planning. Nate blamed Makiko for her spending habits because she was even more extravagant than he was. Finally, similarities can create problems not so much by what they incite as by what they block. If both partners are apprehensive of conflict and thus avoid discussion of difficult topics, they may limit their ability to solve their problems. If both partners are inhibited about physical affection or sex, they may deny themselves sensual pleasures from each other.

In each of these cases a counterbalancing difference in one partner would be a welcome addition to the relationship.

WE COME BY IT RIGHTLY

When faced with differences or similarities that cause problems, your first impulse may be to find fault with your partner. "Why must you be so different from me?" or "Why can't you be different from me?" As we explained in the last chapter, you may view those problematic differences (or similarities) in terms of morality ("It's wrong for you to be this way"), or emotional well-being ("It's a sign of mental illness or emotional immaturity that you're this way"), or adequacy ("If you were a better person, you wouldn't be this way"). You may try to change your partner, and your partner may try to get you to change instead.

In fact, you both come by your qualities rightly. Many forces—including genes, learning, and current circumstances—have determined these qualities, and change is not easy.

It's in His Blood (or Her Genes)

Science is finding more and more evidence for genetic influences on human behavior. Much of what we believed was learned entirely through experience now appears to be influenced in part by our genetic endowment.

One way to study the effects of genes is to look at newborns, who have not lived long enough for the environment to influence them. We now know that newborns start out with different temperaments. Some infants are difficult babies: they are reactive to new stimulation, they are hard to soothe, and they don't sleep regularly. Others are easy babies: they are not easily disrupted by new stimulation, they are easy to soothe, and they sleep regularly. By following infants with different temperaments, scientists have shown that these early tendencies are predictive of later behaviors.

Another way that social scientists investigate the effect of genes on behavior is to compare identical twins, who have 100 percent of their genes in common, with same-sex fraternal twins, who have only about 50 percent of their genes in common. They have found that identical twins show greater similarity in personality traits than do fraternal twins. Even when scientists are able to find twin-pairs who were separated at birth and adopted, they are able to show greater similarity between identical twins than fraternal twins, although the home environments for all members is different from their twin partner.

One group of investigators from the University of Minnesota examined more than 1,500 twin-pairs and found that divorce rates were significantly higher for one twin if the other was divorced. The probability of divorce increased nearly twofold if one had a fraternal twin who was divorced but increased sixfold if one had an identical twin who was divorced. Does this mean there is a "divorce" gene? Hardly. In a later study, the group showed that personality attributes, such as negative emotionality, may be shared by twins, but more so by identical twins, and thus may account for the different divorce rates.

What this research means for you is that your partner's personality and your personality may not be changed that easily.

We Are Our History

> The past is never dead. It is not even past.
> —WILLIAM FAULKNER

The past affects both the present and the future. The kind of marriage our parents had determines to some extent the kind of marriage we will have. The way our parents treated us as children determines to some extent the way we will treat our spouses and our children. The kind of culture in which we were raised determines in part the kind of culture we will try to re-create.

A dramatic example is what has been called the "cross-generational transmission of marital instability." What this means is that children are more likely to divorce if their parents divorced. In one study based on five large surveys, Hallowell Pope and Charles Mueller found that people who had divorced parents were 10 percent more likely to get divorced themselves than people whose parents had never divorced. While this is not a large difference, it is a real difference and one that has been supported by subsequent studies. Presumably this tendency comes from both genetic factors—children inherit the genes of their parents— and environmental factors: the parents' difficult marriage affects the child's own marriage.

Violence in relationships provides another dramatic example of this carryover from the past. Children who witness physical violence between their own parents are more likely to experience violence in their own marriages than children who never witnessed violence in their parents. Children who were abused by their parents are more likely to abuse their own children than are children who were never abused.

But the past doesn't affect us in any simple way. Present experiences constantly modify the effects of past experiences, so that predictability from the past is usually weak. Many children who experience child abuse don't grow up to abuse their own children. Many children who witness violence between their parents don't end up in violent marriages. And many children who witness their parents' own divorce stay with their spouses.

Freudian psychology has popularized the notion that we look for mates who resemble our own parents. We often hear comments like "He married his mom" and "She married her dad." Some of us may notice uncanny resemblances between our own partners and our parents. Connections between our parents and our partners, however, are always complicated. Although there may be some striking similarities between a parent and a partner, there are usually many important differences. Even when one characteristic of our parent influences our choice in seeking a mate, that influence may occur indirectly as well as directly. Consider, for example, a boy who grows up with a demanding mother. He may "learn" emotionally that to get things done you need to have someone around to push you. He may seek a demanding wife and interact with her in ways reminiscent of his relationship with his mother. However, another boy with a demanding mother may experience such negativity from his interactions with her that he seeks a wife who never makes overt demands on him, and he interacts with her in ways that communicate his deep-seated feeling that she better not make overt demands on him. In both cases, the boy's childhood experiences affect his later marriage relationship, but in the first case he re-creates a childhood relationship in his marriage, while in the second case he avoids at all costs the repetition of any semblance of his childhood relationship.

Your experience in your family of origin affects more than just your choice of a mate. The emotional climate in your family of origin or in the larger culture in which you were raised influences what you are comfortable with and thus what you try to create in your own family. If, for example, you grew up in a home where physical affection was expressed freely and openly, while your husband grew up in a family that rarely expressed their love for each other in open physical affection, the two of you will likely have different expectations and comfort levels for physical affection. You may feel neglected and hurt that your husband doesn't put his arm around you more often or hold your hand more frequently. You may often feel disconnected from your husband. For his part, he may feel embarrassed by public displays of affection and uncomfortable with extensive private displays of affection. He likes to watch TV with you but doesn't want to hold your hand the whole time.

The level of open conflict is another aspect of emotional climate that we tend to carry over from our families of origin to our adult families. In Melanie's family, open conflict was suppressed. Her father's motto was "If you can't say anything nice about a person, don't say anything at all." Her mother's view was "most problems solve themselves over time." Both parents avoided confrontation. Harsh words were forbidden. The typical result of parental disagreement was tension rather than open argument. The family achieved respect and consideration for each other, but at some cost in spontaneity and openness.

In sharp contrast to Melanie, Nolan's family of origin had a "let-it-all-hang-out" approach to conflict. Members confronted their conflicts directly, voiced their opinions freely, and rarely suppressed any of their feelings. Both of Nolan's parents were strong-willed and opinionated. The family achieved an open, spontaneous emotional exchange but at the cost of peace.

Naturally, Nolan's opinionated, volatile openness often injures Melanie emotionally and makes her feel disrespected and mistreated. He, in turn, often feels guilty for hurting her feelings. Nonetheless, he often gets angry because she won't speak her mind, and he is frustrated when she simply withdraws at the first sign of conflict. Although their differences are striking and problematic, they could enrich each other's lives. Melanie could learn emotional expressiveness from Nolan, while he could learn respect and restraint from her.

Broader forces from the past than our family history influence us today. The culture in which we were raised may exert powerful pressures on us. If the husband comes from a culture that values close contact with one's family of origin, he may view it as a mandatory responsibility to have his widowed mother live with him. To do otherwise would be disgraceful. If his wife comes from a cultural background that emphasizes separation between generations, she may insist that retirement homes be considered as an option. Why should her mother-in-law invade the privacy of their home? Their challenge will be to meet the wife's needs for privacy and separation in their nuclear family while allowing the husband to fulfill his familial responsibilities.

We Are Both Victim and Architect of Our Current Circumstances

I once heard a social psychologist give a broad and succinct summary of two major findings in the field by saying that (1) situations influence people's behavior and (2) people are not aware of this fact. Study after study has shown that circumstances dramatically affect people's behavior, yet people often explain others' behavior with reference to their personalities alone.

Psychologist Stanley Milgram provided perhaps the most dramatic example of how situations can influence behavior. In the context of a study purportedly designed to explore the effects of punishment on learning, subjects were asked to monitor the performance of another subject in a different room and to press a switch to give the subject an electric shock whenever he made a mistake. In reality the other "subject" was a confederate of the experimenter and was never actually shocked; his reactions were staged. The actual subjects found themselves in a situation in which a scientific experimenter was encouraging them to apply increasingly high and apparently dangerous levels of electric shock to, they believed, a fellow subject. Despite hearing screams of pain from the next room, which they thought were cries from the subject, the great majority of these generally upstanding Americans showed considerable emotional distress but nonetheless complied with the experimenter's directives. Even though they were not people who normally hurt others, they neither refused to give the shocks nor asked that the study be terminated.

Fortunately, most of us will not find ourselves in a situation where we are encouraged to engage in hurtful treatment of others. In fact, even a study such as the one just described could probably not be done today, because of the stress to subjects. But even though we may be spared such a situation, we will be influenced by our circumstances more profoundly than we may believe. Whatever our genetic endowment or historical background, our present circumstances will also powerfully affect our behavior. These present circumstances may minimize or exacerbate personal differences with our partners, differences that initially resulted from our genetic backgrounds and personal histories.

For a positive case in which present circumstances minimize personal differences, consider Dawn and Boris. Dawn is more of a loner than Boris. She came from a small family, feels uncomfortable in crowds, and prefers either solitary activities such as reading and playing computer games or doing things just with Boris. He, on the other hand, comes from a large family, feels comfortable in a group, and enjoys loud parties and team sports. When they finished graduate school and both found a job in Boris's hometown, these differences became less of a problem because Boris could meet some of his social needs through the large network of family and friends in his hometown without either pressuring or threatening Dawn.

Unfortunately, present circumstances may create or exacerbate rather than alleviate personal differences. Consider the stereotypical situation of the traditional breadwinner husband and the mother/housewife at the end of a working day. He comes home exhausted and overstimulated from a day of dealing with people and their problems and wants nothing more than to bury himself behind a paper or in front of the television. She is exhausted from a day of housework and handling their children but has had little adult social contact. She wants to talk with her husband and go over the problems of the day that she has been unable to share with anyone. Whatever their general, personal inclinations to talk over issues at the end of the day, their separate circumstances create different needs for adult conversation.

Daily circumstances can affect not only how *much* we want to talk to our partners but also *how* we talk to our partners. If the breadwinner husband doesn't spend much time with his children, he may not be sympathetic to his wife's difficulties with the children. No one can give advice on child rearing like those who don't have children, and he may almost fall into that category. He may dismiss her problems with them with facile advice about being firm and consistent with them. But let him spend a day with the kids and see how he does! Similarly, because she is not employed outside the home, the mother/housewife may be unsympathetic to her husband's work difficulties. She may express frustration that he won't put some reasonable limits on his boss's demands. Why does he always complain about his boss? Why can't he stand up to him? If only she could spend a day with his boss! Our different daily circumstances may deprive us of our ability to understand and empathize with our partners' worlds, and consequently we don't take their difficulties seriously.

By "present circumstances" we mean much more than simply the daily events in each person's life away from the other. We mean their current position, abilities, and status as well. Roland believes that signing a prenuptial agreement would be a statement of lack of trust between him and Marianne. He urges that they "believe in their love for each other" and go into the marriage without financial preconditions and stipulations. Marianne believes that a prenuptial agreement is a realistic precaution to take in the face of today's high separation and divorce rates. She argues that "love is not incompatible with realism." While there may be personal differences in the level of Marianne's and Roland's romanticism and realism, their different financial situations also led them to their different positions. Marianne comes to the relationship with significantly more assets than Roland and would thus stand to lose more if they eventually divorced. Roland can literally "afford" to be more romantic than Marianne.

Status and ability may affect not only a spouse's reactions to entering a relationship but also his or her behavior in that relationship. Juan and Angela have very different reactions to thoughts and discussion of possible separation and divorce. Juan finds those thoughts and discussions a realistic exercise, given the conflicts the two of them are having. He loves Angela and doesn't really want a divorce, but he experiences the idea of divorce as comforting because he can assure himself that there are alternatives to the painful fights he and Angela have. Angela, on the other hand, finds the discussion of possible separation and divorce threatening. For her, bringing up the topic implies a lack of love and commitment. She asks, "Why are we even discussing this just two years into our marriage?" Although there may be many factors that account for these different reactions, their current ability to attract others is one of them. Juan is a gregarious guy who loved the world of dating and found it very easy to meet others. If he and Angela did divorce, he would find alternative relationships quickly. In contrast, Angela is painfully shy and found the whole world of dating quite unpleasant. She could not easily replace Juan. There is nothing comforting to her about the idea of divorce.

Present circumstances include not only the separate influences of the environment of each partner but also the setup of the couple's own life. These current circumstances of their own relationship may also affect their differences. Barney and Tamera started out with a healthy sexual interest in each other, although Barney had a stronger sex drive than Tamera. Once the two of them began a sexual relationship, they implicitly agreed that Barney was in charge of that area of their lives. He was the one who almost always initiated sex, and when he did Tamera usually consented. Just as it was Barney's role to go to work at 5:00 A.M., and he wouldn't refuse to do that unless there were overwhelmingly good reasons not to, so Tamera would not refuse sexual relations with Barney unless she was really feeling very tired or sick. In the early stages of their sexual relationship, this setup worked well for them. Although Barney was in control, Tamera enjoyed sex with Barney, even enjoyed being the source of his pleasure when she wasn't up for sex herself, and Barney tried to please her also. However, over time, because Barney was in control and Tamera was so compliant, he tended to be driven more by his own interests than by hers. Subtly and without either of them being aware of it, Barney paid less attention to Tamera's needs and Tamera began losing interest in sex. Tamera became more passive and unresponsive during sex, and Barney grew more frustrated. Partly because sex was no longer so fulfilling with Tamera, Barney's own sex drive increased. He pressed on for physical sexual satisfaction because he was getting less and less emotional satisfaction from lovemaking. In the long run, a small difference in sexual drive and interest became a big incompatibility.

A similar evolution occurred in Kristin and Alberto's marriage. When they started out, Kristin tended to be more responsible and Alberto more fun-loving, but this difference was not a serious problem. When they had kids, however, Alberto was so good at playing with them that Kristin naturally took on the role of responsible mother. Over time, they expanded their respective roles and relinquished to the other what they didn't do as well. As entertainment director, Alberto paid less and less attention to such responsibilities as cleaning up after his games or not exciting the kids before bedtime. Now Kristin dislikes always being the bad guy—to the kids and to Alberto; he dislikes her critical interference with what he sees as his wonderful relationship with the kids. As a result, Kristin is more responsible and less fun-loving than she has ever been; Alberto is more fun-loving (with the kids, not her) and less responsible than he has ever been; and both are resentful of the other.

Because we are two different people, we come from different situations and place ourselves in different situations than our partners. These situations can further accentuate our differences or create new differences. When faced with these differences, we can dig in our heels and insist that our way is the only way; either the other person changes, or the relationship is doomed. Or we can take a closer look at the differences and similarities that are causing the conflicts between us. When did they arise? Were they originally points of attraction but now are points of contention? Were they once small stuff but now big issues? How did we come by our differences and similarities: genetics, family history, cultural influences, present circumstances? When examined closely, many of our major incompatibilities reveal themselves as smaller than we thought, understandable, even acceptable. It is only the way that we cope with these differences that turns them into insurmountable problems.

RECAP

In this chapter we have considered relationship problems as incompatibilities. Although we seek out partners who are similar to us in many ways, we also seek out partners who are different from us. Even if we didn't, we would inevitably find others who are different from us. We all have unique genes, unique social histories, and unique present circumstances that shape who we are. Thus we can never find a clone for a partner. Probably we would be unhappy if we could get into a relationship with our clone. More important than finding a clone, we can never find an ideal match for ourselves. Inevitably we will find a partner whose differences from us or similarities with us cause problems.

These incompatibilities are the stuff of arguments. They are the content on which we engage. They are the relationship problems we face. And because the differences and similarities that lead to incompatibilities often represent the result of genetic, historical, and environmental influences, they are not easy to change. In conflict with our partners, we are faced with the dilemma of incompatibilities that are troubling and that may not be easy to change.

Exercise

Think of one area of incompatibility between you and your partner (a similarity or difference between the two of you that causes you problems).

- What is one reason from your partner's history and one reason from his or her current circumstances that might explain why your partner is the way he or she is?
- What is one reason from your own history and one reason from your own current circumstances that might explain why you are the way you are?
- Did you instinctively choose a similarity or a difference between you?

- Do you believe your choice is indicative of the pattern of incompatibilities between you? That is, do problems between you come mainly from being too similar or too different?
- Would your partner agree with your assessment? Does this incompatibility seem as large a problem as you believed before reading this chapter?

Tuck your answers away in a drawer with those you gave for the Chapter 2 exercise.

CHAPTER 4

"Can I Give to You Without Losing Me?"

INCOMPATIBILITIES OVER LOVE AND POWER

Couples can disagree about everything from sex to child rearing to in-laws; from abstract issues in philosophy, religion, and politics to concrete issues of table manners, sleep cycles, and grooming; from the serious issues of life to the trivial. Within this infinite diversity of potential conflict areas, however, many problems sound similar themes that echo the central dimensions of relationships themselves. Not surprisingly, these are our most serious incompatibilities because they threaten the very definition of our relationships. If we accept problematic differences and similarities in these areas, what will we have left? Unlike the incompatibilities discussed in Chapter 3, these may not be so easy to accept, even once we understand them.

THE BUILDING BLOCKS OF A RELATIONSHIP

Two central dimensions can be used to describe all relationships. The first is *closeness* or intimacy—what many of us think of as love. Relationships can range from distant to lovingly intimate, from superficial to profound. This dimension can be measured by quantitative features such as the amount of time spent together and by qualitative features such as the value, intensity, and meaning of that time together.

Over the years, you might log in more time with coworkers than with your own children, yet the parent–child relationship will be closer and more intimate simply because of the type and meaning of the activities in which you have participated together.

The second major dimension of relationships is *power,* or the distribution of authority, dominance, and control. Relationships don't exist only between equals. Many relationships, such as those between parent and child, teacher and student, supervisor and employee, are defined by an inequality between the two parties. Even relationships between equals are not equal in every respect. The members work out patterns of power, authority, even dominance. A husband and wife may see themselves as equals, but the wife is the acknowledged "green thumb" in the family and the husband, a woodworker, is the acknowledged expert in furniture and cabinetry. Thus, when it comes to landscaping decisions, the wife prevails; when it comes to remodeling decisions, the husband prevails.

These two simple dimensions of closeness and power can be used to describe important similarities and differences in relationships. For example, the husband–wife relationship and the parent–child relationship are both close, but the parent–child relationship involves a greater power discrepancy than does the husband–wife relationship. Usually, but not always, parents have more power over their children than spouses have over each other. A friendship and a marriage both assume equality between participants, but a marriage involves greater intimacy than a friendship.

Similarly, these dimensions also describe stages in a relationship. The parent–child relationship advances through stages marked by a decreasing power discrepancy as the child gains greater competency and independence. In some cases, the power discrepancy reverses when the adult child takes care of the ailing parent. Adult romantic relationships progress through stages of increasing closeness as couples advance through periods of acquaintanceship, dating, exclusive courtship, engagement, and marriage. Often marriage is followed by some reduction in intimacy as the couple focuses on careers and child rearing.

Finally, these dimensions describe different subtypes of a particular relationship. For example, traditional marriages and contemporary or egalitarian marriages differ in the way power is divided. In traditional marriages, the husband is head of the household and dominates the relationship, while in contemporary or egalitarian marriages dominance is shared by both partners.

Although conflicts in relationships can erupt over anything, the most serious conflicts develop around closeness and power because disagreements in these areas threaten the very definition of the relationship and of the individuals. If Herb doesn't spend most of his leisure time with Ruth, it doesn't seem like a marriage to him. However, Ruth doesn't feel like her own person unless she has independent friends and activities. To Bill it is obvious that men should be in charge of financial decision making; otherwise it wouldn't be a normal marriage, and he wouldn't be a normal man. However, Shandra won't feel like an independent woman if she lets Bill make all the financial decisions. In these examples, each person's view of the relationship, view of himself or herself, and self-esteem is connected to the role played in the relationship. Although conflict over any topic can be annoying, conflict over closeness and power can threaten a relationship's stability because the conflict challenges the very nature of the two partners and their relationship.

"I WANT TO BE CLOSE BUT NOT TOO CLOSE"

All of us have an intuitive idea of what "closeness" means. We can identify synonyms such as "intimacy," and we can tell when we feel close to someone. But here is the problem: we too often associate *feelings* of closeness and intimacy with intimacy itself. Two people who feel close to each other are certainly likely to be close, but people who don't feel close may be close as well. Couples who have been together for years and have worked out smooth, well-functioning relationships may not experience strong emotions toward each other, such as feelings of closeness. They differ markedly from the romantic adolescent pair, swept up in the strong winds of their passion, and from couples of their own age who, though past the turbulence of passion, still bask in the warm breezes of love, who sit holding hands and regularly express deep affection. Despite their apparent lack of emotion, these couples can be highly interconnected. They are dependent on each other financially and socially. Over the years they have divided up life's tasks so that they can complete them only jointly.

Even in more extreme cases, where strong positive emotion is lacking and a wealth of negative emotion exists, a couple's lives can be strongly interconnected. Jergen and Adele argue constantly, call each other names, and threaten separation and divorce, although neither makes any deliberate move in that direction. Their behavior, as well as their negative emotional arousal, implies anything but closeness. Yet each would feel lost without the other to battle with. Like many other argumentative couples, who seem to experience little or no positive emotion, they would feel uncharacteristically anxious or sad upon the threat of real loss of the other through serious illness, death, or divorce. Genuine separation makes them painfully aware of a closeness they didn't experience emotionally.

A Continuum of Closeness

Closeness, then, can mean not just physical proximity and expressed emotional intimacy, but also emotional and behavioral inter-dependence: what each one does has strong effects on what the other thinks, feels, and does. Defined this way, closeness at the extreme can be so great that one or both people have little existence apart from their relationship. They do nothing without the other person or without at least checking with the other person. The mother–infant relationship is an extremely close one, particularly for the infant. The newborn baby needs the mother or a mother substitute present during most of its waking hours. The mother often finds the relationship extremely close—and demanding—for herself also, leaving little time for anything else.

At the other extreme, so little closeness may exist within a relationship that it can hardly be called a relationship at all. Partners can lead their own lives and "do their own thing" to such an extent that they hardly affect each other. Some married couples grow so far apart over the years that they work and play in entirely separate worlds. They sleep in separate bedrooms, engage in different activities, pursue different hobbies, and take separate vacations. They might more accurately be called joint tenants of the same house than a married couple.

Within these two extremes, which have been labeled by family therapist Salvador Minuchin as "enmeshment" and "disengagement," couples must find their own level of closeness. They must seek a level of relatedness that fulfills their needs for companionship and intimacy without robbing them of their needs for autonomy. Obviously, there is no one "right" level of closeness and intimacy, on the one hand, or of separateness and auton-omy, on the other. One couple's level of closeness might be stifling for another couple. Each couple must seek their own best level.

When Couples Disagree about a Matter of Degree

Working out a comfortable level of closeness would be an easy task if the two people involved had the same needs *and* their needs

remained static. But we all differ in the degree of closeness and autonomy that suits us best, and our preferences may change over time. Generally, Derek wants more time for independent activities, while Mary
wants more quality time together. Even when together, Derek would
prefer to engage in activities while Mary wants to converse, to share feelings, and to express affection. Derek sometimes finds their relationship
stifling, while Mary finds it never "enough." Unlike other incompatibilities that trouble Derek and Mary, this difference in needs for closeness
goes to the very heart of their relationship. Although they could com-
partmentalize a difference over vacation preferences or in-laws, a difference around closeness could pervade their entire relationship.

Consistent personality incompatibilities like those between Derek
and Mary cause the greatest and most immediate problems for couples,
but differences that emerge only on particular occasions can hurt a relationship too. If you want to have a romantic dinner and reflect on your
life together Saturday night, but your wife wants to go a party and see
your friends, one of you may be able to yield to the other without resentment, or you may be able to come up with a satisfactory compromise.
But if the same disagreement comes up weekend after weekend, you
could end up feeling the same way that Mary and Derek have felt right
from the start.

Our needs and desires for closeness with our partners not only
evolve in response to how well they are fulfilled and how much conflict
arises over them but also simply because of the effects of the life cycle.
Early in their relationship Wanda and Ben spent all their free time
together. They both wanted that and both assumed the other did also.
However, after their first child was born, Ben found that Wanda was not
as interested in him or as available for spending time alone with him.
Her attachment to their child limited her own involvement with him.
Ben felt left out, unhappy at being reduced to a second priority in
Wanda's life; he found himself strangely jealous of the baby. Wanda was
incredulous and annoyed that he could not take in stride the fact that the
baby had changed their relationship unalterably.

"Different Strokes for Different Folks"

The crux of the disagreement is pretty clear to Wanda and
Ben and to many other couples struggling with intimacy problems.
Wanda is not able or willing to spend as much free time with Ben as the
couple used to enjoy. The issue is not as clear-cut with other couples.

Burt wants Irene by his side constantly. He hates to do errands without her or to eat breakfast without her or to watch TV without her, yet when they are together Burt prefers light conversation. He discloses little and expresses no strong emotions or intimate feelings. Irene doesn't want to accompany him on every little errand or sit with him for every TV show. She needs some time alone. She also craves more intimate disclosure; she wants an intensity in their time together that is currently lacking. Each wants a high level of closeness, but by "closeness" Burt means mainly physical proximity while Irene means mainly emotional connection. Each ends up dissatisfied and wanting more from the other, but each is able to give only a limited amount of what the other needs.

It's not just our different needs for intimacy that cause problems in our relationships. We all instinctively seek or express intimacy differently, and these incompatibilities can lead to insensitivity to the other. Sex is a perfect example. For one person in a couple, making love is a way to achieve closeness; for the other, it is an expression of closeness that has already been achieved. Ramon wants to make love with Tasha even after an angry scene has distanced them. For him, the arousal and release of sex dissipates tension and brings him closer to her. However, Tasha can't make love unless she feels love. She wants to work out their tensions, feel emotionally close to one another, and then express this closeness through lovemaking. For Ramon, sex is the appetizer that leads to closeness between them; for Tasha, sex is the dessert that follows a full course of closeness.

Partners may use conflict as well as sex to regulate closeness. A good fight may release bad feelings and erase the distance between partners so they can feel close again. However, spouses may also use a fight to create distance if they feel uncomfortably close to one another. Problems develop when spouses use conflict differently to regulate intimacy between them. Nan may pick a fight to get past the distance she feels between herself and Li, but Li may react to conflict with even greater distance.

Most of us get into relationships to achieve closeness and intimacy with another. Incompatibilities in this area are threatening because they make us question our very reason for being in the relationship. If we can't get what we came here for, why should we be here at all? If we have to give up too much of ourselves, shouldn't we leave?

As we shall see later, it is possible to understand, accept, and cope with our differences in ways that not only don't compromise our intimacy with each other but actually enhance it.

"SOME TERRITORY IN THIS RELATIONSHIP MUST BE MINE": POWER, DOMINANCE, AND CONTROL

Each of us seeks some measure of control over our life and the world. To feel good about ourselves we must have the power to affect our own destiny and the destiny of those close to us. As infants we learned that our cries would make the world respond to our needs. As adults we use more mature strategies to exercise power, but we still need to believe our cries will be answered. Without this sense of control, we are likely to feel helpless and depressed.

What gives us power and control as adults? Appropriate resources may grant power. Those with wealth and beauty get their wishes fulfilled more often than those with limited means and ordinary appearances. Knowledge may confer power, in love relationships as elsewhere. If Ella knows more about stocks and bonds than Harry, she will probably make the buy and sell orders. Competency may ensure power. If Grant can get the children to mind better than Susan, he will likely assume the role of disciplinarian. Status may grant power. Claire has advanced degrees, so Sid may defer to her during discussions of political and economic matters. Cultural roles may confer power. Angus and Mary may both expect Angus to make financial decisions because he is the man.

In our social relations, we face an enduring issue of the division of power. Who shall control what? Who will be in charge when? Whether the relationship involves equals, as in marriage, or unequals, as in parents and children, the participants must work out a system of power, control, and responsibility.

Today the division of power and control in relationships has become a more challenging task than ever before. Social and cultural restrictions used to define so many roles for us that our choices were narrow. As long as we were willing to live within the bounds society had drawn for us, conflict over the division of power rarely arose. Now we have choices—and, by extension, conflict.

When Culture Rules

We all learn scripts for social positions such as husband, wife, father, and mother. We know what we should do when we are spouses or parents. Furthermore, we have been trained especially for our roles. Therefore, we can enact them with competence and pleasure. A young husband and wife may come to marriage expecting him to repair the cars and her to prepare the meals. And they may accept these role definitions happily, since their separate training has made him a competent and proud mechanic and her a skilled and proud cook.

Still, trouble can arise in this predetermined paradise. Culturally defined gender roles never go far enough to tell us how to negotiate all the little details of daily life. In the traditional view of marriage, the wife was supposed to handle the cooking, but did she have a right to expect a night or two off from these duties every week? The husband was supposed to help with the dishes and carve the roast, but when and how often? Role definitions leave plenty of room for disagreement over how our roles are to be carried out from minute to minute.

Then there are the "cultural misfits" among us, those who grew up without the necessary interest in or education for enacting our assigned roles. Plenty of women dislike cooking, and the world is full of men who know nothing about car repair. These women and men face a larger negotiation task. They must not only work out the details of their roles but also renegotiate the entire cultural mandate.

Choice and Conflict

In the last thirty years, culturally defined gender roles, particularly for women, have changed dramatically. Not only have women entered the work force in increasing numbers and commanded work and pay on a level equal to men's, but an egalitarian attitude overall is beginning to prevail. The consequences of these changes are sweeping. Money has always conferred power. With greater economic resources, women can command more say in their relationships. Furthermore, the logistics of dual-career couples require some shifts in responsibility. When both husband and wife work full time outside the home, the woman can't also take full responsibility for childcare and the household. In reality, though, these tasks still seem to fall disproportionately to women, because egalitarian ideals, while supported by many, may be achieved by only a few. A husband may believe that he should take on equal responsibility for his infant's care, but his life experiences may not have provided him with either the interest or the skill to fulfill that responsibility well. A wife may believe that she should contribute equally to the family coffers, but her life experiences may have trained her only for traditional "women's work," which offers lower salaries.

Periods of role change, particularly periods when sex roles become less differentiated, may present confusing challenges to men and women. Each may suffer internal conflicts between what they would now like to be and what they feel comfortable and competent being. They may disagree over who does what now that their conduct is "up for grabs" rather than defined by social mores.

The upside, of course, is greater choice and the opportunity for greater individual fulfillment. Couples have the opportunity to divide the power, control, and responsibility for workplace and home according to their own needs, interests, and abilities. People now have new freedoms and new choices. But the choices made by two different free people can often collide. One wants to exercise his or her power in one direction, the other in another direction. If societal roles determine who does what, then there will be little choice but no disagreement. If individuals can choose for themselves, then there will be freedom but frequent disagreement. The price of freedom is conflict.

These conflicts can rightly be called power struggles. Each partner wants to exercise his or her authority and power to determine how things should be between the two of them. To give up power may feel like giving up part of oneself. Some common areas where power struggles emerge are money, housework and childcare, and individual life choices.

Money

> Where there is money, there is fighting.
> —MARIAN ANDERSON (1941)

> He who has the most toys wins.
> —UNKNOWN

It is hardly surprising that power struggles erupt over money. In a society that values consumption, rarely does anyone have enough money to buy all the things she or he desires. So choices must be made about what we can afford and what we cannot afford. He or she who makes those decisions has control.

In some traditional relationships, where husbands were the sole or at least primary breadwinners, women sometimes had no knowledge of how much money the husband made, what savings and investments they had, or what financial decisions were made. He doled out money to her as needed for groceries or clothes, but he retained control. In other traditional relationships, the husband was the sole breadwinner, but he dutifully turned over his paycheck to his wife, who paid the bills and controlled spending.

The great majority of married couples today are both employed. Thus, both are liable to have an interest in and a legitimate claim to control over the finances. However, given the model of his parents, the husband may feel he should control the finances. Given her contribution to the family coffers, the wife may feel she should have equal control. Because of their interests or experiences, each may feel more qualified to handle the money. So for various reasons the couple may have a primary struggle over who will control the finances.

Most contemporary couples are likely to endorse a philosophy of joint control over finances. Both should have a more or less equal say in financial decision making. But such an enlightened view hardly solves the problem; indeed, it raises as many questions as it answers. Does joint control mean that we both decide on every little purchase or only on major purchases? If we decide on joint control for major purchases, what is the cutoff amount for a major purchase: $50, $100, $1,000? Also, might not a plethora of minor purchases create financial difficulties? What about accountability? Does each of us have our own checkbook or our own credit cards, so that we can spend a certain amount privately, away from the scrutiny of our partners' eyes? Or do all purchases come from the same joint checkbook or credit cards and thus are potentially known to our partners? Do we have a source of money that is truly our own, not subject to our partners' control or scrutiny? Some might consider the money they had when they came into the relationship their very own. Others might consider the extra money they made through a side business or by working overtime their very own money.

Incompatibilities between partners can complicate financial decisions between them. One may be a saver and the other a spender, a difference that reflects broader differences about "living for today" versus "preparing for tomorrow." One may be a risk taker, who wants to save money through investment in aggressive stock portfolios, while the other is risk-averse, and wants to make money through insured certificates of deposit. One may be a homebody who wants to put extra money into remodeling the house, buying nicer furniture, and landscaping the yard. The other may be more of a get-out-in-the-world person who wants to put extra money into fun trips and vacations. One may value appearance much more than the other and want to spend money on clothes or jewelry or plastic surgery.

Housework and Childcare

> Few tasks are more like the torture of Sisyphus
> than housework, with its endless repetition: the
> clean becomes soiled, the soiled is made clean over
> and over, day after day.
> —SIMONE DE BEAUVOIR,
> *The Second Sex* (1949)

> Housework's the hardest work in the world. That's
> why men won't do it.
> —EDNA FERBER, *So Big* (1924)

> It's clear that most American children suffer too
> much mother and too little father.
> —GLORIA STEINEM
> in *The New York Times* (1971)

The research is clear about the roles women and men play in housework and childcare. Women do the larger part of both, even when both partners are employed full time outside the home. Psychologists Monica Biernat and Camille Wortman interviewed 139 married, professional couples with young children about how home responsibilities were shared. They chose husbands and wives who were of relatively high and equal job status: the women were university professors or businesspeople. Even in this sample of professional couples, the women did more childcare and household chores than their husbands.

Given this picture of who does what in the household, it is hardly surprising that wives might often complain about their husbands and try to get them to do more housework and childcare. Often the husbands reply that they are willing to help when asked, but they object to the resentful way their wives seek their help. Why can't she ask nicely? The wives often do ask with a chip on their shoulder, because they seek more than a helpful assistant. They would like to have their husbands take some significant responsibility for housework and childcare.

In one couple with whom I worked, the husband was a gardener by profession. He took great pride in keeping his own lawn and garden immaculate. No shoemaker without shoes was he. He described how he would notice if one section of his lawn or garden was drooping a bit from too much sun and too little water, and he would readjust the sprinklers or spray a little water on them as soon as he got home from work. He would notice if an offending weed broke through a crevice, and he would pluck it out by its roots before it could enjoy a full day's sunshine.

He clearly took major responsibility for his lawn and garden, which meant that he noticed when things went wrong and then quickly and independently took action to fix them.

His wife complained that, in contrast, he hardly noticed when things were going wrong with their children. The children could be fighting, and his head would never budge from the newspaper. Their youngest could be climbing on the kitchen counter, and he wouldn't notice. True enough, if she asked him to intervene, and asked him nicely, he would get up from whatever he was doing and faithfully take charge—temporarily. However, she often asked with frustration in her voice, because she wanted him to notice and intervene without her having to call it to his attention. Of course, he responded angrily to her frustration, and tension often ensued. Thus, she often felt angry at him, because, in her view, she always had to be in charge of the kids. In his view, he was living with a woman who was supposed to be his loving wife but was instead constantly "on his case."

Sorting out household tasks and childcare gets complicated because partners often have different skill levels, different standards, and different needs for control. Consider a husband and wife who are mirror images of the usual stereotype. She takes great pride in their sports car, actually enjoys cleaning and waxing it, is careful to park it only next to new or expensive cars (whose owners presumably will be more careful not to nick their car), and notices the first signs of problems— a transmission that runs rough, an engine that needs tuning. He, on the other hand, takes great pride in their home and feels better when things are all organized and in their place, when the counters and floor are freshly cleaned and the carpets just vacuumed. In this situation, the wife should certainly take charge of the car and he of the house. If he tried to take charge of the car, he would not enjoy it as much as she, not do it as well as she, nor do it to her standards. The same could be said of her if she tried to take charge of cleaning the house.

However, what if her skills and interests regarding household tasks stopped with the car? Compared to her, he was more skilled and more invested in cleaning the house, doing the laundry, and cooking. Should he then have to do most of the work, simply because of his greater skill and interest? But if she participates in more housework, so he doesn't have an unfair load, must she do it to his standards? Will he monitor her activities and be critical of her because she doesn't do it that well?

Individual Life Choices

Normally, we can discriminate between decisions that belong to the couple and decisions that belong to the individual. Choices about what house to buy and where to go on vacation are clearly issues in which both members deserve a say. Only the most dictatorial individuals would insist that those decisions be made unilaterally. In contrast, decisions about what career to pursue, what food to eat, what clothes to wear, what friends to cultivate, and what doctor to choose clearly seem to be individual choices. While people often seek out information and advice from others before making these decisions, most would agree that the final decision must rest with the individual.

Couples often get into power struggles over these apparently individual life choices because one person's choices may have a big impact on the other. Consider the issue of career. Seth pushes his wife, Mallory, to go back to school and finish her degree so she can get a better paying job. At times, she resists his pressure: "Whose job are we talking about anyhow? Don't I get to make the decision about what schooling and career I want?" Seth replies that her income has implications for both of them and for their children. He earns much more than she does, but his income will increase only gradually from now on. She is the one who could provide an income jump if she returned to school. He challenges her with accusatory questions: "How are we going to put our kids through college and maintain our lifestyle unless you get off your butt and finish your degree?" She feels guilty about his accusations and comparisons to his salary, but resists his attempts to control her life.

Jodie tries to persuade and at times to pressure Zach to quit smoking. He maintains the view that smoking is his own life choice. "Look, I am a courteous smoker. I smoke only outside so I won't irritate you or put you or the kids in any danger of secondhand smoke."

She replies: "I know, but I am not worried about us—I am worried about you."

He argues: "Look, I like smoking. It's a pleasure I value. My father smoked all his life and died at eighty-one from a fall. I think I can smoke without getting any diseases myself. But basically, it's my decision. I'm willing to take what health risk there is."

Jodie replies angrily: "You may be willing to take the risk, but I'm not. It's not just you who will suffer if you get cancer or heart disease. I will have to care for you. I will have to pay the medical bills. And the children and I will have to live life without you."

RECAP

Someone once said, "A difference that makes no difference *is* no difference." Differences in areas of love and power are differences that *do* make a difference. They are differences that matter. You may not feel that your relationship is deep and meaningful unless your partner values openness and self-disclosure as much as you do. You may not be able to maintain your cherished view of yourself as a free spirit unless your partner allows you the autonomy you desire. You may not feel like a powerful man or an independent woman unless you have a major say over the finances. These issues of closeness and control may define the relationship for you, affirm your self-image, and determine in large part how happy and content you are together.

Incompatibility around closeness may concern not only the sheer quantity of contact you want from your partner. You and your partner may also differ on what you consider closeness to be and how you express it. Incompatibilities over power and control usually center on money, childcare, housework, and individual decision making. Like all couples, you need to work out how you share responsibility and control over these fundamental areas.

Both of you are likely to overreact when even a minor issue tests some relevant principle of closeness or control. The wife who gets furious at her retired husband for going into the kitchen to make himself lunch may just be protecting her territory. He may have retired from his job, but he better not invade hers. The husband who lashes out at his wife for revealing some secret to her friend before she told him may be protecting some boundary around their relationship: disclosures must be made to each other before being made to the world.

Because closeness and power are so fundamental, you may balk at the idea of accepting your partner's differing needs for closeness and power. To "give in" may mean to give up too much of what you wanted in your relationship. But as we will discuss in Part II of this book, acceptance does not mean yielding, giving in, or resigning yourself to something with which you are not comfortable. It is anything but passive. And it offers the promise of even greater intimacy with your partner.

Exercise

Think about closeness and power in your own relationship. Consider the amount of time you spend together, the independent activities you each have (time away from each other to be alone or with friends), the physical affection and sexual contact you have. Under power, responsibility, and control, you might consider money, housework and childcare, and individual life choices.

- What is the most important incompatibility that you and your partner have?
- What does your partner want and need that is different from what you want and need?
- How do these incompatibilities typically show up as conflicts in your life?
- How many arguments over the "trivial" could be reclassified as closeness and power issues?

Put your answers in a drawer with your notes from preceding chapter exercises.

CHAPTER 5

"I Do but I Don't"

CONFUSING INCOMPATIBILITIES

> Go away and stop leaving me alone.
> —Anonymous

Up to now we have been discussing clear differences between partners: One wants one thing, the other wants something else. The wife endorses one set of values, the husband another. No matter how diametrically opposed the positions, such differences present definite, unambiguous goals for the two. They may fight dirty to reach these goals, but the stakes are clear.

Not all conflicts of interest present such clear-cut choices. Sometimes we think we want something and we articulate our desires clearly, but our behavior suggests something else. We send mixed messages, on one occasion pressing in one direction and on another in the opposite direction. Even a partner who is open to changing for us won't know which changes to make.

Edwina says she wants Henry to participate equally in child rearing. Henry reluctantly agrees and genuinely tries to become more involved with their children. However, Edwina's criticisms of his efforts and her unwillingness to relinquish control over the children undermine his attempts. Part of her wants Henry to participate equally, since she finds it difficult to take the primary role in childcare and still succeed at her job. But another part of her wants to stay in charge of bringing up their children—both because she feels she can do it better and because she believes that the mother ought to be the primary caretaker.

In these situations we see both a conflict *within one person* and a conflict *between two people*. Not only do Edwina and Henry disagree, but Edwina herself is not sure what she wants. The situation becomes even more confounded and confusing when Henry also feels ambivalent. Part of him feels he should be an equal partner in raising their children—after all, that is the "modern way"—especially since Edwina spends as much time at work and contributes as much financially to the family as he does. But part of him feels unprepared for the task: he hasn't had as much experience with children as she has. And, to tell the truth, he takes less pleasure in attending to them than she does.

Consider another example of how conflicts within each partner complicate conflicts *between* them. Harold wants Julie to take better care of him. When he feels down or stressed—which is often—he wants to be pampered, drawn out, catered to. Julie often resists his pressure, feeling she shouldn't have to "baby" him. After all, he doesn't treat her that way when *she* feels bad. But there is something about his open anguish, his inability to cover his hurt, his vulnerability that Julie finds appealing. She feels needed, generous, and strong when she takes care of him. But when she's preoccupied with her own concerns, she finds his demands annoying. Thus she alternates between an angry "Oh, grow up" attitude and a comforting "Ah, sweetie, it'll be all right" attitude.

For his part, Harold feels uncomfortable about the level of support he wants and needs from Julie. It doesn't gibe with his ideas about manhood and often makes him feel "one down" in the relationship. Sometimes, when he just wants to withdraw into his own thoughts, he finds her pampering insulting and intrusive. Thus he alternates between a petulant "Aren't you going to help me?" stance and a defiant "I don't need you!" stance.

Given these mixed feelings within each partner, it's not surprising that the conflict between them is confusing. It's no wonder that they can't elicit or implement any change that either of them wants.

MIXED BLESSINGS

> There are no unmixed blessings.
> —JOHN UPDIKE

The personal qualities of our partners are often mixed blessings for us. The presence of any good characteristic is often associated with the presence of a less desirable one.

For example, it's great to have a responsible husband who takes care of business, who is punctual, neat, and orderly. You never have to wait for him, pick up after him, do his chores, check his bookkeeping, or worry whether he'll pick up the kids on time. If he says he'll do it, you know it will get done. But often such husbands demand similarly high levels of responsibility from their wives and children. They may be rigid about following rules and inflexible about adapting to changing circumstances. Their insistence on work before play may create a joyless atmosphere in the household. The "tight ship" they run is rarely a pleasure cruise.

It's also wonderful to have an accepting wife, one who loves you for what you are. She won't criticize you for your inadequacies or pressure you to change. Your foibles create few problems for her. But she may be passive about other aspects of life too. She may not join as vigorously as you'd like in pursuit of the goals you've set for yourself and your family, she may let things slide rather than take corrective action, and her laid-back quality may sometimes feel to you like indifference.

Some positive characteristics are less notable for their other-side-of-the coin association with a negative characteristic than for their failure to include some other positive quality. For example, it's good to have a husband who is devoted to his family, who enjoys spending hours with the children after school and on weekends, playing sports and taking them places. He readily assumes his share of the kids' doctor and dental visits and delights in helping them, playing with them, talking with them. But such a man is unlikely to be a dynamo at work. He may have neither time nor inclination to drive himself to greater heights (and higher salaries) at his job.

By the same token, it may be great to marry a career woman whose prestigious job adds substantially to the family income. Her career provides interesting material for conversation, is a source of pride, and allows upward mobility. However, she may not have the time or the interest to do certain "wifely" things that her husband also desires, such as preparing great meals, taking a personal interest in the laundering of his shirts, and assuming the major role in childcare.

Obviously, it's possible to be responsible without being rigid, to be accepting without being passive, and to combine career, marriage, and parenting successfully. However, the development of one characteristic often precludes or at least limits the development of another. Certainly, limitations of time and energy prevent us from being good at everything. Therefore the characteristics of our partners, though often blessings, may be mixed ones.

Because of this, we may complain that our partners don't help out enough at home, even while we continue to push them to earn promotions at work. We may complain about their being controlling, yet gladly turn over more and more responsibilities to them. We certainly want them to find us sexually desirable but may find their frequent overtures annoying.

YES AND NO

Even if desirable qualities in our partners came unaccompanied by undesirable ones, our incompatibilities might still cause confusion. Often your feelings about a single characteristic are mixed. You may be attracted to your partner because of a particular attribute but at times find the same attribute distasteful. Your ambivalence may arise from your own internal conflicts about a particular characteristic. You may experience certain desires in yourself while finding these feelings emotionally or morally repugnant.

Lucy, for example, has always felt shy and uncomfortable about her sexuality. Discussions of sex embarrassed her, and sexual situations inhibited her. Surprisingly, she found herself attracted to Terry, who seemed just the opposite. He loved to tell ribald jokes, often made suggestive remarks, and vigorously pursued Lucy sexually. Her reactions to his sexual frankness were mixed. At times she found his behavior provocative and arousing, but at other times she found it disgusting.

Jorge has mixed feelings about wealth. Raised in the 1960s when materialism was scorned, he had since tried to lead a simple life. As values changed in the '70s and '80s, he held on to his philosophy, often lamenting society's "conspicuous consumption," "technological fixes," and "insatiable materialism." Yet he also yearned for certain possessions: a "high-end" personal computer, a superb audio system, and a fast car. When he met Wanda, he found himself enjoying her posh condominium and stylish sports car. Even though he teased and criticized her for her materialism, he took full advantage of it himself.

Our desires may create conflicts not because these desires, in themselves, repel us, but because they don't fit our image of ourselves. Consciously accepting these longings would damage our self-esteem. Chim, who wants to be protected and taken care of in a relationship, chose Ben partly because he seemed strong and dependable. Throughout their relationship Ben has come to her rescue financially, taken charge of practical details such as car repairs, and pressured her to do long-range planning for herself (by making investments, buying insurance, and making a will). Such a relationship doesn't fit Chim's view of herself as a liberated, independent woman, so she criticizes Ben for treating her "like a child."

Cecil hates paperwork of any kind. He'll gladly work on the car or in the yard for hours rather than spend ten minutes with bills, budgets, or bank statements. Jessica has taken charge of the paperwork in their relationship, partly because she enjoys it and partly because Cecil avoids it. However, being uninformed about finances doesn't fit Cecil's view of manhood. Jessica's greater knowledge and control over their budget makes him feel weak in the relationship. When she informs him of their financial situation and recommends that they save more or spend less, he often resists, making vague accusations about her inability to control their budget. Sometimes he makes impulsive purchases, partly to demonstrate his financial independence.

Our ambivalence may arise less from internal conflict about a characteristic than from envy and competitiveness. We may seek in our partners those characteristics we lack yet feel angry that they possess those qualities while we do not. For example, James has always had difficulty asserting himself. He went along with the wishes of others, rarely voicing his own desires but often feeling resentful about being "taken advantage of." He found himself attracted to Darlene in part because of her frankness. She spoke her mind and "took shit from no one." James envied this quality in her yet criticized her for being insensitive to others and taking advantage of them.

Ray loved social gatherings of any type: parties, business lunches, dinners with friends. An entertaining conversationalist, he was sought out by others as much as he sought them out. Ray's wife, Tanya, was more reserved and uncomfortable socially. It took her a while to "loosen up" with friends. Tanya envied the social attention Ray commanded but put down his skill as "superficial charm."

Ambivalence may develop over time as you become more familiar with your partner's qualities. As we discussed in Chapter 3 and illustrated with the "Cathy" cartoon, over time, once-appealing characteristics can show a darker side. What you once saw as unkempt charm now seems more like sloppiness; what you once viewed as a relaxed, easygoing attitude toward life now looks like laziness; what you once regarded as loving caretaking now seems like controlling behavior. You're finding fault and demanding change, and your partner quite naturally cries "Foul!"

Whatever its source, ambivalence adds confusion to any conflict with your partner. You generate mixed messages, sometimes supporting a characteristic of your partner, sometimes complaining about it. These changing responses cause confusion not only because they are contradictory but also because you present them *indirectly*. If you directly told your partner, "I don't like this" and then said, just as directly, "I do like this," he or she could comment on the contradiction and attempt to clear up the confusion. But you may not be fully aware of the ambivalence and present at least one side of the contradiction indirectly.

Lucy may criticize Terry's sexual vulgarity as bad taste yet actually reward his suggestive comments and jokes by making ineffectual protests that draw attention to his antics. Cecil may complain about Jessica's financial management and control but continue to force her to take charge by refusing to get involved with their finances himself. Tanya may minimize Ray's social skill by labeling it "superficial charm" yet depend on him to "break the ice" and bring her into the social swim. As these examples illustrate, we directly communicate the negative side of our ambivalence: don't do that or don't be that way. Yet at the same time we often indirectly communicate the positive side of the ambivalence—by acting in such a way as to reinforce the characteristics in question.

Ambivalence in *both* partners about the *same* issue creates even greater confusion. Each one has mixed feelings about an issue, has limited awareness of the confusion, and sends contradictory messages. No wonder they fail to resolve their conflict.

Consider, for example, Chim's ambivalence about being taken care of by Ben. She wants to be an independent woman, and so she criticizes Ben for treating her like a child. Yet she makes impulsive financial decisions that get her into situations from which she needs Ben to rescue her, and she avoids practical planning for her life, depending on him to do it for her. For his part, Ben wants her to need him, enjoys taking care of her, and seeks opportunities to exercise his considerable abilities in attending to the practical side of life. Yet he wants her to express appreciation for his efforts, insists on control of these practical areas if he has to take responsibility for them, and expects her to carry out the tasks he allocates to her without giving him any static. When she does give him static—which she often does when she sees him assigning her errands to take care of *her* life—he complains about her lack of responsibility. Or, when he is overwhelmed by his own responsibilities and finds the addition of hers a burden, he may tell her to "grow up." Thus Chim accuses Ben of treating her like a child and Ben accuses Chim of acting like a child; both are genuinely angry at each other's behavior, but both support and maintain these characteristics in each other. Their conflict is confused by the ambivalence of both about the issue of caretaking.

THE MENTIONABLE AND THE UN-

Sometimes our incompatibilities cause confusion because we focus on the wrong ones. Our arguments camouflage rather than illuminate the real issues between us. We can't hope to resolve genuine problems if we waste our energy battling over false ones.

We may feel uncomfortable or embarrassed by some differences with our partners. Rather than voicing these feelings, we may discuss other unrelated, minor, or irrelevant differences. Rather than telling Neil about her sexual inhibitions, Rachel criticizes his sexual abilities. They argue about his experience and skill rather than finding ways to make her feel more satisfied.

Rather than telling Gayle about his social discomfort, Mark refuses to go to parties with her, on the pretext that such events are exercises in superficiality. They fight about the inherent value of parties instead of dealing directly with his shyness.

We may feel our partners would be hurt by knowing about our differences with them. And so we "protect" them by camouflaging real issues with false ones. Because Maria doesn't want to confront Tony about his tendency to be domineering in a social situation, she withdraws from joint social encounters. Tony is denied important feedback about himself, and they argue about her lack of social participation.

Bruce isn't satisfied with his and Sara's sexual routine. He wants her to dress more provocatively and to try different positions, yet he protects her from his feelings, afraid that knowing about his dissatisfaction would hurt her. He withdraws more often into his sexual fantasies, enacted through masturbation, while she complains vaguely about how little they make love.

When you've been hurt by your partner, you may express anger over a related but irrelevant issue. Expressing genuine pain is scary, because it makes you vulnerable to more pain. To express anger over the true issue may also feel uncomfortable, because the hurt might be transparent. So we often take the safe way and fight over an incidental issue.

Rather than express his feelings of hurt and jealousy over Martha's long conversation with Ernie at the party, Bill criticizes Ernie to Martha. She then defends Ernie, and they have a major argument about Ernie's personality, which is not an important issue for either of them. Rather than comment on Eric's lack of interest in her achievements at work, Susan interferes with Eric's disciplinary actions with the children, causing a heated but irrelevant conflict between them.

Sometimes we are unaware (or only dimly aware) of our feelings toward our partners. We experience dissatisfaction, but its origin is unclear. No wonder we can't voice our feelings clearly. For example, Donna may feel irritated with Fritz but fail to understand clearly that her reaction stems from his apparent lack of interest in her. He has done nothing specifically wrong, but his kisses feel perfunctory, his participation in conversation seems merely polite, and his interest in her appears lukewarm. Since she is only vaguely aware of the source of her dissatisfaction, she couldn't articulate the problem even if she wanted to. So she expresses annoyance at his choice of clothes and his table manners—which irritates him and encourages him to withdraw further.

In each case, we disguise the real issues. Whether out of embarrassment and shame, protectiveness toward our partners, protectiveness of our own hurt feelings, or unawareness, we focus on minor, tangential, or unrelated differences. While our discussion of these differences may serve to vent our anger and dissatisfaction, it can never lead to a resolution of the problem. And the ensuing exchange may also elicit reactions from our partners and ourselves that further confuse and intensify the conflict.

IT'S NOT US

Instead of finding a convenient scapegoat *in* the relationship, we can sometimes achieve a better disguise by finding a red herring *outside* the relationship. There is nothing wrong with *us*, we insist, but this thing outside the relationship is causing us no end of grief. We have a perfect relationship except for . . .

Bruno and Ivana seem exceptionally well matched. They rarely differ on anything except Bruno's work. Ivana fears that Bruno's long hours at work may be driving him to an early death; Bruno insists that his work schedule is no different from that of his peers in high-pressure careers. Ivana pushes Bruno to relax and spend more time at home with the family, while Bruno insists that he can't stay home because of various work deadlines. If only they could resolve this difference, they feel, their marriage would be virtually perfect.

A closer examination suggests that they do experience other difficulties but attribute them all to Bruno's job. When Bruno is unresponsive to Ivana's sexual overtures, both blame his fatigue on work. When Bruno is distracted in conversation with Ivana, both insist his inattentiveness is caused by his preoccupation with work. When he doesn't want to participate in household tasks, he can always claim he has work to do. By placing the entire fault on Bruno's work, they both avoid dealing with the very real difficulties in their sexual relationship, their communication, and their allocation of household responsibilities. Their avoidance of these issues makes it safe for them to disagree but prevents them from solving major problems, among which Bruno's work is only one.

Safe problems may absorb dangerous ones. By storing threatening problems under the umbrella of a familiar difficulty, we can cushion their impact. But why are some problems safer than others? Why is it so much easier for Bruno and Ivana to lay all their problems on Bruno's work rather than confront their difficulties over sex, communication, and household tasks? The answer is simple: direct confrontation over an incompatibility between two people threatens their relationship. Attributing problems to some third factor separate from both partners allows them to join forces against this disruptive element. Bruno and Ivana can discuss his work problems comfortably because they define his work as something separate from them as a couple. They define his job as high pressured, rather than defining him as more stimulated by his work than by his home life; they define his work as exhausting, rather than defining their sex life as boring; and they define his work as preoccupying rather than defining their conversation as dull. Of course, Bruno's job may actually be high pressured, but by ignoring his part in choosing and maintaining his high level of work performance, husband and wife avoid the inadequacies in their relationship and limit their ability to improve it.

By attributing problems to *people* outside the relationship rather than to things outside it, we can even more effectively avoid threatening difficulties. If Bruno had a demanding boss who pressed relentlessly for greater effort by Bruno, then Ivana and Bruno could blame their difficulties on him rather than on the vague concept of Bruno's "demanding work."

The effectiveness of outsiders in detouring conflict and emotion away from the couple can be seen most clearly in jealousy over extramarital affairs. Spouses may direct all their emotion toward the "spaceheaded bimbo" or the "slick-talking hunk" who stole their partner's affections—as if their mates were helpless victims. The extramarital lover gets the felony conviction, the partner gets away with misdemeanor charges of weakness and poor judgment, while the relationship escapes all charges and gets away scot-free.

In-laws often serve as useful targets for marital problems. A demanding, intrusive mother-in-law can take the heat off a couple's relationship difficulties. By arguing about her, they manage to avoid their conflicts with each other. Children may serve a similar purpose, since conflicts about offspring between parents may mask difficulties in the marriage. A mischievous or rebellious kid has preempted many a marital struggle.

When couples argue over a third party, the content of their argument may reveal important clues about their dissatisfaction with each other. Debra and Vic argue about their son, Derick's, school problems. Debra insists that Derick is a lazy underachiever who needs motivation and positive examples from his parents; Vic argues that Derick is a good-natured, relaxed, "true-blue" American boy who should be left alone to be what he is. Not surprisingly, Debra feels Vic is not achieving his potential at his job, while Vic views himself as an easygoing guy who is not caught up in the "rat race." Their struggles over their son mask their disagreement about Vic's role in the work world.

IT'S NOT THEM

Scapegoating can also go the other way. Rather than real incompatibilities in the relationship generating heat for tangential issues, frustrations outside the relationship can be taken out on the relationship or on your partner. If you're comfortable with some level of negative emotion and the issues targeted are not threatening to your relationship, you may release some of the stress generated from the outside world on your relationship.

Each of us suffers from temperamental bosses, financial strains, traffic jams, and bad weather—to name but a few of the myriad frustrations of modern life. We cope with these irritants not only through direct problem-solving actions but also through indirect strategies of release, escape, and rejuvenation. We may "space out" in front of the television, get sick, pursue sex, indulge in drugs or alcohol, or just go to sleep. One common strategy involves fighting the battle again, but on the home front, where victory is more likely.

Our partners represent safe and easy targets. Even if we criticize them unfairly or pick fights over minor issues, we are safe from such major consequences as missing out on an important sale, being denied a promotion, or losing our job. We may risk temporary alienation from our partners, but not an enduring loss. As long as we don't bring up a truly threatening issue, our spouses may be able to absorb the disruption. We are immune from disastrous fallout. Furthermore, on the home front we feel safer. Here we are accustomed to airing strong emotions. For many couples, intimacy gives license for emotional expression; even inappropriate feelings can erupt without embarrassment or shame.

At its best, this process provides for a working through of conflict. Your partner helps you unload your struggles without him or her being victimized. You show some restraint in your unloading; your partner tolerates some injustice out of love for you. For example, Mike sometimes comes home from work exhausted by his efforts, pressured by deadlines, and frustrated by his inability to "get more done." He greets Dawna with a scowl and launches into various diatribes about the people at work, people on the highways, and her. Yet he never attacks the children, and he avoids Dawna's sensitive areas. He may criticize her cooking and her failure to do errands but not her appearance or her parenting. For her part, Dawna tolerates his rages with a few comments about his "rare mood," brings him the newspaper and a drink, and goes on with her activities. Before long his anger has spent itself. Now calm, he realizes that the issues he raised with Dawna are not important, and he tries to make up to her with an apology. No love is lost between them.

At its worst, this displacement of your anger at the outside world onto your partner victimizes your partner and, by causing a conflict in your relationship where none existed, becomes a self-fulfilling prophecy. You know your partner's weaknesses and soft spots. Thus you can execute more effective attacks on your lover than on the outside world. Unable to do battle where the real war is being waged, you fight where you can win, where you can provoke a reaction denied to you by others. The world may have demonstrated your impotence, but your partner reaffirms your power.

When Rhea gets frustrated about not having an impact at her job, she attacks Vadim mercilessly, pointing out his lack of ambition, his "soft" and low-paying job, and his long hours in front of the "imbecile box." In his defense Vadim tries in vain to prove his adequacy to her. Later he gets furious at the unfairness of her attacks and her unwillingness to "accept me for what I am" and withdraws from her. Rhea finds some relief in his strong reaction but feels guilty about her attacks on him. Yet she finds herself angry at his inability to stand up for himself. Faced with this complex of feelings, she too withdraws from Vadim. Thus, Rhea's frustration with the outside world and Vadim's inability to absorb some of that frustration lead to a personal conflict that is more serious than the job stress that led to the conflict in the first place. They get drawn into a struggle that was not genuine in its origins but becomes genuine in its unfolding.

Whether or not these conflicts cause damage, they are confusing because you and your partner are fighting over an irrelevant issue. The overt conflict doesn't mask any hidden conflict; it simply expresses dissatisfaction that has no other outlet. The incompatibility is confusing because it is more apparent than real. It is the world, not your partner, that is the problem.

RECAP

Although some incompatibilities with your partner are defined and clear-cut, others may be more nebulous and slippery, adding confusion to your conflicts. The good qualities you like in your partner may be part of a natural constellation that includes some qualities that you don't like. Your partner's personality is inevitably a "package deal," and you have no "line-item veto" whereby you can cancel some qualities but keep others. Even a single quality in your partner may evoke complex and ambivalent reactions in which you are drawn to the quality at times but bothered by it at others. At times confusion arises because you argue over a false incompatibility and disguise the real one. Whether out of embarrassment, a desire to protect your partner or yourself, or unawareness of what your true feelings actually are, you scapegoat an irrelevancy in your partner or in the outside world and fight the wrong battle. Finally, if your relationship is a comfortable one for negative feelings, your scapegoating may go in the other direction. Rather than displacing an issue in your relationship onto the outside world, you may take your frustrations with the outside world into your relationship.

Socrates declared that "an unexamined life is not worth living." Although you can never understand your own mixed feelings and motives completely, calm reflection can lead to a more enlightened, complex, and accepting view of yourself and your partner. A living relationship is worth examining.

Exercise

When you are not upset at your partner and are thus better able to sort out confusing feelings, consider one or two of your partner's qualities that trouble you.

- Is that quality associated with another characteristic that is more appealing to you?
- Is that troublesome quality sometimes attractive to you?

Sorting out real issues from false issues can be challenging, but there are important clues:

- Do you and your partner sometimes argue intensely over issues that later seem trivial—of little meaning to either of you? What might be the real issues behind the false ones?
- Are you aware of sometimes holding back your real feelings about something to protect your partner or yourself? If your partner knew of your genuine feelings, how might he or she react?
- Do your frustrations with the outside world spill over into your relationship, so that you make relationship molehills into mountains? What typically happens in these situations?

Store your answers with your answers to preceding chapter exercises.

CHAPTER 6

"You Know How to Hurt Me"

RELATIONSHIP PROBLEMS AS VULNERABILITIES

> You always hurt the one you love.
> —DORIS FISHER and ALLAN ROBERTS
> (song title, 1944)

> A Roman divorced from his wife, being highly blamed by his friends, who demanded, "Was she not chaste? Was she not fair? Was she not fruitful?" holding out his shoe, asked them whether it was not new and well made. "Yet," added he, "none of you can tell where it pinches me."
> —PLUTARCH, *Parallel Lives: Aemilius Paulus* (circa 100 A.D.)

*I*n the early years of their marriage, Susan spent most of her time raising three children. Tom was heavily involved in his work as an architect. When their youngest child was eight, Susan started law school in the evenings; five years later she got her degree. She was offered a job with a fine law firm and wanted to take the position, but Tom asked her to postpone it for a while. He had taken on extra responsibilities as head partner and needed help from her at home to entertain colleagues and clients. She agreed. Here is how she describes her reaction to that decision and subsequent events:

"I was relatively satisfied with my decision. I was able to help Tom and at the same time do interesting law work. My volunteer work was well recognized in the legal community. A year and a half later, I was to receive a special award for my contribution to Legal Aid. I was really happy and looked forward to the award dinner, which many lawyers I respected would attend. But that evening, I was very embarrassed when Tom never showed up at the banquet; the chair reserved for him next to me near the center of the table stayed empty all evening. I was even angrier when I returned home that night to discover him watching TV and to hear him tell me that he had been just too tired to attend the dinner.

"That incident brought matters into focus. It forced me to realize how much the two of us had been drifting apart. I realized how much effort it now took me to ask Tom about his work and how rarely he inquired about mine or even listened when I did tell him about an experience. I also realized there wasn't much of a spark in our sex life. I started actually reveling in my extra 'space' when Tom was away on a trip. I began to feel resentful about the imbalance in our lives: Tom, at the peak of his career, expecting me to continue making sacrifices while giving me little in return. I became resentful about doing the bulk of the housework; resentful about Tom's taking me for granted; resentful that, after all the years I'd listened to his stories and supported his career, Tom now didn't give a damn about my career." (Levinger, 1983, pp. 317–318)

This incident—Tom's failure to attend the banquet—set off a train of events that ultimately led to the failure of their marriage.

"Finally, I figured I'd had enough. I received another good job offer and decided to take it without consulting Tom. I also told Tom that I'd probably want to separate from him. When I told him that, he seemed stunned. He said I was the most important person in his life and asked what he could do to keep me. I was so shocked at his insensitivity, though, that I blurted out: 'Nothing. There's nothing you can do to keep me, if you can't even figure out how unhappy I've been.'

"After I moved into my own apartment, I began to feel a lot better physically. The headaches and backaches I'd been having went away, and I felt good to be on my own. At the same time, I felt bad about the breakup and felt bad for our kids. Sometimes I worry about my future alone. But I think I made the right decision." (Levinger, 1983, p. 318)

When probed after the separation, Tom revealed that on the day of the banquet he had lost an important competition for a major design contract, yet he insisted at the time that the only reason he had skipped the banquet was that he was tired. He did not seem to understand that his absence had hurt Susan or that he may have been threatened by an award for her on a day of failure for him. Susan, too, was incredulous at the suggestion that Tom might be threatened by her success. She saw Tom as being so far ahead of her professionally as to be invulnerable.

This true story dramatically illustrates how relationship problems—and in this case relationship dissolution—are created when one partner fails to come through for the other. This failure to be there when it counts most causes the other embarrassment and humiliation and makes him or her feel unimportant. Our story also illustrates how partners can have limited understanding of their own motives or of the other's reactions, a lack of knowledge that allows them to attribute the other's behavior to the worst instincts. Tom had no sense of how important this recognition dinner was to Susan; she had no sense that he could feel threatened by her success.

"YOU WEREN'T THERE WHEN I NEEDED YOU MOST"

You are more likely to need your partner during moments of despair than during moments of glory. When threatened with illness, coping with the death of a loved one, or dealing with a failure, you feel most vulnerable and in need of your partner's help and support. At these crisis points you may need heroic actions from your partner. His or her failure to come through for you may leave you wounded deeply and angered inconsolably. The experience may etch a memory that won't be easily erased.

Gerard had chest pains late one night when Delia was on a business trip. When he called her at 3:00 A.M. and told her of his pains, she encouraged him to go to the emergency room but assured him that his pain was probably due to stress or possibly just in his head. Reminding him that he often had various aches and pains, she said, "Don't let your hypochondria get the best of you." Gerard took Delia's reassurances as veiled attacks on him and asserted that he had never awakened in the middle of the night with chest pains and had never before called her about them. When he got off the phone, he wasn't sure whether he was more upset with Delia or with the threat to his health. Impulsively he called for an ambulance—*someone* had to take seriously the pains that scared him so much. After all, his father had died of a heart attack at fifty-nine. In the ambulance and at the emergency room, Gerard was struck by the irony of his feelings: hoping on the one hand that his pains were nothing, and on the other that something was wrong with him so he could justify his call to 911 and vindicate himself with Delia. He got a little of both: the doctors found some irregularities in his heartbeat that required follow-up but no evidence of a heart attack. Now Gerard felt justified in being furious at Delia: she hadn't been there for him when he really needed her, when something really was wrong with him.

When Mara's mother died, Walter decided not to go to the funeral. He had an important business meeting that day, one that could lead to a new and large account for him. He explained to Mara that he had never gotten along with his mother-in-law, so to attend the funeral would be sort of a sham. Furthermore, he hated funerals. Mara was surprised and hurt by his decision but could not argue with his logic. Walter's decision not to go to the funeral was just another upset that got muddled in with all the rest, and it was only at the funeral that she realized clearly that she needed him there for her. Whatever his feelings toward her mother had been, it was her feelings that mattered now. She was terribly hurt by his absence at this difficult moment for her.

"NOT ONE BIG THING, BUT A THOUSAND LITTLE THINGS"

We can understand and perhaps excuse powerful and dramatic reactions to stunning events, such as a failure to show up at an honorary dinner or a funeral. Fortunately, such events in marriage are rare. More common are daily slights, ordinary injustices, and routine disrespects that hurt and anger us. He doesn't respond when she reaches for his hand. She shows little interest when he talks about his day. His kisses seem perfunctory. She seems bored by his stories.

At times we voice no overt reaction. Surprised by the intensity of our response, we try to convince ourselves we are overreacting and end up suffering these hurts in silence. At other times, however, we react strongly. We make sarcastic comments: "I didn't realize I was so boring to you." We accuse: "You don't care about me. You can't even bring yourself to touch me." We make attacking suggestions: "Maybe you should find someone who will capture your interest better than me." We storm out of the room: "I don't want to be in the presence of someone who has no interest in or love for me."

When we do react strongly, our partners are likely to respond in kind, either defensively or offensively: "Is it a crime to yawn?" "Look,

I'm tired tonight." "We are not adolescent love birds." "Here you go again!" "You are so demanding." "You can't take not being the center of attention."

Why such seemingly small actions can provoke such big reactions may be explained by our history. A chronic pattern of daily neglect, in which each single incident might be easily explained, can eventually create powerful reactions of hurt and anger. In John Updike's novel *S.*, Sarah Worth leaves her physician husband of more than two decades not because of any egregious actions on his part but because of his "genteel atrocities of coldness and blindness toward me." In a letter to him, she describes the "nearly twenty-two years of mental and emotional cruelty you with your antiseptic chill have inflicted on me." In a letter to her adult daughter, she tries to justify her leaving: "Well, I recently tried an experiment. I didn't tell your father a thing about my day. And *he never asked*. Not once, day after day of biting my tongue—he utterly didn't notice. That settled it. So absent from his perceptions, I might as well be absent in fact." A long history of neglect—of inattentive acts, each one small and easily dismissed if considered in isolation but powerful in their totality—led Sarah to leave her husband and the material luxury they had.

"MY SENSITIVE SPOT"

Sometimes we react strongly to small events even in the absence of a history of neglect. All of a sudden, seemingly out of context, we explode emotionally, as if some combustible material inside us, some personality plutonium, reached its critical mass and blew up.

Although *explosion* is an appropriate analogy for the force of our reaction, the connection between the precipitant and our response suggests something more akin to an allergic reaction. What is to most a mildly negative experience, such as a bee sting, or a curative one, such as penicillin, or even a pleasurable one, such as the smells of spring or the taste of a particular food, can cause strong negative, allergic reactions in others. Their bodies react with fits of coughing and sneezing or with rashes and itching or much worse. One person's meat is truly another's poison.

Viewing some of our emotional reactions as "psychological allergies" is appropriate for at least two reasons. The precipitating event is an innocent one, or at most a mildly annoying one, for many people, whereas we have a special sensitivity to that kind of event. Similarly, just as the body's exaggerated, protective response to an allergy can create difficulty and in some cases threaten life itself, so our efforts to defend and protect ourselves from psychological allergies can create difficulty and in some cases threaten our relationships.

In the midst of an argument Hector mentions that he and Clarice ought to divorce. For him, this statement merely indicates his anger at the time; he has no intention of divorcing Clarice. For many couples such comments would be unpleasant and might be responded to in kind ("Yeah, well why don't you just move out?"). However, for Clarice, such a comment is deeply troubling. Her sensitivity to abandonment and rejection makes it impossible for her to dismiss Hector's remark. She is hurt and scared but mostly furious. Her reaction is to pack up and leave that very night. She will protect herself by rejecting him. She will implement his plan before he can. It takes Hector several difficult days of coaxing before she returns. But her strong reaction to his comment makes Hector genuinely question their marriage much more than the argument that led him to suggest divorce.

Our reaction in these situations is so intense because we take the precipitating event so personally. Like a heat-seeking missile that finds the engine of an aircraft, the seemingly innocent event finds our hot button. It exploits our vulnerability. It finds the weak spot in our defenses, where we lie openly exposed. We expect our partners to be sensitive to this vulnerability, even though we may be taken by surprise by it ourselves. We are offended; they are remiss. They simply *must* change their egregious acts, yet we can't explain the subtext we expect them to perform to.

COMMON VULNERABILITIES

The crimes of the heart are usually misdemeanors. Although partners will sometimes do horrible things, most of the events that create conflict in relationships are relatively small infractions. Yet the reaction can be intense, because the infraction touched on a vulnerability. There are a number of common vulnerabilities in people that can help explain their strong reactions, their psychological allergies. These sensitivities occur around universal themes of security, freedom, admiration, approval, and control.

"Don't Ever Leave Me"

Compared with animals, we humans have an exceptionally long period of dependency on our parents. We are born totally dependent, unable even to roll over or raise our heads. Even after a year, we can barely walk or feed ourselves. It takes almost two decades before we are recognized by society at large as adults capable of handling our own affairs.

Developmental psychologists have studied the attachment of infants to their primary caretaker—usually the mother. Because infants' physical survival depends on their caretaker, they have an automatic reaction to separation from her. They don't take it lightly if she leaves them alone, particularly in an unfamiliar place. They use her as a secure base from which to explore the world; if anything scary happens to them, they rush back into her arms. Psychologists speculate that if the caretaker is responsive to distress, if she handles separation sensitively so that the infant is familiar with his or her new surroundings and new caretakers before she leaves, then the infant develops "secure attachments." The infant learns that others can be trusted, that others will be there when he or she needs them; he or she will not be abandoned.

On the other hand, if the caretaker is not responsive to distress, if she does not handle separation sensitively, and especially if she is rejecting, the infant will not develop a secure attachment. He or she will *not* learn that others can be trusted, that others will be there for him or her—because they weren't. Some genetic predisposition may amplify these distressing experiences for the infant.

Psychologists tend to weight early experiences more heavily than later ones, because these early experiences are the foundation of learning on which the infant builds its model of what the world is like. However, later experiences certainly modify earlier ones. Infants exposed to inconsistent caretakers early on may later be exposed to more reliable ones and learn greater trust and confidence. Unfortunately, early experiences tend to predict later ones. Children don't have the luxury of "trading up" their caretakers. Usually the one who was inconsistent and rejecting when they were infants is still around to be rejecting and inconsistent when they are older.

If you emerged from a history of caretaking that didn't inspire trust or confidence and had perhaps a genetic predisposition that magnified these unfortunate experiences, you may be an adult with a vulnerability to signs of abandonment or rejection. Separations from your partner may be difficult for you. The simple business trip that takes your partner to another state for a week may be threatening to you. Reunions may be tinged with anger: "Why did you leave me in the first place?" You may be especially sensitive to signs of love or commitment. Your partner's temporary preoccupation with other matters may feel like a message of rejection. Your partner's desire for time alone or time with friends may feel like abandonment. You may have exquisite radar that detects your partner's slightest interest in potential rivals. Your partner's mild flirtation or sidelong glance at an attractive other may feel like betrayal. Your partner, unfortunately, did not grow up like you and is mystified by your attitude.

Current circumstances can exacerbate, perhaps even create, feelings of vulnerability to abandonment and rejection. Having a partner who is not committed to the relationship or one whose love is inconsistent or one who pursues others may generate a sense of vulnerability and distrust in you even if you were not scarred by your history.

Now here is the complication. A vulnerability to abandonment and rejection may, in part, *create* circumstances that trigger that vulnerability. Reacting strongly to any signs of rejection or lack of commitment may create or intensify doubt in your partner. As a result of this doubt, your partner then shows less commitment, which in turn retriggers your vulnerability. So the process works like a feedback loop: rejection and lack of commitment by one may stimulate a vulnerability in the other, which in turn may cause further rejection and lack of commitment, and so on.

Consider an example. After the early stages of their relationship, when Dylan pursued Shawna intensely, Shawna was usually the more involved and committed one in the relationship. She was the one to press for marriage with a reluctant Dylan. Now, two years into their marriage, Dylan is voicing greater doubts about their relationship. He misses the freedom of the single life. He is attracted to many other women. He is frustrated by the daily grind of their relationship. His vocal doubts and his wandering eye create anxiety in Shawna, even panic at times. She loves Dylan and has come to depend on him, but she has always felt some insecurity with him. In her anxiety, she pushes Dylan for reassurance; she becomes clingy at times, and at other times she attacks him for his immature desire for the single life at thirty-five. Dylan loves Shawna and reluctantly gives her reassurances, but they feel phony to him. He tolerates her clinginess at times, but it feels uncomfortable to him. He hates her criticism, although he fears it may in part be accurate. All of her reactions combine to make him even more doubtful about the relationship, and his growing doubts, in turn, create greater anxiety in her.

"Help, I'm Trapped"

The trouble with wedlock is that there's not enough
wed and too much lock.
—CHRISTOPHER MORLEY

A vulnerability to feelings of entrapment, like a vulnerability to feelings
of abandonment, makes love a fearsome activity, but for very different
reasons. Those with a sensitivity to entrapment are on guard for signs
that their partners may smother, overwhelm, or intrude on them.

This pattern of vulnerability may also begin early in life. Perhaps
you had a parent who showered you with love, but the hugs and kisses
and expressions of love were triggered by your parent's needs rather
than your own. So you often got hugs and kisses whether you wanted
them or not. And if you resisted, maybe you got messages that made you
feel guilty, as if you didn't love your parent or weren't a good, grateful
child. Maybe reciprocity of love was demanded. Thus your early experiences showed you that love has claws. Closeness with another is a
needed but troubling experience.

Apart from your own childhood experiences, you may have developed or aggravated your sensitivity to entrapment through your adult
romantic relationships. Through some combination of chance and
design, you had a partner who intruded on your space, demanded your
love, overwhelmed you with his or her feelings, and made guilt-inducing
comments about your failure to reciprocate. Closeness with another
raised danger signals even as it provided love and support. Closeness
seemed to offer a luxuriously furnished prison, golden chains, a velvet
coffin.

Love consistently raises the question "How much of me do I have to
give up to be with you?"

"I Am Somebody"

I want to be somebody to somebody.

As children we seek recognition from our parents. We look expec-
tantly for the "Good girl!" and the "That-a-boy!" for our accomplishments. We want attention for the pictures we draw, applause for the
balls we hit, laughter for the jokes we tell, and compliments for the
grades we get. Although most parents naturally provide this kind of
recognition to their children, some may be so preoccupied with their

own lives that their child gets little notice. These parents may experience their children's bids for attention as irritating annoyances. As a result, the children get little concrete evidence that their achievements really matter to anyone. It is not clear that they are special in anyone's eyes.

The presence of more than one child in the family complicates the recognition of children. Parents' attention, compliments, and applause must be shared. Children inevitably compete for this parental recognition. But often the playing field is not level. One child may be more verbal or more athletic or more humorous or more social or more physically attractive than the other and therefore may have a built-in advantage for recognition. Parents may favor a particular child because he or she looks or acts like them or otherwise has some attractive feature they value. As a result, parents will never mete out exactly equal doses of recognition to their children. In some families the inequities may be obvious and dramatic.

Little overall parental recognition in childhood, or little recognition relative to a sibling, may sensitize you to issues of recognition in adult relationships. If your experience throughout childhood was that others in the family were getting an unfair surplus of attention, you might be on guard to see that the same doesn't happen in your marriage. The opposite is true too: an overdose of attention and recognition in childhood may lead you to expect a heavy diet of attention and recognition in adulthood.

Sensitivity to recognition may spring from adult relationships as well as childhood ones. If you have been with unresponsive partners, who have been stingy with their praise, you might well be on the lookout for personal slights. If your partner seemed to hog the attention, you might have felt hurt and jealous. If your partner seemed to value his or her own accomplishments and to slight yours, you may have felt competitive.

Whatever its origins, some of us will be sensitive to recognition in our relationships. We may feel hurt if our partners are not enthusiastic about our successes or make too much of our failures. We may need our partners to serve as cheerleaders for whatever we attain. We may want to be looked up to and honored for our accomplishments. We may want our partners to listen to our stories of what we have done and the clever way we did it. We seek admiration as much as love from our partners. When we don't get it, we seek change in our partners, a request that may feel like a significant imposition to them.

"Tell Me I'm Okay"

Carl Rogers, one of the early giants of psychotherapy, told a story about a preschool girl with whom he had worked. To start a conversation with her, he asked her what her name was. She replied: "Alice Don't." Rogers surmised that she had been told "Alice, don't!" so often that she had incorporated that parental warning not only into her self-concept but into her very name.

One of the main tenets of Rogers's theory of personality development was that children need validation and approval from their parents. They need messages that they are okay children. According to Rogers, if they get many messages that they are not okay, or if they have to do everything just so, or if they have to do everything right to get approval, then their development will be harmed.

Whatever the merits of Rogers's theory, experiences of approval and disapproval with our parents early in life and in other close relationships later in life will likely affect our concerns about approval in our adult romantic relationships. Those of us sensitive about approval may seek reassuring messages from our partners that we did or said the right thing. We may have difficulty taking action without approval from our partners. We may feel upset if they do not support our actions or are irritated by the pressure we put on them to express approval. We may also confuse legitimate disagreement with disapproval. If our partners disagree with our views or our actions, we may experience such disagreement as disapproval of our very selves.

If you are vulnerable about receiving approval from others, you may be especially sensitive to criticism. For you, criticism represents obvious disapproval. You may have thin skin. You can sense the implied criticism even in an innocuous remark. If your partner sighs and says, "Well, I better do the dishes now," you may hear the overtone "You should have already done them." If your partner voices frustration that he or she has too much to do, you may hear an implication that you should have done more. Your antenna is tuned to the criticism frequency, and you can pick up even the weakest signal. However, your response to the criticism "Why did you have to say that?" may elicit yet another criticism, "Why are you so sensitive?"

"I'm in Charge"

An older couple I once worked with described the following incident. The husband had recently retired from his job of some thirty years and was having difficulty finding daily activities to keep himself occupied and interested. One day, late in the morning, he wandered into the kitchen and began fixing himself a peanut butter sandwich. His wife noticed what he was doing, rushed into the kitchen, and ordered him out. It was not yet time for lunch, which she had already planned. Furthermore, if he was hungry now, she would fix him something. But above all, he should get out of *her* kitchen!

The husband was a bit dumbfounded by the strength of her response. After all, he was just trying to fix himself a simple sandwich. He certainly wasn't trying to take over food preparation in general or her kitchen in particular. However, she saw his action as an incursion into the territory she had controlled all of their marital life. She was also anxious about his difficulty in finding meaningful retirement activity and hoped he would find something soon, but not the activities that were hers. He may have lost his territory through retirement, but he was not to take over hers.

Issues around control come up from time to time for all of us, particularly when an area of control that we cherish seems threatened. However, some of us may be especially sensitive about power and control. We may feel threatened even when the challenge to our control seems less obvious. We don't want to appear weak or under someone else's thumb, particularly our spouse's thumb. Our anxieties about life are soothed whenever we are in control but ignited whenever others are. We want to be in the driver's seat, literally and figuratively. If our partners express a strong opinion, we may feel they are trying to take over. If they assert their rights, we may view the assertion as an attempt to abridge ours. Delegating work to others may be difficult because we fear that they won't do it as we would—indeed, they often don't.

In the process of raising children, parents must constantly make decisions about how much control to maintain and how much to relinquish. It is the job of parents to protect their children, both physically and psychologically. Therefore, they must limit their children's independence until their children can manage particular situations on their own. When and in what situations can toddlers play by themselves or bathe by themselves? When can you let children walk to the store by themselves? When can teenagers be allowed to take the family car out for the evening?

Human beings desire some measure of control over their lives. Such control is important to their well-being. This principle was illustrated dramatically in a study of ninety-one elderly nursing home residents, who often have little control over their lives. Psychologists Ellen Langer and Judith Rodin divided the residents into two groups. One group was given information emphasizing their responsibility for themselves; then they were given the freedom to make choices for themselves and assigned responsibility for caring for a particular plant. In contrast, the other group of residents was given information emphasizing the staff's responsibility for them; the staff made all their choices for them, and the staff took care of their plants. Not surprisingly, the group that was given responsibility and control exhibited greater alertness, more active participation, and better general well-being than the group without responsibility and control.

Even little children want control. They want things their way. They want to do things by themselves. Some appropriate measure of control is certainly important for children's well-being and their appropriate development. It is clearly important to their satisfaction. Once my wife and I allowed our toddler son to maintain control of some M&M candies we bought for the family. We assured him that he could be the "boss of the M&Ms." He beamed with the pride of ownership and power. Carefully and judiciously he passed out the candies to his parents and his sister. After that incident he would occasionally ask, "Can I be the boss of the _____?" He wanted to reexperience the power of having control.

Given the struggle between parents, who must protect their children by exerting control over their behavior, and children, who want independence and control for themselves, it is not surprising that some people might emerge from this struggle with sensitivities about control. Perhaps an overprotective parent exerted excessive control that created anger and rebellion. Perhaps a permissive parent failed to exert sufficient control so the child became used to little accountability and maximum independence. Experiences such as these might lead one to exert control over a partner or to fear and rebel against such control by a partner.

As we discussed in Chapter 5, power and control is a central dimension of relationships and is crucial for our definitions of ourselves and our relationships. Thus we all resist what appear to be excessive attempts to control us.

As noted earlier, this list of psychological vulnerabilities is intended simply to illustrate the kinds of sensitivities people may bring to or develop in their relationships. The list is certainly not meant to be exhaustive. Nor are the categories mutually exclusive. It is possible for someone to have sensitivities in more than one of the areas. Furthermore, there are many specific sensitivities that may trouble partners in relationships. For example, one member may be embarrassed about how little formal education she has had, another may be sensitive about his hair loss, another about his weight, and another about how poorly her children have done in school.

It is impossible to get through life without becoming sensitive to certain issues. People who never overreacted or underreacted to any event, who took all the vicissitudes of life in stride, who had only the reactions that make logical sense and seem conventionally appropriate would be strangers to all of us who must struggle daily with the "slings and arrows of outrageous fortune." And these automatons would probably not be very sympathetic to our struggles.

VULNERABILITIES AND INCOMPATIBILITIES

Some of the common vulnerabilities we have discussed may have sounded familiar to you. Themes common here are similar to themes common in the incompatibilities discussed in previous chapters. In fact, vulnerabilities provide the driving emotional force for our incompatibilities. If a husband prefers more closeness in the relationship while his wife prefers greater independence, but neither is particularly sensitive about these issues, accommodation is relatively easy. They might be able to adapt to each other's needs and meet in the middle. If, however, the husband is easily threatened by possible neglect and abandonment and the wife feels easily suffocated, their differences will be explosive. Their incompatibilities will create turmoil. And it will be unclear whether their love is troubled because of the starvation rations she provides or because of his insatiable appetite.

Similarly, if wife and husband both prefer to handle the money in the family, but neither is particularly sensitive about issues of control in relation to money, they will have an easy time coming to some compromise. However, if husband and wife are both sensitive about control, if each would feel powerless or less of a man or woman without a major say in the finances, their efforts to solve this incompatibility may be complicated indeed. For it is not just a difference in preferences but a difference in ideology that is driven by passionate emotions. A compromise may seem less like accommodation and more like loss.

Vulnerabilities provide the emotional fuel to our incompatibilities. They make our disagreements so difficult, our differences so divisive.

HANDLE WITH CARE

> The finest qualities of our nature, like the bloom
> on fruits, can be preserved only by the most
> delicate handling.
> —HENRY DAVID THOREAU, *Walden* (1854)

In our areas of vulnerability we will be especially alert to how we are treated. Our feelings are close to the surface and easily disturbed. So we are vigilant, lest those feelings be ignited.

A fascinating study by Dartmouth College researchers Robert Kleck and Angelo Strenta illustrates how we can be hypersensitive to other's behavior when we feel vulnerable. They told a group of women that they were interested in studying how other women would react to them if they were disfigured by a facial scar. With the women's permission, they used theatrical makeup to create an authentic-looking scar. Then they had the women examine the scar with a hand mirror so they could see how authentic the scar appeared. After the women had finished examining the scar, the experimenter applied a "moisturizer" to "keep the makeup from cracking." In fact the so-called moisturizer actually removed the scar, but without the women's knowledge. Then each of these women, thinking she was showing a disfiguring scar, talked with another woman who saw no disfigurement and had no idea of what had gone on before. The conversations were poignant. Thinking they looked horrible, these "scarred women" were very self-conscious. Compared to a control group of women, who were led to believe that their conversational partners merely thought they had an allergy, the "scarred women" rated their partners as more tense, distant, and patronizing. Neutral observers who watched the videotapes of these interactions could see no difference between how the "scarred women" and the "allergy women" were treated. Clearly a sensitivity about the scar made these women interpret the behavior of their conversational partners differently.

Something analogous to what happened in this experiment may occur with psychological vulnerabilities. A heightened sensitivity may lead us to misinterpret our partner's response or lack of response to us. If, for example, a husband is sensitive about the interest and attention his wife gives to his accomplishments, he may react angrily if his wife does not ask him about his job interview as soon as he gets home from work. She may reply honestly, albeit defensively, that she has been both aware of and concerned about his interview, but given her own frustrating drive home from work, she was not at that exact moment thinking of his job interview. An argument might easily ensue in which he claims she doesn't really care about his efforts to find a better job and she claims he is overly sensitive.

When we are sensitive about some issue, we want to be handled with care. Our fragile feelings need to be cushioned from the bumps and jolts of normal handling. We expect those who love us to treat us with special consideration.

Our partners may feel we are asking too much. They may invoke a fairness argument: "I don't ask you to treat me that way." They may list instances in which we were not so sensitive to them and they didn't get upset. The wife who forgot to ask about her husband's job interview may charge, correctly, that he often forgets to ask her about important events at her job and certainly doesn't do so immediately upon his entry into the house. Such reactions, although understandable, fail to acknowledge that one is sensitive in a particular area while the other is not. It is a bit like someone with a normal ankle saying to someone with a sprained ankle: "I don't have to limp. Why should you?"

WHEN VULNERABILITIES COLLIDE

Dealing with sensitive areas can be challenging under the best of circumstances. We may feel burdened by the demands of handling our partners' feelings with such care. We may feel like parents dealing with an immature child. We may fear that accommodating them will increase their demands so that we, like they, become slaves to their sensitivities. For example, the wife who was scolded by her husband for failing to ask about his interview may fear that if she makes an effort to show him extra attention, his needs for special consideration will increase, his demands for immediate response will become insatiable. However, often the special care that we can give our partners may soothe their vulnerabilities and make them more responsive. They may become more giving to us because they feel cared for and want to reciprocate. Their sensitivities may, paradoxically, be less of an issue for them than for us.

As challenging as it is to handle a partner's area of vulnerability when we are doing well, it becomes even more formidable when our own sensitivities come into play. If a particular incident or issue taps both of our sensitivities, then conflict is liable to result. Consider, for example, a wife, Ruth, who is sensitive about abandonment (Don't ever leave me) and her husband, Gaylord, who is sensitive about entrapment

(Help, I'm trapped). If each of their sensitivities gets aroused by the same incident, emotional turmoil will likely result. Let's say that the stressful circumstances of his life at work and with Ruth have made Gaylord feel a strong desire for space, for separateness from Ruth so he can calm down, while similar stressful circumstances have aroused fear in Ruth that their relationship is falling apart. She needs the reassurance of closeness with Gaylord. When Gaylord informs Ruth that he is making plans to spend the weekend hiking with his best friend, she may explode: "How can you leave when things are so bad between us?" He replies, "That is exactly why I want to leave." And a battle ensues.

Consider a second example, but one in which partners share the same sensitivity. Clayton and Carmen are faced with a cross-country move that must be completed by the end of the month so they can start their new jobs. Both are anxious about whether they can accomplish all that they need to do in that time frame. Clayton in particular fears that the furniture he inherited from his parents may get damaged during the move. Carmen is especially worried that the files from her home office will get lost or disorganized in the process. Both cope by taking charge, by exerting control. But theirs is a divided command. They argue about which mover to choose, about who should do what, and about why the other is being so resistant. The stress of their communication equals the stress of their move.

STRESS AND VULNERABILITIES

As the two previous examples illustrated, stressful circumstances expose vulnerabilities. Increased demands on us activate our sensitivities. When things are under control and we feel comfortable, our sensitivities often lie dormant. Even though we may be vulnerable to feelings of abandonment, in good times we can encourage our partners in their separate pursuits. Even though we may be vulnerable to feelings of entrapment, we can enjoy intimacy and commitment. Even though we may often want to be in charge, we can be loose and casual.

Psychologists typically divide stress into two major categories: major life stressors and daily stressors. *Major life stressors* include important transitions that happen to most of us: for example, having a child, moving, getting a new job, retiring, or suffering the death of a parent. Life stressors also arise from unexpected negative events, such as an illness, accident, disability, business failure, and financial loss. *Daily stressors* are chronic conditions we have to deal with, such as a difficult child, a contentious boss, noisy neighbors, limited financial resources, or a long commute.

Both kinds of stress typically train our attention on the stressor and how to cope with it. If we are faced with an imminent business failure, we go over and over in our minds what went wrong, what we are going to do next, and how we will make ends meet financially. If we have a difficult child, we may struggle with our mixed feelings of love and anger toward the child, we may think about how to handle him or her, and we may wonder about what the future will bring. This narrowness of attention means that we neglect other aspects of our world. We may ignore our partners or be unresponsive to another child's needs. The stressor has commanded most of our psychological resources, so we have less to give to anything else.

Stressful events may activate well-learned patterns of coping. If we have learned to cope with stressors socially, we may want to share our problem with others, to elicit reassurance and support from them, and to feel that we are not alone in this. If we have learned to cope independently, we may pull back from others and become totally preoccupied with our own thoughts as we try to work it through. In this case, social contact is a burden, not a relief. If we have learned to cope with anxiety by exerting greater efforts to order and control our life, we may map out plans, make lists of things to do, and organize the papers on our desk.

Stressors may affect our vulnerabilities in two ways. First, a stressor may directly hit our vulnerability, like an arrow into Achilles's heel. If Donna is sensitive to feelings of abandonment and rejection, an incident at work in which a coworker snubs her may be especially difficult for her. It raises her fears that people won't be good to her. If Michael is sensitive to issues of control and has a boss who breathes down his neck and gives him little independence, he may react strongly because he feels like he has no power of his own.

Second, a stressor may affect our vulnerability indirectly. It doesn't hit us in our weak spot, but by hitting us at all it weakens us and makes us cope in ways associated with our vulnerability. For example, even when Donna has a stressor that has nothing to do with interpersonal rejection, such as the stress of an oncoming deadline, her needs for interpersonal support may increase. She may need increased love from her husband not because her own vulnerability to rejection has been challenged but because she can cope better with any challenge if she gets support from those close to her. Similarly, any anxiety that Michael faces, whether it involves control or not, may increase his own efforts to exert control. An upcoming deadline may make him organize and schedule because he then reduces his own anxiety about the deadline.

Thus, stressful events, particularly those that hit us in a weak spot, increase our needs even as they make us less able to accommodate the needs of those around us. This double-barreled effect may be manageable if only one of us is under stress. When we both are under stress, conflict may be inevitable. Rather than living up to Hemingway's ideal of "grace under pressure," we may grate under pressure. And the grating may be with our partners, who love us most and who could support us most—if they weren't also so stressed.

PROVOCATION OR VULNERABILITY?

Between the obvious cases of provocative action that would upset most of us and the obvious cases of psychological allergies in which only those with a particular sensitivity would get upset, there is a vast, unmarked land of mildly provocative actions and well-tuned vulnerabilities. Which is the most important cause of the hurt and anger: the mildly provocative action or the reactive vulnerability?

Couples often battle over this issue in the "action–reaction conflict." You blame your partner for a particular action that triggered upset, but your partner suggests that it was your reaction, not his or her action, that was the problem. For example, you charge your partner with being "too critical," and he replies that you are "hypersensitive." Or your partner accuses you of not being affectionate, and you reply that she is "too insecure." When one of you charges the other with being impolite, the accused replies that the accuser is "too uptight."

Who is right?

Both are. For an interpersonal problem to occur, one partner must do something or not do something that has the potential to sting. But the other must have some exposed skin tender enough to respond. Without a provocative action (or inaction), there would be no problem. However, even if there were a dastardly act, if there were no tender, exposed skin, it could be sloughed off and no problem would occur.

For June to be critical of Ward, she must make a statement that could be interpreted as critical. She might say something obviously critical, in an angry tone, such as "You don't do your share of work at home." Or she might say something more innocent, such as "I've got to clean up the mess the boys made," which carries the implication that Ward should have cleaned up after them. But her statement by itself, even the obviously critical statement, is not sufficient for Ward to feel criticized. He could respond to her statement about not helping out at home as if June were upset and simply "blowing off steam." Ward might experience her comment as "She is not primarily attacking me but simply expressing her frustration." Or Ward might agree that he does in fact not help out enough at home and that she is merely stating, albeit harshly, what they both know to be true. "She is simply pointing out a characteristic of mine," Ward says to himself, "that I don't spend enough time doing household chores and leave them to June. And she is really frustrated by it now." He might even openly agree with her and validate her view of him. If Ward responded in any of these ways, we might say that criticism didn't even occur between them. Or, at the very least, the critical comment did not create an interpersonal problem.

If, however, Ward was sensitive about approval from June or was sensitive about how much he helps out at home, he would respond very differently. He might defend himself by listing all the things that he does at home or by describing all of his other responsibilities. He might counterattack her for what she doesn't do at home. Even if June made the more innocent comment that "I've got to clean up the mess the boys made," Ward could respond with defensiveness and counterattack. If Ward responded in these ways, we would know that criticism had occurred. And that an interpersonal problem had been created.

Who is responsible for this conflict between Ward and June? Clearly, both are. Ward's sensitivity to criticism combined with June's critical comment to create their struggle. And so it is with most conflicts: they start from a volatile combination of a provocative behavior and an exposed vulnerability.

But just because partners share responsibility for an interpersonal conflict does not necessarily mean that they share this responsibility equally. Mutual responsibility does not necessarily imply equal responsibility. A problem may result more from the husband's criticism than from the wife's hypersensitivity. If the husband's friends, family, and coworkers all experience him as critical, but none of the wife's friends, family, and coworkers experience her as hypersensitive, we could confidently place more of the responsibility on the husband.

Spouses cannot easily obtain information about how most other people respond to their mates. Even if they could obtain this information, it would never be as clear-cut as in the preceding example. Even people who are critical in many of their relationships show considerable variability. With some people, they criticize a lot; with others, they criticize very little. Some people handle their criticism well, and it does not create problems; other people handle it poorly, and it creates serious problems. Therefore, to accept that both are responsible for a problem, but to argue over who is more responsible, is to quibble over a fruitless question that is virtually impossible to answer.

RECAP

Our vulnerabilities are often the powder keg for conflict. Dramatic incidents of neglect, when our partners are not there when we need them, or stunning examples of provocation, where our partners do something that embarrasses, humiliates, or betrays us, will certainly create conflict. But the more common, everyday instances of neglect and provocation, many of which are suppressed or ignored, can eventually cause conflict as well. The power of these events lies not just in the actions or inactions of our partners but in our own sensitivities to these events. We may have vulnerabilities that, like psychological allergies, make us especially reactive to possible threats of abandonment or entrapment, lack of recognition or approval, or loss of control. We want to be handled with care in these special areas of vulnerabilities. However, when our vulnerabilities collide with our partners' vulnerabilities or when stress activates both of our vulnerabilities, we may be unable to provide care for our partners but need extra care ourselves. At those points conflict may be inevitable. We argue over incompatibilities that get their power from the vulnerabilities in each of us.

Exercise

Consider the list of common vulnerabilities described in this chapter: (1) Don't ever leave me; (2) Help, I'm trapped; (3) I am somebody; (4) Tell me I'm okay; and (5) I'm in charge.

- Which of these is similar to your own vulnerability?
- Which of these is similar to your partner's vulnerability?
- Are there other, special vulnerabilities that you or your partner have?

- Can you identify times when your vulnerabilities collide?
- What kind of stress typically activates your vulnerability?
- If you can recognize vulnerabilities at work at the beginning of a conflict, will you be able to handle the argument differently than in the past?

Put your answers in the drawer with your other exercise answers.

CHAPTER 7

A Cure Worse
Than the Disease
RELATIONSHIP PROBLEMS
AS SOLUTIONS

Bad solutions don't merely fail; they create an even
bigger problem.

Anika felt neglected by Ralph because he was preoccupied with his
new computer software and unresponsive one evening when they were
alone together. She had wanted to discuss a problem she was having at
work with him, but his disinterest killed any desire on her part to pursue
the topic with him. She was upset by his inattention but also upset that it
aroused such strong feelings in her. She was unsure about how to handle
the situation but decided to share her feelings with Ralph. Because of the
way she expressed her feelings, because of the history of this problem in
their relationship, and because of Ralph's state of mind at the time, he
felt unjustly criticized when she disclosed what was going on with her.
He tried to deal with the situation by explaining to Anika that she gets
upset too easily and should relax and learn to "go with the flow." Anika
felt patronized by Ralph's message and responded with a defense of herself and an attack on him for being "insensitive." She supported her
view that he was insensitive by providing confirming evidence in the
form of provocative examples of his insensitivity, such as the time his

mother was upset with him for how he mishandled his father's terminal illness. He countered with evidence of her "gross overreactions," such as the incident just yesterday when she yelled at the kids over nothing. She claimed that living with Ralph was like living in an emotional desert. He countered that maybe she should find someone else, and then he stormed out of the room.

Clearly, as we discussed at the end of Chapter 6, both partners had a hand in this conflict. Just as clearly, their efforts at dealing with the initial problem of Ralph's inattention to Anika created an even bigger problem. In fact, in the turmoil that was generated during this argument, they temporarily forgot the initial problem.

A slogan of the 1960s, based on a speech by Eldridge Cleaver, charged "If you are not part of the solution, you are part of the problem." In relationships, it is somewhat different. Even when you are part of the solution, but an ineffective one, you are part of the problem and often part creator of an even bigger problem.

Throughout Part I of this book we have seen couples encounter problems, make efforts to cope with these problems, and then face reactive problems, that is, difficulties created as they try to solve the initial problem with which they were confronted. In the preceding example, the initial problem was an incompatibility in desire for closeness, triggered in part by Ralph's focus on his new software and Anika's desire to talk about a work problem, all of which led to hurt and angry feelings. Perhaps the initial problem was emotionally fueled by Anika's vulnerability about being abandoned or neglected and Ralph's sensitivity to criticism.

In response to the initial problem, the couple made efforts to solve the difficulty. Anika tried to solve the problem by sharing her feelings with Ralph and later by presenting evidence of his "insensitivity"; Ralph tried to solve the problem by pointing out to Anika that her emotions are too intense and later by presenting examples of her overreactivity. These efforts at coping were not only unsuccessful, they created a reactive problem, a subsequent problem that was bigger than the initial one. Now they must cope with the hurt and anger that each feels as a consequence of the other's attacks, specifically, with Anika's sense that Ralph really doesn't care about her feelings and with Ralph's sense that Anika will hurl unjustified accusations at him at the slightest provocation, and with the breach in their relationship that this argument created—Ralph's vague suggestions that maybe Anika "should find someone else."

THE INITIAL PROBLEM:
THE CONTENT OF CONFLICT

As we've already discussed, our incompatibilities and vulnera-bilities are like flammable material. If kept in a cool, dark place in separate containers, they create no problems. But if exposed to the heat or friction of a provocative incident, they ignite. With Ralph and Anika, the combina-tion of his new software and her problems at work, as well as the fact that they were both tired from a long day at work, triggered the combustion. The immediate consequence when vulnerabilities and incompatibilities are triggered is negative feelings such as anger, hurt, and disappointment. Anika was first hurt and then angry that Ralph was inattentive to her.

The initial problem that a couple faces—a triggering event or cir-cumstance, the activated incompatibility or vulnerability, and the imme-diate emotional reactions—provides the *content* of their interaction. The initial problem is what each thinks about during conflict, what they dis-cuss during argument. These initial problems set the early agenda for conflict discussions.

Typically, couples focus on the triggering situation rather than the broad incompatibility between them or the vulnerabilities within each partner. For example, even though Gary favors a relaxed, take-it-easy lifestyle while Jana is ambitious and wants to get ahead financially, they rarely if ever discuss this broad difference between them. Instead, they are much more likely to discuss disturbing incidents that reflect this incompatibility. They may disagree about whether to take an expensive vacation, which Gary prefers, or to do something more economical and save their money, which Jana prefers. A conflict may get started when Jana gets up early on a Saturday morning to get a head start on what she wants to accomplish rather than spending the morning lazing around in bed with Gary. Gary's comment that his sales record this year is going to be lower than last year's may precipitate an argument about how much effort he is putting into work. In each of these three instances, Gary and Jana are discussing a *triggering event*, which is a manifestation of their somewhat incompatible approaches to life.

COPING WITH THE INITIAL PROBLEM:
THE PROCESS OF CONFLICT

Any particular initial problem can be coped with in a variety of ways. Gary and Jana could debate their choices of vacation, with each presenting the advantages of his or her own point of view. They could bargain and negotiate their choices, for example, by proposing that one choose the kind of vacation they take this year and the other choose it next year. Jana or Gary could unilaterally make plans and inform the other of what was done. Jana could criticize Gary for his irresponsibility in proposing to deplete their savings with one vacation. Gary could criticize Jana for her stinginess and inability to enjoy life. Gary could withdraw in anger until Jana supports his point of view. Combinations of these and other approaches are also possible. The point is that the *content of conflict*, provided by the initial problem, is distinct from the *process of conflict*, which is how couples cope with the initial problem.

This distinction between content and process is like the distinction between the words and the melody of a song. Like the words of a song, the content of conflict represents what it is about. Like the melody of a song, the process of conflict represents its sequential patterning. Just as different words can be written for the same melody, so different content issues can fit the same process. Marilyn may pressure Rod to help out more with childcare, paying the bills, or sending holiday cards, and Rod may resist. Even though these issues seem unrelated, the process of pressure and resistance may be identical. Furthermore, just as different melodies may be written for the same words, so different processes may be enacted over the same content. Both the Barclays and the Williamsons may have differences in which the wives value religious affiliation more strongly than the husbands. However, the Barclays argue endlessly over theological and philosophical issues while the Williamsons avoid such discussions but belittle each other's behavior, such as her "silly superstitions" and his "base materialism." While the content of conflict is identical for the two couples, their process of conflict differs.

The process of conflict—the way couples cope with their initial problem—is the way they try to find a resolution for the initial problem. Anita wants to spend much more time with her aging parents than does her husband, Sean. Anita tries to solve the problem by calmly persisting in her desire that she and Sean spend more time with her parents; Sean tries to solve the problem with emotional objections, for example, that they are "being held hostage" by Anita's parents and that her parents "aren't emotional invalids yet!" Although theirs is not an ideal solution, Anita's calm persistence leads to a measure of contact with her parents, while Sean's objections impose some limits on that contact. Their way of coping provides a partial, but sometimes painful, resolution of their conflict.

Gayla and Josh disagree about housekeeping. Gayla feels comfortable only when her home is completely organized and spotless. Also, her self-esteem is tied up with the state of her home: if friends dropped by and her home was less than spotless or disorganized, she would be embarrassed. But Gayla believes in equality, and so she wants Josh to share in the housework. In contrast to Gayla, Josh finds clutter somewhat comforting. If he lived alone, his house would have to be positively unsanitary for him to feel embarrassed about it when others visited. Although he generally endorses the ideology of equality between men and women, he certainly doesn't want to do half of the housework, especially if it means doing the housework to Gayla's high standards. Furthermore, he feels his work on the cars should count in the housework equation. All of these differences define the initial problem that Gayla and Josh have about housework.

Gayla and Josh could cope with this problem through different kinds of communication. They could negotiate detailed schedules of who has to do what when. They could tease each other about her compulsivity and his slovenliness. Or, in a more complicated scenario, Gayla could do most of the housework herself but experience a building resentment that eventually leads to an emotional outburst that spurs Josh, already feeling guilty, into action. He helps a lot for a while but then drifts back to doing little until Gayla takes over completely and the pattern repeats itself.

The existence of an initial problem—an activated incompatibility or vulnerability and the resultant negative feelings—does not necessarily mean that open conflict such as an argument will occur. Partners may cope with an incompatibility by ignoring it, hoping it will be resolved over time. Or they may suppress their hurt and angry feelings. For example, during a visit to her parents, Beth was hurt because Harry seemed to ignore her mother and father and watched TV as a way to avoid talking with her family. She chose not to mention her feelings, fearing that any discussion would lead to an unproductive conflict between her and Harry at her parents' house. She reasoned that Harry was tired from a stressful week at work and probably needed to retreat.

While not necessarily leading to open discussion, an initial problem will lead to actions within and between partners. One or both partners go through some process of thinking and feeling as a means of coping with the problem. For example, when Beth felt angry with Harry for watching TV at her parents' house, she thought about why he was watching TV and whether she should mention her feelings to him. These thoughts and feelings led to subtle communication between the two that were their attempts to solve the problem. For example, even though Beth decided not to mention her feelings to Harry, she was somewhat distant with him and asked him about the TV program in a tone of voice that alerted him to her dissatisfaction with his TV viewing. Given the history of difficulty over his level of involvement with Beth's family, he felt guilty about his TV watching and tried harder to relate to Beth's parents. In this example, even though the couple did not openly discuss the content of their conflict, their thinking about the issue and subtle communication around it, of which both may have been only dimly aware, provided a solution to the problem. He got to watch TV, but she then got some extra effort on his part to converse with her parents.

The process that goes on within and between partners may represent more than just the means for coping with a problem: it may be the solution itself. To resolve their incompatibility over how much Gordon should participate in parenting, Jenna criticizes Gordon for being a poor father and Gordon tolerates but doesn't respond to this criticism. Jenna's criticism is aimed at increasing Gordon's involvement, and Gordon's tolerance of her criticism is aimed at increasing her acceptance of his level of involvement. Neither of these efforts is successful, but the interaction itself is a kind of solution. Jenna still handles most of the childcare, but she gets to relieve her frustration by criticizing Gordon. Gordon has to tolerate Jenna's criticism, but he doesn't have to increase his participation in childcare. Obviously, this solution is not ideal, but it is the only one they have.

We care about the content of our conflicts. We are invested in having sex tonight, in not going to the in-laws' house this weekend, and in getting more attention from our partners. We want the freedom to take the weekend off for a hike with a friend or the power to buy the new sofa for the living room. We care because the content of the conflict represents the problem we face: a mate who differs from us on an important matter, a mate who mishandles our vulnerable side and creates hurt and angry feelings.

We may recognize but ignore or we may lack awareness of the process of our conflict. Fixated on our angry and hurt feelings, we don't attend to the way we cope with these problems. Given our problems, we can't imagine other ways of interacting. Carlos knows no other way to deal with his greater sexual appetite than to keep the pressure on Jan. If he doesn't push, he fears, they will have no sex life at all. Lori knows no other way to deal with Manny's lack of involvement with the kids than to criticize his lack of involvement and complain about being a "single mother." If she didn't complain, she fears, he would forget about his role as father entirely.

THE REACTIVE PROBLEM: A WORSE PROBLEM, AN ADDITIONAL PROBLEM, A RELATIONSHIP RIFT

Escalation

As we cope ineffectively with the initial problem, created when our incompatibilities and vulnerabilities are triggered, we often generate a worse problem. The argument escalates: our tension increases, our voices become harsher or louder, our emotions are amplified. The volume goes up, literally and figuratively. We started out with a small conflict; now it is a big conflict.

Arguments can escalate not only vertically, with an increase in tension, but also horizontally, with an expansion of focus. New issues are raised during the conflict, some legitimately related to the original topic, some brought in just to "get back" at the other. In Anika and Ralph's argument, Anika brought up Ralph's handling of his father's terminal illness; Ralph brought up Anika's handling of the kids. In what is often called "kitchen sinking," everything but the kitchen sink is brought into the discussion.

A common direction in which arguments escalate is toward the process itself. Although couples are often focused on the content of their incompatibilities and hurt feelings rather than the process by which they cope with these problems, at times their interaction becomes so painful for one or both of them that it becomes a focus of discussion. At times when Lori criticizes Manny for not being involved with their children, he may criticize her for her criticism: "All you do is complain and criticize. Can't you think of something better to do with your time?" She may defend her behavior—"I wouldn't have to complain if you would do something around here"—or she may attack him: "You can't take any criticism, can you, even when it is 100 percent deserved?" At this point they are arguing about the way they argue. They are criticizing each other for being critical. Now the process of their interaction, the way they cope with their problem, has become the content of their discussion. Their solution to the problem has become the problem. The "cure" has become the disease.

Polarization

When we cope with our problems ineffectively, we often become polarized in our positions. We get more rigid, fixed, and extreme in our views. Although we might have been open to listening to and trying to understand our partners' position prior to the argument, once the argument gets under way we stop listening. Instead we become more convinced of our own positions. In the heat of an argument, we engage in what psychologist John Gottman has called the "summarizing self syndrome." We restate our own positions or we state them somewhat differently, and then we summarize all that we have said. As we listen to ourselves making repeated arguments in favor of our own views, we become more and more convinced of the correctness of those views.

Not only do we become more convinced of our own views; we may also become more extreme in those views. Although early in the discussion we may feel justifiably that we have an important point to make, as the argument progresses we may feel that our point is the only point worth making. Our point is self-evident. Only a fool would argue against it. Any other ideas are at best irrelevant and at worst a devious attempt to undermine truth.

Sometimes the argument itself provides us with evidence that makes us more convinced about the rightness of our views. As the argument between Anika and Ralph escalated, Anika became more convinced that Ralph cares little about her. He certainly showed no caring during the argument, instead, he completely dismissed her concerns. For his part, Ralph found incontrovertible evidence that Anika overreacts to problems by the fact of her increasing upset during the argument. So both found evidence in the argument that polarized their positions.

Alienation

After conflicts escalate and positions become polarized, partners may eventually end the discussion in despair. They can't get through to each other. The other doesn't "get it." Further conversation about the matter is hopeless. Each retreats to his or her own corner. Further conversation, if there is any, is tense and stilted. Partners have become alienated from each other.

Sometimes in the heat of the argument comments are made that trigger alienation. Right before he stormed out of the room, Ralph suggested that both he and Anika should find someone else. This comment catalyzed her concerns about his commitment to the relationship. Consequently, she withdrew from him for days.

Although alienation often occurs after escalation and polarization, it can happen much earlier in the conflict. When partners avoid dealing with an important problem, they often end up feeling distant from each other. They have prevented an open argument from erupting, but they haven't given themselves a chance to air their feelings or to express their views about an important matter. Because the issue is important to them, they think about it. They make conjectures about the other's motives and reactions. They have conversations in their head rather than with each other. Any actual discussion between partners often feels distant and ingenuine.

A BROAD LOOK AT THE ANATOMY OF AN ARGUMENT

The accompanying diagram summarizes how we move from an initial problem to coping efforts that are so misguided that they cause reactive problems.

Every conflict described in Chapters 1–6 of this book fits this definition of the anatomy of an argument. So far, however, we have concentrated mainly on the initial problem: provocative actions or inactions that trigger incompatibilities or vulnerabilities and lead to emotional upset. We have also seen how most people focus on trying to change their partners when incompatibilities cause conflict and vulnerabilities wreak emotional havoc. In this chapter we've seen what happens when changing our partners is our only approach to conflict resolution: we

ANATOMY OF AN ARGUMENT—I

INITIAL PROBLEM (THE CONTENT OF THE ARGUMENT): Provocation → Incompatibility/Vulnerability → Anger/Hurt
↓
UNSUCCESSFUL COPING (THE PROCESS OF DEALING WITH THE INITIAL PROBLEM)
↓
THE REACTIVE PROBLEM: Escalation creates a more intense and/or a new problem. Polarization creates more rigid and extreme positions on the problem. Alienation creates a rift in the relationship.

create reactive problems, problems that are bigger than and sometimes different from the initial problems.

Why can't we see the error of our ways? Sometimes our ways of coping are so habitual and reflexive that we're not conscious of what we're doing. In this case it can be useful to categorize the ineffective ways we try to solve problems and create change.

TOXIC CURES

Toxic cures are solutions that make the problem worse. They are treatments that aggravate the disease. Their intent is often to create change for the better; their result is to create change for the worse.

Accusation, Blame, and Coercion

The classic ABCs of heated argument are accusation, blame, and coercion. We hold our partners responsible for the initial problem, and we pressure them to change as a means of fixing the problem. We could also add a D to the ABCs, for defensiveness. If our partners should charge us with any complicity in the problem, we defend ourselves. But primarily we attack them.

One common focus of blame is the "action–reaction dilemma," introduced in Chapter 6. We blame our partners for a particular action, perhaps the triggering action. But they in turn suggest it was our reaction, not their action, that was the problem. Rather than accusing them of specific behaviors that may have triggered an initial problem, we may also charge them with broad, negative personality characteristics. We engage in the fault finding described in Chapter 2, analyzing our problems and concluding that they are caused by the moral weaknesses, emotional limitations, or personal inadequacies of our partners. Then we accuse our partners of being bad, we blame them for emotional instability, or we chastise them for incompetence. Of course, they may defend themselves and countercharge us.

Coercion goes beyond mere attack of our partners. In coercion, we force our partners to do what we want by barraging them with aversive behavior. We make demands, threaten, nag, criticize, complain, and induce guilt until our partners give in. Then we get what we want, and they get peace. Our coercive efforts are reinforced because our partners comply with our demands. Our partners' compliance is reinforced because we cease our coercive actions.

Coercion has a seductive appeal because it produces such immediate responses. But like an addictive drug that requires increasing dosages to achieve the same effect, higher levels of coercion are required to get our partners' response. During the early stages of romance, slight indications of dissatisfaction may have drawn our partners' attention and prompted them to try to right the situation. But over time our partners may habituate to our coercive attempts, they may deliberately ignore them, and they may even actively resist them. While an edge to the voice was all that was necessary early on in the relationship, now screams and yells may be required to get a reaction.

The immediate rewards of coercion are often dwarfed by the ultimate costs. Although our partners get peace by giving in, they may find our demands more and more onerous. They may become upset with themselves for being weak, for complying with our demands. They may become more and more angry and resistant when we push them.

Coercion breeds countercoercion and punishment. Our partners don't just respond to our coercive attempts, they initiate their own. And they punish our failures to satisfy their own needs. A vicious cycle of mutual coercion and punishment quickly develops. However successful these coercive and punitive efforts are in the short run, they erode the positive feelings and loving atmosphere in the relationship.

Avoidance, Denial, and Minimization

Avoidance is a time-honored method for dealing with problems. Look the other way. Get involved in something else. Problems are unpleasant, so don't face them; they will probably clear up on their own. Discussing them directly might make matters worse.

Avoidance works in the short term. What we choose to do when we avoid problems gives us more pleasure (and is easier) than facing problems. No matter what the program, watching TV will provide more relaxation than discussing incompatibilities or soothing vulnerabilities. However, we often carry with us a nagging sense of discomfort about the problem when we avoid it.

We can achieve the benefits of avoidance plus weaken the nagging discomfort if we deny the very existence of the problem. There is nothing wrong. Everything is fine. Therefore, there is nothing to discuss.

Avoidance and denial may work in the long term as well as in the short term. Sometimes problems develop from some unique combination of circumstances; discussion might complicate or prolong a problem that will disappear with changing circumstances. Mary notices Lou's excessive flirtation with another woman at her company picnic. She feels hurt by his actions but avoids discussion. Then she denies to herself that his actions were even inappropriate. He is just a solid all-American man, one who had a couple of drinks in him and a pretty woman in front of him. Since he doesn't repeat his behavior at future parties, Mary's (and Lou's) avoidance and denial are innocent enough. Discussion might have increased the tension between them, although it might also have led to greater understanding and appreciation between them.

Sometimes long-standing problems improve over time. Changing circumstances and individual growth lessen the problems that were once avoided and denied. Dave often resented Lena's attachment to her mother, but except for some occasional sarcasm and innuendo, neither brought up the matter for discussion. However, as they developed their individual careers and their own life together, her attachment to her mother and Dave's resentment about it lessened. The avoided problem did improve on its own.

However, avoidance and denial are more likely to nourish problems than to stifle them. Changing circumstances are not so fortuitous or individual growth so benign as to erase long-standing difficulties. More often, tension and resentment rise in both partners. Even though they may refuse to discuss a problem and deny that it exists, their emotions force a discussion of sorts. Indirectly, through their moods or through unrelated minor arguments, they communicate their dissatisfaction. However, without direct discussion, the partners may easily miscommunicate, get confused, and make the problem even worse.

Barbara feels unhappy about her sexual relationship with Sol. She sees him as a selfish lover, insensitive to her needs but vigorously pursuing his own. She doesn't discuss her dissatisfaction directly with Sol but withdraws from sexual interaction with him. She shows less interest in making love and is not responsive when she does. Sol feels distressed by her withdrawal and disinterest and wonders if she is "frigid," but he too avoids discussion. He reacts with more forceful initiations and more vigorous pursuit, which provides further evidence for Barbara that he is a selfish lover. She withdraws even more, which provides further evidence for Sol that she is "frigid." Their avoidance of the problem makes it worse.

Overreaction

> When in danger or in doubt
> Run in circles, scream, and shout.
> —UNKNOWN

At the other end of the continuum from avoidance and denial is overreaction. Responding catastrophically to problems may be as destructive as denying their existence. *This is horrible. This means our relationship is no good. How can we go on when we are so different?* These reactions create a cloud of emotion that may confuse any attempts at resolution.

Catastrophic problems demand catastrophic solutions. If we perceive dramatic difficulties, we will propose drastic solutions: personality change in our partners, affairs, separation, and divorce. The threat of drastic solutions drives discussion away from the initial problem and into conflict about the drastic solutions.

In our overreaction to a problem, we often resort to the toxic trio of accusation, blame, and coercion. For example, Roland overreacts to Martha's flirtations by calling her a "slut," accusing her of being unfaithful to him, and threatening her with affairs or separation. She reacts with threats of her own: *Go right ahead. You're so insecure, you could never find a woman you could trust anyway.* In the midst of these challenges, criticism, and counterchallenges, the problem of Martha's flirtations gets hopelessly lost.

At other times overreaction may lead to dramatic, unilateral self-protective actions. When Miguel seeks Gabriela's support for a problem at work, he finds her disinterested and unresponsive. In his hurt and anger, he vows to himself never to share any problems with her again. When Joan dresses provocatively for Matt but finds him unresponsive to her, she feels rejected and rebuffed. She vows never to wear her sexy clothes for him again. In each case one makes a unilateral decision based on his or her hurt and anger that will make the initial problem even worse.

Overreaction in one is often met with avoidance and denial in the other. One member may overreact as a means of jolting the other to face the problem. Sometimes this works: overreaction often garners attention. But those who overreact ultimately lose credibility. Their partners may discount their feelings and use their overreaction to justify a denial of any "real" problem other than hysteria. Through mutual escalation, the denial drives hysteria and hysteria drives denial.

Jim complains about the lack of physical affection, intimate disclosure, and simple time spent together between him and Tammy. Overreacting to the situation, he proclaims that Tammy doesn't love him and probably never has. She denies any problem and attributes his concerns to his immature desire for adolescent "puppy love." At times their behavior escalates until Jim makes outrageous threats that he cannot live without more love, while Tammy claims that they have nothing but a normal relationship but Jim is too blind to recognize it. Locked in a vicious cycle of overreaction and denial, they lose sight of their initial problem: an ordinary difference in the level of closeness they want.

ALLIANCES AND COALITIONS

Russ found it hard to talk to Shanna about any problems between them. Being uncomfortable with such discussions, he came on critically, and she then reacted coolly, showing no interest in pursuing the matter. Her attitude could be summed up in her favorite cliché: Let sleeping dogs lie. Since Russ had always had a close relationship with his mother, he started telling her about his problems with Shanna. His mother made some discreet but pointed suggestions to Shanna, who initially responded with polite tolerance. Then, as the suggestions kept coming, Shanna became colder and colder toward her, finally telling her mother-in-law to keep her nose out of other people's business. Russ and Shanna began fighting about his mother, with Shanna criticizing her and Russ defending her. Russ and his mother preoccupied themselves with laments about Shanna's problems and inadequacies. Shanna felt ganged up on; Russ's mother felt rebuffed; and Russ felt caught between his wife and his mother. What had been an ordinary problem between Shanna and Russ became an entangled conflict among the three of them.

When we experience difficulties of any kind, but especially interpersonal difficulties, we seek the support and counsel of others. We want an ally to listen to our point of view, to validate our position, to support our efforts, and perhaps to give us advice. This universal tendency to seek personal cover in a storm can restore calm to our emotions, give reassurance to our shaken confidence, and provide direction and motivation for our efforts to deal with the difficulty.

But this alliance in the face of adversity may become a coalition against the supposed cause of the adversity. The one experiencing difficulty may initially seek an alliance for individual support, but then he or she enlists the new ally in the struggle against the other. When the other is a spouse, this kind of alliance often makes the problem worse. The alliance with the supporter disturbs the alliance with the spouse.

How do these understandable efforts to seek support from others when faced with marital difficulties go awry? First, others may fuel the fires of discord. They may encourage our tendencies to blame and punish our partners for difficulties that are caused mutually. Second, they may actively interfere in our relationships with our partners. However well intentioned, they may take it upon themselves to assist us directly through words or actions to our partners. Usually these efforts backfire: our partners get angry at us and our allies for "butting in." Third, others may provide substitute benefits that weaken our relationship. The husband who seeks reprieve from the troubles with his wife by having intimate conversations about his marital problems with another woman may find temporary solace and comfort. However, the intimate conversations with the other woman may lead to a closeness that excludes his wife. If his wife discovers this other relationship, she may be angered by the betrayal of their confidential marital problems and suspicious that something else is going on. Even if she never discovers his other relationship, the fact that another woman is meeting his needs weakens his relationship with his wife. Fourth, the involvement of others may create problems for these unsuspecting supporters. The most obvious and frequent example occurs when parents use children as allies in their marital difficulties. The alliance may put the children in a position of divided loyalty, which leads to anxiety and stress. The children may feel that they must "choose sides" in the conflict. They may feel that they have to see one parent as good and the other as bad. If parent–child alliances become too intense, the closeness may inhibit the children's development. Children need time with peers and emotional freedom from parents to develop attachments with their peers. If children spend most of their time with a parent or if they worry about a parent or their parents' marriage, they will not experience enough freedom to develop independence.

Our understandable and human efforts to reach out for family and friends in times of relationship struggle may relieve our stress and ease our difficulties. We may find temporary solace from our troubles and strength to renew our efforts at solving the problems. We may gain emotional release from the tension, new perspectives on the problems, and new ideas for solving them. However, if our family and friends directly interfere with our relationship, if they promote adversarial views of the problems, and if they offer a continual source of benefits and satisfactions that we should be receiving from our partners, these well-meaning supporters may make our relationship problems worse.

A MORE DETAILED PICTURE
OF THE ANATOMY OF AN ARGUMENT

You probably recognized the toxic cures just discussed, either as coping efforts made in your own relationship or as patterns of interaction you've seen in other relationships. All of these toxic cures have one thing in common: they reflect a lack of acceptance of the initial problem. As we've seen, we come by many of our incompatibilities and vulnerabilities rightly, and they're not so easy to change. Still, we struggle with our partners over them. In other cases, we simply misunderstand or misinterpret the initial problem. Faced with a confusing incompatibility, we end up focusing our efforts on a nonissue, the wrong problem, or a red herring. We generate toxic cures for confusing and undefined problems. A resolution in these cases is especially unlikely. In any case, we end up hurt, angry, defensive, and frustrated. Worst of all, our conflicts perpetuate themselves and spawn new reactive problems, and our relationship spirals downward.

The coping segment of the accompanying diagram captures the major categories of "cures" we have discussed and demonstrates the part they play in the painful transition from the initial problem to the reactive problems.

ANATOMY OF AN ARGUMENT—II

INITIAL PROBLEM (THE CONTENT OF THE ARGUMENT):
Provocation → Incompatibility/Vulnerability → Anger/Hurt

↓

UNSUCCESSFUL COPING
(THE PROCESS OF DEALING WITH THE INITIAL PROBLEM):

Accusation	Avoidance	Overreaction	Alliances
Blame	Denial		Coalitions
Coercion	Minimization		

↓

THE REACTIVE PROBLEM:
Escalation creates a more intense and/or a new problem.
Polarization creates more rigid and extreme positions on the problem.
Alienation creates a rift in the relationship.

VICIOUS CYCLES OF INTERACTION
(REPEATED APPLICATIONS OF A TOXIC CURE)

If at first you don't succeed, try, try, again.

The model we've been discussing describes a single argument. Depending on how serious an argument is, we may ignore it and move on, or it may cause a major rift in our relationship. Fortunately, major, serious arguments are few and far between for most of us. What we have to deal with instead are smaller but repetitious arguments. We go over (and over) the same or similar issues; we do our usual dance.

One incident between two people, by itself, rarely constitutes a relationship problem. A single argument may be unpleasant, but it won't propel a couple onto the therapist's couch or send them to divorce court. Repetition transforms arguments into relationship problems. We use the same toxic cures to try to solve the same problem—again and again.

Repetition does not necessarily mean that the problem occurs the second time exactly the way it did the first time. As we flounder around in the problem, we will enact many variations on the same "solution." We repeat the same dance but with different steps. Consider Valerie and Brad's jealousy problem. Brad tries to cope with his jealousy of Valerie in several different ways: sometimes he interrogates her closely about her actions ("So what were you and Bill discussing at the party?"), occasionally he barks out a demand ("I want to *meet* these so-called business partners before you have lunch with them"), or sometimes in the presence of others he hovers over her, trying to be a buffer between her and other imagined suitors. These are his attempts to solve the problem of jealousy. For her part, Valerie often evades his accusing questions, tries to escape from his hovering presence, and occasionally in anger at Brad flaunts her attractiveness and provocatively seeks the attention of other men. However varied, his behavior reflects a hovering, heavy-handed, suspicious watchfulness, while her behavior varies between avoidance of Brad and his questions on the one hand and taunting, angry flirtatiousness on the other. Their attempted solutions to the problem of jealousy have created a vicious cycle of interaction that, far from solving the problem, sustains it.

Who Started It?

If we realize, even dimly, that we are in a vicious cycle of interaction, we may focus on the question "Who started it?" We both got caught up in a negative pattern, but who started the thing in the first place?

Naturally, we disagree. We each see ourselves as reacting to the other's negative behavior. I think it started with your ignoring me; you think it started with my criticism. I think it started with your coldness; you think it started with my preoccupation. But who is right?

We are both right and both wrong. Once we are in a relationship, we can never "start fresh." Our current discussions are affected by our past ones. We may decide that a particular argument has nothing to do with any dispute from the past, but that simply isn't true. What past event we choose as a starting point will be somewhat arbitrary.

WIFE: I come home, I greet you happily, and you scowl at me.

HUSBAND: You don't call all day, and then you come home and give me this "innocent" greeting. And you expect me to respond?

In this example, the husband and wife see the argument beginning at different points. The wife thinks the argument started when she got home. He thinks it began earlier in the day, when he expected a phone call. She didn't think she had to call. She was not attempting to appease him with an especially cheerful greeting. Furthermore, she didn't leave that morning ruminating about any unsolved problem from the past. She had no hangover from any previous interaction. For her, the argument really did start when she got home. But for him the argument started when she failed to call. He expected her to call, and when she didn't he got upset. So, there are two beginnings to this argument: his and hers. The interaction genuinely started at different points for them.

The problem of deciding when an argument begins and ends gets even more complicated when the arguments are repetitious, when they are part of vicious cycles of communication. The preceding example was an isolated instance. But consider Phillip, who often nags Jennifer to pick up her things and keep the house neat and orderly. She often resists his efforts and complains about his "nagging." He says to himself, "I have to nag her because she resists doing what she ought to do. If she wouldn't resist, then I wouldn't need to nag her." In his view the problem begins with her resistance and is followed by his nagging. Of course, she says to herself, "I resist him because he nags at me. If he didn't nag, I wouldn't resist." In her view, the problem begins with his nagging and is followed by her resistance.

We can think of our relationship as a long, continuous film. When we discuss it, we show parts of the film. We can't show it all, so we select portions. But this editing of the film—these decisions about where to start and end the episode—are up to the editor. Every editor chooses a different beginning and a different ending. We usually start the film with our partners doing something to us and end it with our justifiable reaction. We are good; they are bad. Not surprisingly, our partners start the episode with our behavior and end with their understandable reaction. They are good; we are bad.

Impact of Vicious Cycles

Escalation, polarization, and alienation can occur gradually over time rather than in a single argument. As we repeat the same unsuccessful solution to our problems, persisting in wanting our partners to change, our tensions may escalate, our positions may become polarized, and we may become alienated from each other.

Escalation often occurs through a kind of "short-circuiting" of the interaction. As we experience a vicious cycle of behavior repeatedly, we tend to anticipate its occurrence. Then we sometimes respond to our anticipation as much as we do to our partners and get into the cycle more quickly and intensely than we would have otherwise. For example, consider a pattern of criticism and defensiveness. Erik is often critical of Alicia, particularly concerning her messiness and lack of organization. She tends to respond with defensiveness, trying to convince him that she has been too busy to put away things or trying to show him that she has her own organization system that is different from his. As this pattern repeats, Alicia will anticipate Erik's criticism and become defensive even before he has been critical. For example, she may try to explain why her papers are on the couch even before he has noticed them there. For his part, Erik may anticipate that things will be out of order and get angry at Alicia even before he has seen anything out of order. When their responses are short-circuited like this, they are primed for emotional reactions. They may have a more intense encounter than otherwise because their anticipations have set them up for it.

Polarization may occur over time as it does in a single argument. We repeat our own positions and get more convinced of them and more rigid in them. However, polarization over time may also occur in more subtle ways. Repeated conflict over an issue and pressure about an issue may squelch our inherent interest or spontaneous desire. Consider

Enrico and Rosa's differences in desire for sexual contact. Because of these differences, Enrico initiates sex with Rosa far more than she does with him and more than she would like him to. Often Rosa declines, but his hurt response makes her feel guilty. Over time, she gets apprehensive about his requests, at times even dreads them. She begins to question her own sexual interest, particularly her interest in Enrico. All of this dampens whatever inherent, spontaneous sexual interest she had in him. When she forces herself into sexual contact with Enrico even when she doesn't want to, the whole experience takes on a negative emotional tone for her. Thus, as a result of their repeated conflict over sex, Rosa's interest in sex decreases and their incompatibility increases.

Deprivation may also play a role in polarizing a couple. As you are both unable to get your needs met, those needs can become intensified. For example, if sexual contact happens less and less, Enrico may find his desires for sex increasing. Apart from simple deprivation of this special experience, Enrico may find his desires for sex increasing simply because it is being denied to him—a pleasure denied is a desire intensified. Meanwhile Rosa finds her sexual desire decreasing because of Enrico's pressure. Their persistent attempts to solve their sexual incompatibility have made the incompatibility greater. Their repetitious solutions have created a bigger problem.

As our problems escalate and become polarized over time, we may feel trapped by these problems. How can we ever solve them? Even if our "solutions" don't create a bigger problem, their ineffectiveness can create despair. We may question our relationship. Are our partners really right for us? We may say things in anger—a threat to leave, a harsh accusation—that create a rift in the relationship. Feeling trapped and hopeless about ever solving the problem and angry with our partners for the problem, we become alienated from them. It is not just a problem we have in the relationship. The relationship itself is now a problem.

RECAP

In this chapter we put together the pieces of conflict discussed in earlier chapters to create a complete anatomy of an argument. Earlier, in Part I, we saw how provocative actions by our partners are often readily understandable if seen in the light of the incompatibilities and vulnerabilities that trouble our connection with one another. In our effort to cope with these initial problems, we respond reflexively with dubious methods that only cause further problems. These methods tend to get reinforced because they all provide some occasional benefits. Avoidance, denial, and alliance provide temporary refuge from the problem; accusation and blame may vent angry feelings; overreaction and coercion force an immediate reaction and sometimes a temporary solution to a problem; alliances and coalitions provide some immediate support for a problem. However, far from solving the initial problem, these strategies are often toxic cures that escalate the conflict, polarize our positions in the conflict, and lead to alienation between us—largely because they focus our efforts on changing our partners rather than on first looking clearly at the incompatibilities and vulnerabilities that affect us both. Repeated use of these toxic cures leads to more serious "reactive problems" and, over time, to vicious cycles of interaction. In turn, these cycles of interaction may escalate the conflict, polarize and alienate us, and eventually cause us to question our relationship. The solutions that were designed to "cure" the initial problem finally undermine our very relationship.

Exercise

Think about the ways that you cope with conflict with your partner.

- What are the most common "toxic cures" that you use to solve problems between you and your partner?
    1. Accusation, blame, and coercion?
    2. Avoidance, denial, and minimization?
    3. Overreaction?
    4. Alliances and coalitions?

Think of a recent example in which you and your partner tried to solve an initial problem, but the effort only led to a bigger "reactive problem."

- What unsuccessful strategies did you use?
- Which unsuccessful strategies did your partner use?

Identify one "vicious cycle of interaction" between you.

- What role do you play?
- What role does your partner play?

Now collect all the answers you gave to the exercises in Chapters 1–6 and read them over.

- If you did the exercises again right now, would you give the same answers?
- Would you characterize your partner as having the same flaws as you did when you began the book?
- Has there been any discernible change in the level of conflict between you and your partner?
- Do arguments unfold with the same cycles of interaction as they always have?

You won't necessarily see your relationship transformed just because you have a new understanding of the anatomy of an argument. You may, however, see glimmerings of change between you and your partner. Perhaps you view your partner's foibles a little more philosophically than in the past; maybe you have a sharper awareness of your own vulnerabilities and how they contribute to conflict with your partner. Maybe you even catch yourself occasionally nipping an argument in the bud, or your hot buttons aren't quite as sensitive as they used to be.

How much (if any) improvement you already notice in your relationship may depend on whether you and your partner have been reading this book together. Because all conflict between partners takes two, improvements may be greater when both of you are altering your perspective. If your partner is not reading the book along with you, you may want to encourage him or her to read Part I before you move on to Part II. However, if your partner is unwilling to read the book, it is still helpful if you go it alone.

Understanding is the first step toward acceptance in relationships. At this point you should understand not only the general anatomy of conflicts but also much more than before about your own specific brand of argument. Part II will show you how to use this information to accept the vulnerabilities and incompatibilities that trouble your relationship. In so doing, you may lessen the conflict that plagues your relationship, particularly the reactive conflict. Equally important, you may increase the intimacy between the two of you. And, as an added bonus, your partner may spontaneously make some of the changes you were unsuccessful in producing with your toxic cures.

PART II

From Argument
to Acceptance

CHAPTER 8

The Delicate Balance

ACCEPTANCE AND CHANGE

*I*n the movie *Blue Sky*, for which she won an Oscar, Jessica Lange portrays the emotionally volatile wife of an army nuclear radiation expert (Tommy Lee Jones). In one scene, they and their two daughters enter the dilapidated house that will be their new home on an army base in Alabama. Upset at the move and the condition of the house, Lange has a major emotional outburst. She tears down the curtains, storms outside, jumps into the car, and screeches away. Tommy Lee Jones runs after her, eventually rescues her, and brings her back home. The next morning, as she sleeps, the girls are still upset about the incident. Jones tries to comfort his daughters and explain his perspective to them. He assures them of his own and their mother's love for them. He uses the metaphor of water to explain their mother. Just as water can be liquid or steam or ice, so their mother has many shifting properties. He tells them, "I made a decision a long time ago just to love her basic properties."

This movie dramatically illustrates what we mean by acceptance. Jones clearly experiences pain from his wife's emotional outbursts, yet he is able to tolerate that pain, recover from that pain, and accept that pain. He is even able to make humor out of the situation with a pun about nuclear fishing (fission) in the water that is his wife. He sees her specific behaviors in the larger context of her whole life—as just one of her shifting properties. And he sees her behaviors in the context of their life together: her emotional dynamism has made her the provocative, charming, and challenging person she is. In his dealing with her emotionality, he never seems weak or submissive, but strong and loving.

You may have heard people say lovingly, "I accept her completely," or say with exasperation, "I guess I have to learn to accept him." In these cases acceptance sounds nebulous and global. But we mean something much more specific and concrete: "to accept" means to tolerate what you regard as an unpleasant behavior of your partner, probably to understand the deeper meaning of that behavior, certainly to see it in a larger context, and perhaps even to appreciate its value and importance in your relationship.

Acceptance does *not* mean being submissive to that behavior. In the movie *Mr. and Mrs. Bridge*, Paul Newman's and Joanne Woodward's characters are having dinner together at a country club when a tornado threatens. Everyone seeks shelter in the basement except Newman and Woodward, because Newman wants to finish his dinner. Distressed by the danger, Woodward wants to seek refuge but waits as her husband eats. As the wind wails and crashes outside, Newman comments, "They never give you enough butter." Woodward anxiously searches at other, now abandoned tables for more butter for Newman's bread. Finally, when her fear of the tornado surpasses her fear of offending him, she hesitantly questions, "Don't you think we might be better off downstairs in the basement?"

Newman replies, "Now look here, for twenty years I've been telling you when something will happen and when it will not happen. Now, have I ever, on any significant occasion, been proved wrong?"

The tornado subsides, and Newman is proved right again, but Woodward's weak voice of hesitant protest is muffled further.

Newman's stubbornness in the face of the tornado and his insensitivity to Woodward's anxiety are painful for her and dangerous to them both. However, she submits to his control and suffers with only the weakest of protests. Hers is not acceptance but submission.

Submission comes from a position of weakness, acceptance from a position of strength. Submission means enduring aversive behavior from your partner because you have or believe you have no alternative. Acceptance, in contrast, is tolerating aversive behavior because you see that behavior as part of a larger context of who your partner is and who you are. Acceptance does not mean that you lack power to protest or are fearful of protest. Rather, acceptance means that you regard the negative behavior, as Jones did, as part of the many shifting properties of your partner. Your partner's scalding steam is just another manifestation of the water that he or she is.

In its highest form, acceptance can promote more than just tolerance: it allows you to see beyond your partner's negative actions in the moment to the good intentions from which they spring or the positive consequences they sometimes have. This does not mean that you never resist your partner's aversive behavior, never argue about it, or never try to limit it. But it does mean that you can go beyond it.

Sarah wants to be updated on important developments in Jack's job, a desire that Jack would accept, but she also wants to express her opinion about these developments and encourage actions that she deems appropriate, two desires that upset Jack. She is particularly interested in how Jack is being treated by his superiors at work, and she often nags him to stand up for himself and demand his due. Her involvement in his work annoys Jack and causes many arguments. It also makes Jack feel devalued, as if he can never do enough to satisfy her perceptions of what is right. And he recoils from the idea that he should be fighting at his workplace to meet *her* expectations for *his* job.

Yet he also knows that were it not for Sarah, he would have accepted job assignments without insisting on the necessary support to carry them out. He would have gone several years without a pay increase simply because he was hesitant to ask for one. And he might even have lost his job to another. He knows that without Sarah's discriminating judgment, his naive trust in the goodwill of others would have gotten him into considerable trouble. So Jack has mixed feelings about Sarah's critical questions and nagging concerns. Jack often disagrees with Sarah's comments and must take care to maintain a boundary defining what Sarah can and cannot control, but he has learned to listen to her opinionated views because he knows she usually has his best interests at heart, she understands his weaknesses, and she has insight into others' attempts to take advantage of him. In short, he accepts her criticism, nagging, and pressure about his work.

ACCEPTANCE VERSUS CHANGE

Acceptance and change are fundamentally different but linked events. A conflict ignites for a couple when one member, the *agent*, does something undesirable to or fails to do something desirable for the other, the *recipient*. Sarah was the agent of the problematic behavior of nagging and pressuring; Jack was the recipient of this behavior. *Change* occurs when the agent performs the unpleasant action or inaction less frequently or less intensely—for example, when Sarah does not nag or question or criticize Jack's work as much as usual. In contrast, *acceptance* occurs when the recipient reacts less negatively to the agent's behavior, is more tolerant of it, and has greater perspective about it. Acceptance occurs if Jack develops more tolerance for Sarah's behavior, perhaps because he sees its importance for their relationship and for him personally. The roles of agent and recipient shift back and forth as couples engage in conflict. Although Sarah is the agent of the problematic behavior of nagging and pressuring, were Jack to accuse Sarah of interfering in his work, then Jack would be the agent of this accusation, and Sarah would be the recipient of it.

Acceptance and change represent two ways to solve relationship problems. Although they are very different strategies, they can achieve the same goal: ending the conflict. For example, Denise is distressed because Frank rarely initiates any affectionate physical contact. If she sits beside him on the sofa, he will instinctively move away, as if to provide them both with more space. Yet the space in between them is precisely what Denise wants to bridge. One way to resolve this problem would be for Frank to become more openly affectionate with Denise, by holding her hand more often, kissing her more frequently, hugging her more intensely, and cuddling with her at night. These changes would all solve the problem, especially for Denise. If Frank felt comfortable with these changes and if the changes endured, then the problem of lack of physical signs of affection would truly be eliminated from their relationship. In a second possible solution Denise could become more accepting of Frank's difficulties with physical affection. She might see that he expresses his love for her in other ways than through physical affection: he works hard for her and the family, he is available to help her in times of need, and he listens attentively to her concerns. She might realize that he was raised in an unexpressive family, that he has never been very affectionate to anyone, and that he feels uncomfortable giving and receiving physical affection. This greater acceptance would certainly solve the problem, especially for Frank. If Denise were truly accepting, so that Frank's lack of physical signs of affection was comfortable for her on an ongoing basis, then the problem would be solved for her as well.

If Frank and Denise solve the problem in the first way, then Frank makes a change: he becomes more physically affectionate. If they solve the problem in the second way, Denise makes a change: she becomes more accepting of Frank's lack of physical affection. Her change is not so much a behavioral change—although she may respond differently when Frank is not affectionate—as it is a change in how she receives or reacts to his behavior. It is a change in her attitude about his behavior, in her emotional reaction to his behavior, and in her interpretation of his behavior. We call this significant change she has made *acceptance* and reserve the term *change* for the type of specific behavior change Frank would make if he increased his affection. In an important sense both are changes, but we will use the terms *change* and *acceptance* to distinguish them.

This leads us to principle number 1 for solving problems: *A relationship conflict can be solved through either change or acceptance.*

But which solution should couples choose? Frank would, of course, choose that Denise accept him as he is, and Denise naturally would choose that Frank become more affectionate. Each would prefer that any movement toward a solution be made by the other.

Most of us would like to hear the message "I love you the way you are" from our partners. They should see our foibles as endearing, or at least, in the shadow of our strengths, easily forgivable. Alongside the fantasy of being accepted exactly as we are, we may also harbor the fantasy of changing our partners. Our ideas for change would improve them and make life easier for us. This fantasy is captured in the old joke that asks what three things the bride thinks of as she walks down the aisle in church on her wedding day. The answer: Aisle, altar, hymn (I'll alter him). Therefore, each of us sends out the message "You should accept me as I am, but you should change to accommodate my needs." In our view, this message carries a justifiable demand because "your negative features are deeply disturbing; mine are merely inconveniences."

Let's suppose that Frank and Denise, after open communication about their affection problem, agreed on either change by him or acceptance by her. Would that be the end of the issue? Only if Frank's new affectionate behavior felt comfortable to him or Denise's new acceptance could be reconciled with her need for open signs of affection. Otherwise, given Frank's history, he might have a hard time keeping up his new level of affection, and after a few days or weeks of effort fall back into his old patterns. Similarly, Denise might make a good start of accepting Frank the way he is, but end up feeling resentful and returning to her old angry pursuit of greater physical affection.

Theoretically, relationship problems can be solved through unilateral change by one person or unilateral acceptance by the other, but that kind of one-sided solution often does not work. Fortunately, there is a third solution.

THE THIRD SOLUTION

The third way to solve this affection problem and most other human relationship problems is through a combination of acceptance and change. Frank could make some changes regarding his infrequent displays of affectionate behavior *and* Denise could become more accepting of Frank's ways of showing love, which often don't include physical affection. This third possibility offers a number of advantages. The burden for solution falls on both partners: both give, but both also receive. Their actions may create a positive cycle that encourages and motivates each. If Denise sees some change on Frank's part, some effort to be more openly affectionate, she may find it easier to accept his overall limited ability to provide physical affection. A lack of any change in one partner, however, often proves to be a barrier to the other's acceptance of problematic behavior. Likewise, if Frank experiences Denise as being more accepting of his lack of open affection—as less negative and applying less pressure about it—he may find it easier to be somewhat more affectionate. Often another's pressure to change becomes a major barrier to change, whereas another's acceptance facilitates and even encourages change.

Frank and Denise have one other big area of conflict. Frank complains that Denise criticizes him too much, that she constantly monitors and evaluates him, usually negatively. Clearly Denise could cut back on her surveillance and criticism, or Frank could become more accepting of Denise's criticism. But because either unilateral approach could foster resentment in the party making all the changes, the third option might be best: Denise becomes less critical *and* Frank becomes more accepting of Denise's criticism. Denise's change would thus encourage Frank's acceptance, and Frank's acceptance would encourage Denise's change.

The benefits of this double-barreled solution go beyond their problem of criticism. Often relationship problems are linked: one person's problematic behavior is intimately connected to the other person's problematic behavior, such that solving one has mitigating effects on the other. Denise's criticism and Frank's lack of affection are linked in a vicious cycle of communication. Denise is often critical of Frank because of his lack of affection. Likewise, Frank finds it difficult to be openly affectionate with Denise because of her criticism. A solution to one problem would go far in solving the other one.

Frank and Denise started out their life together with differences in their desire for and need of physical affection. This incompatibility may have been fed by vulnerability in one or both—perhaps a fear in Denise of being neglected or abandoned or a fear in Frank of being suffocated or overwhelmed. Denise tried to solve this initial problem by being critical of Frank, and Frank reacted by being even less affectionate. Therefore their initial problem of an incompatibility about affection grew into a bigger incompatibility.

In addition, Denise started out their relationship being more outspoken, more likely to voice her likes and dislikes, than Frank. Because of his own sensitivity to criticism, this difference was a problem for Frank. He tried to solve the problem by withdrawing from Denise, but that made her even more critical of him. If Frank and Denise tackled their affection and criticism problems through the bilateral, third alternative solution, they might gain greater improvements in both problems than they could expect for either problem with a unilateral approach. Solving the criticism problem will leave Frank less "on guard" with Denise, and thus he might be more physically responsive to her. Solving the affection problem will neutralize at least one major criticism of Denise's.

This brings us to principle number 2 for solving problems: *The best solutions to most problems involve acceptance by one member and change by the other.* This two-pronged approach not only makes both partners part of the solution and serves to motivate both partners, but may affect the solution of other, linked problems as well.

But aren't there some problems that shouldn't be accepted, where change should be the only solution? And aren't there certain problems that can't be changed, where acceptance should be the only solution?

WHAT *SHOULD* BE CHANGED BECAUSE IT *SHOULDN'T* BE ACCEPTED?

Is there anything that should *not* be accepted? Are there any behaviors that should and must be changed, no matter what? Physical violence—battering—should not be accepted in any couple. It can and does bring about physical injury and sometimes death. Even if it doesn't cause physical injury, it can inflict serious emotional damage on both the victim and the perpetrator.

Many spouses, particularly wives, do endure physical violence. Their response is not acceptance but submission. They often feel they have no choice; many may have little power to stop the violence they endure. Ending physical violence, either by leaving the relationship or by stopping it from happening in the relationship, is no simple matter. Chapter 16 will address violence. For now, however, how do you determine what else is unacceptable?

Many would put emotional, psychological, and verbal abuse together with physical abuse as unacceptable behaviors for any couple. Even though these actions cause no physical harm, at the very least they can be emotionally distressing, and at the worst they can be emotionally damaging. Because of the importance of emotional, psychological, and verbal abuse and its association with physical abuse, we discuss it further in Chapter 16.

Emotional, psychological, and verbal abuse is harder to define than physical abuse. Some language, such as threats and degrading names, is clearly abusive. No one should accept comments such as "You do that again and I will bust your face" or "You worthless bitch." Beyond these obvious examples of verbal abuse, however, it is impossible to establish clear-cut, universal criteria of what is abusive and what is not. A shouting match with name calling may feel abusive to some couples but may be merely a heated argument to others. What seems like criticism to one member may feel like abuse to the other. To define emotional, psychological, and verbal abuse, we need to take into consideration both the actions of the agent and the reactions of the recipient.

In fact, other than physical violence and obvious cases of verbal abuse, it is difficult to list specific acts that no one should accept. Most might argue that no couple should accept infidelity, yet even this is not a universal rule. Some couples accept extramarital sex openly and others accept it implicitly. Many spouses have learned to forgive a partner who was unfaithful. Thus, the list of unacceptable actions must be individualized. Each spouse has the right to identify the actions that are totally unacceptable to him or her.

The danger is that a list of unacceptable actions will grow to the point that it includes every negative or unpleasant behavior. Melinda may insist that disrespect, rudeness, coldness, public humiliation, insensitivity, dishonesty, and selfishness (to name a few) are all unacceptable to her. Such a list mixes what is truly unacceptable to Melinda with what is merely unpleasant for her. This kind of list defeats its own purpose: it makes it less likely that Manfred, her husband, will make changes in either group. The list is so long that it implies that he is a major villain, perhaps the sole villain in their relationship.

A declaration that some action is unacceptable carries with it a moral force. When Joe tells Patrice that he can no longer accept her "public humiliation" of him, he is telling her that her actions are morally wrong, that she is at fault for taking these actions, and that she must change unilaterally. He frames his declaration in such a way that his reaction to her actions is not relevant. Whatever he might have done to provoke her actions is immaterial. Her public humiliation of him is so onerous that it dwarfs any negative actions of his. She must stop it forthwith.

Change by the perpetrator is the only antidote for so-called unacceptable behavior. Yet this antidote is often a cure worse than the disease. Describing behavior as wrong and thus unacceptable often creates barriers to change rather than facilitating change. The perpetrator often does not view the behavior in question as wrong, resists being accused of wrongdoing, and rebels against the notion of making unilateral change. A perpetrator who does change may resent the initial accusation and subsequent pressure that forced the change. Also, the communication sets up an inequality, with the partner "in the right" occupying the high moral ground and the partner "in the wrong" in the moral swamp. Such a position is not comfortable for the "lesser" partner and not likely to be tolerated well.

A story about Abraham Lincoln and his volatile wife, Mary Todd, illustrates that even behavior that might be defined conventionally as unacceptable does not have to be viewed in that intractable way. As we have explained, an interpersonal problem depends not just on some provocative behavior but also on a vulnerability to that behavior. Lincoln was outside talking to a congressman about the important political matters of the day. Mary Todd stormed out of the house, ruthlessly castigated Lincoln for something he had done, and then stormed back inside. Aghast that a wife would behave so outrageously in public, the congressman looked to see Lincoln's reaction. Lincoln was undisturbed by the incident and explained to the incredulous congressman that such outbursts made his wife feel so much better that he hardly wanted to put a stop to them.

This kind of action by a wife would have certainly been considered "public humiliation" by most of Lincoln's male peers and thus deserving of the most serious sanctions. Most men today might also experience such an act as public humiliation. Lincoln, however, was not humiliated, either publicly or privately. His reaction made Mary Todd's action something therapeutic for her rather than something bad and unacceptable for him.

Not only must "negative actions" be defined in terms of the recipient's vulnerable response as well as the perpetrator's provocative action, but negative actions must be considered in context. People are rarely disrespectful, rude, cold, insensitive, or selfish "out of the blue." Often their behavior is part of a vicious cycle of negative behavior. As we saw in the last chapter, partners may differ on where they define a starting point for a conflict. The victim may feel that the partner "attacked out of the blue," while the partner may view his or her attack as simply a reaction to some previous behavior by the other.

When viewed in this way, much of what partners call "unacceptable behavior" in the other can be described more accurately as components of the negative cycles between them. Certainly, spouses have the right to declare specific actions of their partners "unacceptable." In a later chapter we will describe ways to create change in unacceptable behavior. However, "unacceptable behavior" is harder to change than merely problematic behavior that is part of a vicious cycle between a couple. Problems are more manageable, more solvable, and more changeable when they are not defined as unacceptable behavior. The more powerful combination of change and acceptance can work with these problems.

WHAT *SHOULD* BE ACCEPTED BECAUSE IT CAN'T OR *SHOULDN'T* BE CHANGED?

Are you obliged to accept some aspects of your partner? Does love create a moral imperative to accept some of your partner's features?

Some would say that to love, and certainly to marry, you must accept the essence of the other person. To pressure your partner to change some central characteristic would be asking your partner to be untrue to himself or herself. By choosing to love and marry this person, you have accepted who he or she is. You have forfeited the right to question your partner's central essence. You can push for change at the periphery, but not at the core.

A related notion is that people cannot change their basic essence even if they try to do so. Whether or not it is morally wrong for partners to press for change, it is futile to do so. People cannot alter what is at their core. Only the periphery is amenable to change.

We can call these two notions the "leopard argument": you shouldn't and can't ask the leopard to change his spots. It is wrong to ask. Even if you do ask, the leopard won't be able to change his spots.

Even if both partners accept this position, there is plenty of room to disagree about what is essence and what is not, about what is core and

*"I'm not asking you to change your spots. I'm just
asking you to take out the garbage."*

what is periphery. Denise may see Frank's inability to make affectionate gestures as just some learned behavior that he can change, while Frank may view his physical reticence as a central part of himself. Frank may view Denise's criticism as simply an annoying habit of hers, while she may view her discriminating high standards as an essential (and admirable) characteristic.

Sometimes such a disagreement may reflect genuine differences in how each views what is essential and what is not essential. At other times the issue can be raised simply to deflect a request for change. Like the leopard in the cartoon, one invokes the "essential characteristics" notion—You can't ask me to change who I am—as a way of thwarting any change at all.

Our core characteristics are certainly difficult to change. Indeed, many may be impossible to change. However, that doesn't mean that it is wrong to ask for change. Antonio has been a risk taker all his life. He has always enjoyed challenging and dangerous sports, such as hanggliding and rock climbing. He chose a career on the police force because of the danger and thrill it provides, and he regularly volunteers for assignment to the most dangerous areas of the city. Anna was attracted to Antonio in part because he was so wild and reckless. Far from being something she wanted changed, she found his risk taking a source of excitement. She even joined Antonio in many of his risky leisure-time activities. But now that they have settled down and have two small children, she fears for Antonio's life on and off the job. His partner was recently killed by a gang, and she wants him to seek a safe desk job with the police or change his occupation entirely. She also wants him to stop his dangerous hobbies.

Antonio may reasonably protest that Anna is asking him to change who he is. She has always known that he lives dangerously. How can she request that he change what is basic and essential about him? If she loves him, she must accept him as he is.

Anna may just as reasonably respond that she does love Antonio, but now they are at a different stage of life with different responsibilities. Their children need them both. Love for her and the children demands that he change.

Appeals to either acceptance or love are unlikely to solve Antonio and Anna's dilemma. She has the right to ask; he has the right to refuse. This dilemma will challenge them and their relationship.

Although couples may disagree about whether a particular psychological characteristic is an unchangeable core feature of personality or merely an annoying habit, they are likely to agree that physical characteristics are largely unchangeable. Isn't it necessary to accept the physical characteristics of your partner because they cannot be changed? Even here the answer is not clearly a yes. First of all, some physical characteristics can be changed. While we can't change our age, we can try to lose the extra weight that we have gained with age. We can even treat the wrinkles that come with age, whether that be with makeup, skin medications, or plastic surgery. As medicine advances, what seemed to be unchangeable physical characteristics are being subjected regularly to change. For example, infertile spouses can receive a variety of medical treatments to increase the chances of their bearing children.

Even when some physical characteristic is truly unchangeable, there can be genuine disagreement about whether it must be accepted. After years of trying to have a child, Malcolm and Darlene discover that Darlene is infertile and that no existing treatments can help. Both are understandably disappointed, since having children was one of their major goals. Darlene is able to shift to adoption as an alternative way to have children, but Malcolm cannot make this shift. Having a biological child is a core life goal for him. In her anger at his inflexibility and her fear that he might leave her, Darlene tells Malcolm he *must* accept this condition of hers and not make her feel so bad about it. He must change his attitudes about adoption and pursue that option with her. Malcolm resists her moral imperative and now ponders the issue of whether he has the right to pursue a central life goal even if it means ending his marriage.

There is one final area in which one partner may argue that there is a moral obligation for acceptance. If partners have in good faith worked out an important agreement dealing with their differences, one may argue that they are both obligated to accept its terms unless both agree to change. Certainly, everyone would expect couples to honor their agreements with each other. However, changes may take place that make it difficult or impossible for one to follow through on an agreement. Mike and Beth handle their religious differences by pursuing their faiths separately. At the beginning of their marriage she attends mass at the Catholic church sporadically, while he attends the synagogue regularly. They agree even before their marriage that they will not raise their children as either Catholics or Jews. Rather, they will expose the children to both faiths and allow them to make their own choices. However, as their marriage progresses and they actually have children, Beth's religious faith deepens. She cannot bear the thought of her own children not being baptized. Mike points repeatedly to their agreement: "This is what we decided on; you must abide by it." Beth acknowledges that she made the agreement in good faith. However, she argues, the agreement was made years ago and now she has changed. She should not have to accept conditions of an old agreement that no longer works for her.

Obviously, there is no universal list of what should or must be accepted in relationships. Both partners can request or demand that the other accept certain aspects of themselves. Both can certainly refuse to make any changes in those characteristics for which they seek acceptance. However, whether the partner actually accepts those characteristics is another question entirely.

Demanding acceptance, like demanding change, can decrease the likelihood of its occurrence. Pressure, demands, and moral imperatives are barriers to acceptance just as they are barriers to change. In fact, they may even be greater obstacles to acceptance than they are to change. While it is possible to make some changes on command, it is not possible to alter acceptance on command. Acceptance is in part an emotional reaction that is not under voluntary control. One can no more create acceptance by demanding it than one can create love by commanding it.

HOW CAN WE CREATE ACCEPTANCE?

In the next three chapters we will discuss ways in which you and your partner can promote acceptance in each other. Because acceptance is in part an emotional reaction not under voluntary control, we cannot provide recipes or formulas; we can only describe the kind of experiences that may promote acceptance and offer guidelines for generating those experiences in your relationships.

Promoting acceptance in relationships is a little like promoting trust. Exhortations and pleas, evidence and argument don't go very far. Steve entered a relationship with Joan bothered by questions about her trustworthiness, not because of anything Joan had done, but because his own history had engendered distrust: previous girlfriends had lied and cheated on him. How can Steve learn to trust Joan? It will do little good for Joan to command or demand trust; these actions would merely create resistance or, worse, suspicion in him. It might be useful at times for Joan to reassure Steve that she loves him, but he still might be wary because his other girlfriends had also professed their love. Joan could tell him of her history of honesty and monogamy in relationships; intellectually he might believe her, but emotionally he still may distrust her.

Experiences that demonstrate her faithfulness will help most. Situations like a party in which a man shows interest in her, a visit by her old boyfriend, and the development of a close relationship with a male colleague at work would challenge Steve's trust in Joan but also offer an opportunity for her honesty and faithfulness to be demonstrated and his trust to develop. If she is open and honest about these events, and if she maintains appropriate limits on all of these contacts, Steve's trust in Joan might grow—as might her confidence in his trust.

However, these situations could clearly challenge them both and exacerbate the trust problem. Because of his distrust, Steve could accuse Joan of having feelings about these men that she doesn't have. He could demand unreasonable limits on her behavior: that she refuse to meet with her old boyfriend, that she shun her colleague at work. In response, she could withhold information from him to prevent his unreasonable accusations and demands. Yet her lack of openness could fuel his distrust. She could rebel against his prohibitions about contact with these other men and provocatively increase her contact with them. She could show him that he can't control her, but in so doing increase his anxious and distrusting efforts to try to control her.

Thus, the very occasions that offer the opportunity for trust to grow also generate the risk of trust deteriorating. How the couple handles these situations relevant to trust determines the experience they have of trust in their relationship. These experiences around trust influence the feelings and attitudes of trust, for good or bad.

As with trust, acceptance cannot be commanded or demanded. There is no recipe to make it happen, no formula to call it into being. Acceptance develops based on the particular experiences a couple has as they cope with their differences. These differences offer the opportunity for acceptance-enhancing experiences but also the risk of rejection-inducing experiences. For example, an evening in front of the TV, in which Frank sits at one end of the sofa away from Denise and she feels unconnected and lonely, offers both of them an opportunity for either acceptance or rejection of the other. Depending on whether and how they discuss her desire for affection, they could on the one hand come to a greater understanding and appreciation of each other, perhaps even create greater intimacy between one another, or on the other hand get angry and grow more distant from each other. The very situations that may promote acceptance may also make matters worse. Conflict situations offer not only the risk of alienation but also the possibility of acceptance and intimacy. It all depends on how the discussion and the experience of it go.

WHAT ABOUT CHANGE?

Acceptance is important in its own right because it makes us feel comfortable and "at home" with our partners. We are loved, flaws and all. We can drop pretense, relax, and just be ourselves. Somewhat paradoxically, however, acceptance is also important as a major route to change. As we discussed earlier in the chapter, the kinds of experiences that promote acceptance also promote spontaneous change in couples. When we feel accepted, when we don't feel defensive, we are better able to hear our partners' concerns and appreciate their struggles. We may change to accommodate our partners, not out of force or pressure or coercion, but because we see and experience them differently. We change because we care for them and want them to feel better. When they feel accepted by us and hear our concerns, they may do likewise for us.

Because it requires less effort and comes naturally, spontaneous change can be more gratifying than deliberate change. You don't feel as if you've given up something by compromising. You avoid the work of negotiation. Spontaneous change feels inner-directed: you change because you feel like it, because you want to. It is given freely, without strings.

Planned, deliberate change is more complicated. Sometimes easier to achieve than acceptance in the short run because much behavior is under our voluntary control, planned change may be tough to sustain because it often comes with tangled emotional strings. You may, as we've discussed, be able to see the sense in making a change and appreciate the fairness of it, but if it treads too heavily on your core characteristics and ingrained vulnerabilities, you could resent and regret it in time. Or you could simply return to your old ways.

So we strongly advocate working on acceptance first, not only to promote acceptance, but also because acceptance may generate spontaneous change and thus reduce the need for planned change. Who knows? Maybe you won't even need to read Part III of this book, where we offer suggestions for successful planned change.

RECAP

In this chapter we distinguished between acceptance and change. Change occurs when the perpetrator of some offensive behavior (or the partner who lacks some desired behavior) does something differently. A criticizer lowers the frequency or intensity of criticism; an unaffectionate partner becomes more affectionate. Acceptance takes place when the recipient of the offensive behavior or lack of behavior responds in a different way. The recipient of the criticism or the partner of an unaffectionate mate is less affected by the criticism or the lack of affection and is not so hurt by the offensive behavior (or lack of behavior). Problems in relationships can be solved, at least theoretically, by complete change on the part of the perpetrator, complete acceptance on the part of the recipient, or a combination of the two. The third solution, a combination of acceptance and change, is clearly the most viable path.

Certain behaviors, such as physical abuse, should never be accepted. Also, certain characteristics of the other, such as an unchangeable physical characteristic or a core personality characteristic, may need to be accepted. However, there are precious few universals that absolutely must be changed or must be accepted in all couples for a good relationship to exist. In fact, each of us must decide what is unacceptable to us in our partners and what we are unable or unwilling to change in ourselves (and thus may need to be accepted by our partners). The danger is that the list of what is unacceptable in our partners may grow too long and the list of what we are open to changing may come up short.

In this book we focus first on promoting acceptance in relationships, not only because it is important in its own right, but also because it can often lead to spontaneous change. When there is greater acceptance in a relationship, both partners will be less defensive and more open to hearing what the other needs and wants. Both may respond to those needs and wants simply because they care about the other.

Exercise

Think of some of the core characteristics of your partner.

- What are some specific aspects of him or her that you have, over time, come to accept?
- What are some specific features of your partner, including ones from the previous question, that you could become more accepting of?
- What are some characteristics of yourself that your partner has come to accept?
- What specific characteristics would you like your partner to be more accepting of?

CHAPTER 9

A Story of Our Own

ACCEPTANCE THROUGH
UNDERSTANDING

> To understand all is to forgive all—and to accept
> all.
> —Variation on an old adage

> Narrative is radical, creating us at the moment it is
> being created.
> —Toni Morrison,
>   in *Book of Nobel Lectures* (1995)

*T*he definition of a problem contains the seeds of its solution. How we understand a problem determines the way we cope with it. As we have reported throughout this book, most of us try to resolve marital conflict by demanding an overhaul of our partners. Why? Because we have defined the problem in terms of the other person: *I have problems because of you. I have problems because of the way you are.*

We have also seen—many of us firsthand—that such solutions usually fall short and often even cause problems of their own. Defining relationship problems in terms of your partner can create destructive conflicts over who is bad or mad or inadequate, and thus over who should seek medical or psychological help. Even the ultimate solution to marital conflict, separation or divorce, often causes more problems than it solves—as many couples know.

Our goals in this book are twofold. We want to help couples deal with everyday relationship problems constructively, and we want to help couples deal with these relationship problems in ways that actively bring them closer together. The first goal is simply to manage a problem effectively; the second, more far-reaching goal is to create greater intimacy in the face of problems. To give you the greatest chance of devising solutions that work in achieving these goals, we want you to define the problem accurately. The method we have devised for doing so is to create a true and workable "story" about your problems.

In our couple counseling, we spend three or four sessions evaluating the problem and then provide couples with our feedback. An important part of this feedback is the story we tell about their problems, which must meet demanding criteria. First, the story must be true in the sense that it fits all the facts we have learned about the problem. Second, it must be unique in that it captures the particular experience of each partner and of his or her relationship. Third, it must be original and realistic. And fourth, it must be a story to which both can agree. This last criterion is the most difficult to meet. Usually a couple comes into treatment with different and incompatible stories about their problems. He sees the problem as resulting from something in her; she sees the problem as resulting from something in him. Our goal is to create a common story.

This problem story is essential because it provides the framework for our intervention efforts. It is the foundation for both acceptance and change by both partners. We know that couples spend time thinking about their problems and why they have them. We want them to incorporate a common story into their thinking.

WHAT A PROBLEM STORY SHOULD AND SHOULD NOT INCLUDE

A good problem story is based on the analyses in Part I. It is the "anatomy of argument" for one unique couple. Like any good story, it emphasizes certain features and neglects others, as will be illustrated by three couples with common relationship problems. Chuck and Grace's problem is sex: they cannot agree on how and how often to have sex. Janice and Leif have a responsibility problem: they argue over who does what in the household. And Jacob and Carmen have an in-law problem: they argue about his mother. Even though each couple has unique circumstances, their conflicts may sound familiar.

Differences Rather Than Defects

A good problem story will emphasize *differences between* partners rather than *defects in* either of them. It focuses on incompatibilities between partners rather than faults in either partner. In our story of the sex problem, we would focus on the fact that Chuck has a different sex drive than Grace. He prefers frequent sex involving a great variety of positions, and he likes to begin lovemaking with Grace dressed provocatively in sexy underwear. Grace usually prefers physical affection to sex, feels uncomfortable in sexy underwear, and feels most interested in having sex after a romantic evening, with the lights off and in the missionary position.

It would be easy to find defects on either side of this story. We could label Chuck an oversexed husband who treats Grace like a sex object rather than a wife and lover; we could label Grace a sexually inhibited wife who is uncomfortable with her body in general and sexuality in particular. Instead our story will emphasize the simple differences in what Chuck and Grace find comfortable and pleasing in their sexual relationship.

In our story of the responsibility problem, we would focus on Janice's need for order in her environment and on her preference for equality between husbands and wives both inside and outside the home. Our story will acknowledge Leif's comfort with some level of disorder in people and things and his belief in equality in theory, if not according to the same exact standards held by Janice. We will resist the temptation to label Janice as compulsively neat and controlling or Leif as slovenly and passive–aggressive.

In developing a story about Jacob and Carmen's in-law problem, we will emphasize the difference in their attachment to their mothers rather than exploring whether Jacob is a man who has "never cut the apron strings" from his mother or whether Carmen is insecure and jealous of Jacob's relationship with his mother.

But what if there really are defects in one or both members of the couple? Should we paper over these deficiencies by euphemistically calling them "simple differences" rather than facing them squarely? Shouldn't we make a clear distinction between what are defects and what are differences?

Except in the extreme, such distinctions are almost impossible to support, because all behavior falls somewhere along a continuum. Who is to say where "normal" differences end and pathological defects begin? Even if we had reliable data on the sexual responsiveness of women or the disorderliness of men, and even if we could prove that Grace was below average on the former and Leif was above average on the latter, any decision about a cutoff point for "defectiveness" would clearly be arbitrary.

And even if we could make reliable distinctions between differences and defects, what end would be served? A focus on defectiveness often leads to blame and accusation on the one hand and defensiveness on the other. As we have seen, this does not lead to solutions but often to reactive problems that are even more intense than the original problems.

Vulnerability Rather Than Violation

In our stories about our problems, we are likely to focus on the violating behaviors that offend us, the provocative acts that upset us. Grace may focus on the aggressive way that Chuck grabs her. Janice may focus on the inconsiderate way in which Leif leaves his clothes scattered over their bedroom. Jacob may focus on the coldness with which Carmen responds to his mother.

This focus on the violating behavior that offends us often leads to disagreement and argument. Chuck views his sexual initiatives toward Grace as simply showing a healthy sexual interest in her. In his view, she should be flattered rather than offended by his behavior. Leif regards Janice as compulsive rather than his own behavior as inconsiderate. Carmen cannot imagine how she could respond differently to a mother who has fostered such an unhealthy dependency in her son.

To build a common story, it is better to focus less on the violating behavior and more on the vulnerability that the behavior triggers. However we might describe Chuck's sexual initiatives, to Grace they feel more like an assault than an invitation. They touch a sensitivity in her to being physically invaded. Janice feels anxious and out of control when her surroundings are in disarray. A vulnerability about control and disorder is triggered when there is clutter around her. Finally, Jacob feels supremely protective of his widowed mother. As an only child, he knows she has no one else to care for her. He feels torn between his wife and his mother when Carmen reacts to his mother in ways that don't seem friendly to him.

Description Rather Than Evaluation

A good problem story includes a description of how each partner copes with the initial problem created by their differences and vulnerabilities. How a couple tries to solve their problem is as important as its content. But the description of the coping process must focus on the prominent thoughts, feelings, and behaviors of each partner without judgments about whether the thoughts are distorted, the feelings over-blown, or the behaviors appropriate. Getting caught up in mutual evalu-ation as you construct your story will only distract you from your goal of trying to understand the problem.

A nonjudgmental description of Chuck and Grace's coping process might go like this: Because of their history of conflict over sex, Chuck approaches Grace half in hopeful desire and half in irritable anticipation of a negative reaction from her. Grace often feels guilty and inadequate because she is not more sexually responsive, but she also feels strongly that it is not her role to service Chuck's sexual needs. If she senses any negativity in his sexual approach to her, she finds responding even more difficult. She resists his efforts, which of course confirms his fears. Some-times, to avoid an argument, they both back off tensely. Other times they engage each other in an acrimonious dispute, in which Grace accuses Chuck of being insensitive and he accuses her of being frigid.

Chuck's accusations of frigidity are not likely to promote a loving response in Grace. Nor are her dismissals of him as "insensitive" likely to stimulate satisfying intimacy or productive discussion. If their story focuses on what each does wrong, it will not capture the dilemma in which they are caught. A portrayal of wrongdoing will become another piece of their struggle over the problem rather than a story *about* their problem.

A good, nonjudgmental story captures the process by which Chuck and Grace try to deal with their sexual difficulty, but it does not con-demn either one for the desperate measures they sometimes employ. There is a world of difference between saying "You are frigid" and say-ing "When I get frustrated, I accuse you of being frigid." The first is a judgment that will perpetuate the problem; the second is a descriptive account of the problem that may lead to understanding.

Valid Rather Than Invalid Aspects of Each Partner's Experience

In any serious dispute in a close relationship, coping will involve distortions, exaggerations, denials, miscommunication, misper-ceptions, and the like. A good problem story will emphasize what is true and valid in each one's experience rather than what is distorted or exag-gerated. Often exaggerations, denials, and distortion come about be-cause partners aren't being heard or they are feeling attacked. If you sense that your partner understands the truth in your experience, you may not need to exaggerate or distort information.

Consider Jacob and Carmen's conflict over his mother. In their many arguments about this issue, Carmen often exaggerates Jacob's dependency on his mother, caricaturing him as a little boy afraid to leave his mommy. Conversely, Jacob will deny that *any* dependency exists and will distort Carmen's position, depicting her as a pathetically insecure and jealous wife. A good conflict story would focus on what is valid in each of their positions: that Jacob has an important connection to his mother that he wants to maintain and that Carmen feels that his connection to his mother interferes with their own connection to each other.

In describing how each partner copes with the problem, a good conflict story centers on the understandable emotions that motivate exaggerated claims or wholesale denials. When Carmen feels that Jacob's concern about his mother takes precedence over his concern about her, she gets angry and hurls assaults at him or his mom. On the other hand, when Jacob feels Carmen is attacking him or his mother, he gets furious and responds with either wholesale denial or defensive counterattacks. In each case, our story focuses on the valid feelings of each person. To the extent that a good story focuses on "invalid behavior," it describes that behavior as arising from valid feelings that get frustrated or threatened.

Complex Dilemmas Rather Than Simple Solutions

A good conflict story stresses the complex dilemmas that long-standing problems present rather than offering simple solutions to them. Simple solutions usually derive from a limited understanding of the difficulties that a problem presents, particularly of how one's own behavior contributes to that difficulty. These simple solutions focus on "the obvious things that *you* can do to solve this problem." They are often solutions that further complicate the problems, cures that exacerbate the disease. Therefore, somewhat paradoxically, couples can resolve complex dilemmas more easily than they can implement simple solutions.

Leif's simple solution is "Look, I am cooperative and want to help. Ask me for help when you need it and ask me nicely, not in an irritated, angry way, and I will usually do what you want done." This simple solution ignores at least two major issues. Janice wants Leif to be a copartner, not just a helper. She wants him to notice when the children have needs, to notice when the house needs picking up or the dishes need to be done, and then to take action. Instead, he withdraws into his own world, reading the paper or watching TV, and she is left with the responsibility. When she gets overwhelmed with the household responsibilities and sees him "in his own world," she is too irritated to ask nicely and sweetly for his help.

Janice's simple solution to their problem is for Leif to "stand up and take an equal role in the family. Look around, see what needs to be done, and do it. Don't wait for me to tell you or for things to get out of hand. Just do it." Janice's simple solution also ignores some major facets of their problem. Leif has different standards for the household and for the kids than Janice does. For Leif to act on his own, the kids have to be louder and more boisterous and the household has to be in greater disarray than Janice can tolerate. So Janice wants Leif to take action according to her standards rather than according to his own, which would of course be much more difficult for Leif. Furthermore, when he does take action, whether it be with the kids or with the household, he often doesn't do it as well as Janice. She then criticizes him, which makes him feel that she won't be happy unless it is done her way. He reacts by withdrawing from household responsibilities altogether; he is not eager to take them on in the first place, especially if he gets criticized for his efforts.

Thus, the simple solutions proposed by each will not succeed. They lay full responsibility on the other, ignore each one's own role in the problem, and ignore the emotional barriers to their implementation. As Leif and Janice argue about these "simple solutions," they will likely create reactive problems that will, at the very least, complicate their initial problem. A story that describes their complex dilemma, rather than "obvious solutions" to it, may create more acceptance in each and possibly even more realistic opportunities for change.

Conscious Consequences Rather Than Unconscious Intent

In a conflict, each partner's behavior usually has important consequences for the other—often strong, negative emotional consequences such as hurt, anger, and disappointment. Earlier we described how conflict starts when some provocative event, usually one partner's behavior, triggers an incompatibility or vulnerability in one or both, which then leads to emotional reactions. Because these emotions can be so powerful, the one experiencing them may assume that it is the other's intent to create them. The logic goes something like this: "If you are doing something that creates a strong negative reaction in me, then you must *want* to create that reaction in me."

Chuck often feels a mixture of anger and hurt because, in his view, he can so rarely express his sexual feelings for Grace. Even on those occasions when they do have sexual relations, he feels limited in his sexual expression. Beyond his immediate emotional reactions, he feels emasculated by the whole situation. In his thoughts about the problem, he entertains the idea that maybe Grace wants to emasculate him; maybe she is threatened by his masculinity and is trying to cut him down to size. Maybe unconsciously she wants him to be impotent!

For her part, Grace feels such pressure and dissatisfaction from Chuck that she questions her own sexuality. She vacillates between feeling angry at Chuck for his advances and feeling inadequate as a wife and lover. In her anger, she may think that only a porno star could satisfy Chuck. Yet she knows that she has always been shy and inhibited sexually. Unfortunately, her sexual relationship with Chuck is distorted by so much pressure that her inhibitions have increased, not decreased. Maybe he wants her to feel inadequate. Maybe unconsciously he is taking out some kind of anger toward women on her.

An ideal conflict story emphasizes what each partner experiences consciously, not what might be motivating them unconsciously. Chuck does experience sexual deprivation, he does feel less of a man because of their sexual problems, and he does feel emasculated because of what he considers the sexual limitations in their relationship. However, Grace experiences no desire to hurt him, except perhaps in moments of frustration. While she may wish that his sexual desire was not so intense, she does not consciously wish to emasculate him.

Does she have an unconscious motivation to emasculate Chuck? By definition, she is not aware of this, if she does. Given his emotional involvement in the situation, Chuck is not a good candidate to make that determination. No spouse could be trusted to be objective in determining the partner's unconscious motives. Even the psychological experts would have difficulty sorting out unconscious motives. Many have abandoned the notion of unconscious motives entirely as a useless construct.

For Grace's part, she does feel bad about their sexual relationship and she does feel inadequate as a sexual partner. As a result of her sexual relationship with Chuck, she has grown more inhibited, not less so, about sexual expression. But it is certainly not Chuck's conscious desire to make her more inhibited, even though his behavior has contributed to greater inhibition on her part. His fond hope is that she become less inhibited! In moments of anger, he may want her to feel bad about her inhibitions, but only as a means of spurring her to change. He wishes she felt good about sex and her sexuality so it could play a more prominent part in their life together.

And what about possible unconscious motives on Chuck's part? Does he secretly want her to be inhibited? Is he playing out with Grace his anger toward someone else, such as his mother? As we said before, he cannot know, by definition, what his unconscious motives are, and she is not an objective judge. The experts, were they called to testify, would disagree.

When the notion of unconscious motivation comes up in the context of a couple's conflict, it is usually a source of accusation and blame. Chuck may accuse Grace of having an unconscious desire to emasculate him. He may charge that she wants to psychologically castrate him. Since she has no sense of wanting to emasculate him, she will respond incredulously to his accusations. She may charge that his accusations are outrageous, that he has been reading too much pop psychology, and that his mental faculties are in question. She may charge that he wants her to feel inadequate more than he wants a good sexual relationship. She may accuse him of taking out his anger toward his mother on her. He is also likely to respond incredulously to her charges and reciprocate her attacks. Such charges and countercharges will divert the two of them from the difficult sexual problem they face and lead to angry and hurtful exchanges.

A good problem story, therefore, stays with the present experience of each partner but does not jump from this experience to accusations of negative intention, whether unconsciously or consciously driven. We can genuinely "feel controlled" without our partners consciously or unconsciously "trying to" control us. We may feel deeply hurt without our partners "wanting to" hurt us. We may feel powerless even though our partners are not "trying to" disempower us. We can feel inadequate without our partners "trying to" make us feel bad.

Emotional Reactions Rather Than Motives

> No one can love anyone the way that everyone
> wants to be loved.
> —MIGNON MCLAUGHLIN,
> *The Neurotic's Notebook* (1963)

Even if we don't assume that our own strong emotional reactions implicate unconscious, negative motives in our partner, there is another way that the emotional consequences of conflict can affect our stories about those conflicts. We may find, in the presence of our own strong emotion, evidence for an absence of motivation in our partners. "If you are doing something that creates such a negative reaction in me, then certainly you couldn't care about my feelings. If you do things that hurt me, how can you possibly respect me? If you take actions that make me feel unloved, how can you really love me?"

Carmen wants a closer relationship with Jacob. She often feels neglected by him, particularly when she sees the amount of contact he has with his mother and senses the intimacy they must have together. She wonders whether Jacob really loves her. In her anger, she accuses him of lack of love. In dramatic moments, she takes off her wedding ring and offers it to him with the challenge, "Why don't you give it to your mother? She's really your wife, not me!"

For his part, Jacob feels hurt by and defensive about Carmen's frequent attacks on his mother and his relationship with his mother. He tells Carmen that he is not asking her to love his mother, only to accept her as she is, or at least not to attack her. Yet, much to his dismay, Carmen can never seem to say a positive thing about his mother and highlights all of her shortcomings instead. Jacob counters Carmen's charge that he doesn't really love her with charges of his own: "How can you love me when you constantly attack someone who is so important to me?"

Accusations about lack of love are double-edged swords. Jacob can question Carmen's behavior as emanating from lack of love just as easily as Carmen can question Jacob's behavior as stemming from lack of love. Jacob can argue that love of a husband would imply acceptance of his mother. Carmen can argue that love of a wife would imply putting her first, before his mother.

A challenge lies within the accusation of lack of love: *If you really loved me, you would do . . .* Carmen challenges Jacob with the charge that if he really loved her, he would turn away from his mother and put more energy and effort into their relationship. Jacob's challenge is that if Carmen really loved him, she would support his contact with his mother.

We would all like our partners, out of love for us, to put aside their own self-interests and address our own, to put aside their needs and nurture our own. Carmen wants Jacob to put aside his own attachment to his mother and devote himself more fervently to her. Jacob wants Carmen to put aside her feelings of neglect and accept, if not actually encourage, his close contact with his mother.

Sometimes couples are able to put aside their immediate interests and meet their partners' needs. And to the recipient, and even the giver, that feels like love. But when the stakes are high, when important needs clash, when giving to you means giving up something for me, then it is difficult to be responsive. When these discussions about clashing needs occur in a context of accusation and blame, our partners will not even hear our needs, much less attend to them.

The motives that Jacob and Carmen discuss are ones that they attribute to each other. Because each experiences painful emotional reactions from the other, each accuses the other of unsavory motives, such as lack of love. These accusations, just like accusations of unconscious motives, become an additional source of conflict and thus create much more difficulty than they solve. Therefore, a good problem story will describe the emotional reactions that we and our partners experience from the problem without speculating on possible motives in our partners that led to their actions.

The Big Picture Rather Than the Little Behavior

As we already discussed, conflicts often begin with specific, provocative incidents. One partner does something or fails to do something that triggers a vulnerability or an incompatibility that generates a strong emotional reaction in the other. During the course of an argument about this incident, feelings may escalate on both sides until one or both partners do something especially negative, such as insult the other or refuse to listen. In our stories about our problems, some of us focus on specific, negative behaviors of our partners, behaviors that initiated a conflict or served to escalate it. We hold up snapshots of their doing something particularly onerous. But the snapshots don't give the context, the interaction that preceded and followed the onerous behavior that makes that behavior at least understandable, if not acceptable.

For example, in arguments about their household responsibility problem, Janice may mention the time that Leif blurted out in anger "Well, you should do it—you're the woman." She may use this statement as evidence that Leif really is a "sexist pig at heart" and doesn't endorse the goals of equality that she cherishes. However, when Leif made that statement, he was so angry at Janice that he was trying to say something to upset her. For his part, Leif may mention the time Janice blurted out "You can't do anything right." He may use that in his own defense: "Why should I even try to help you? You said I can't do anything right."

A good problem story attends not to the little behaviors that show our partners in the worst possible light, but to the big picture, the theme of our conflict. A good story describes the problem in broad strokes but may illustrate those broad features with specific examples. For example, the themes of Janice and Leif's conflict center on responsibility, competence, and control. Janice wants Leif to take on more childcare and household responsibility because a disproportionate amount of both falls on her shoulders. She not only wants his greater involvement, she needs it. She got in that position partly because she was more interested in childcare and housework, was better at it, and desired more control over it. Leif deferred to her because of his own lesser interest. Now he finds that his efforts at childcare and housework often do not meet her standards; he comes off as inadequate and feels inadequate yet resents her control. In these areas she is in charge and regularly gives him unsatisfactory grades for his performance. He resents her judgments, doesn't feel good about his contributions, and often rebels against her control. She finds herself stressed out by the responsibility because she has a partner who doesn't initiate, often doesn't do a good job, and gives her a lot of static in the process. Part of her wants to leave him out of the process entirely, but another part realizes that then she would be even more stressed.

A SAMPLE STORY

Up until now we have examined bits of conflict stories, snippets of each couple's struggle. Now we present one complete conflict story: Chuck and Grace's sexual difficulty.

The differences between Chuck and Grace's interest in sex and their ways of expressing it have multiple origins. In part, they represent stereotypical sexual differences between males and females in America, and thus may reflect the ways that boys and girls are socialized. In part, they may represent biological differences between men and women. But, their differences also reflect their own personal histories.

Grace came from a more religious home than Chuck, where modesty was the norm. She learned about sex from her parents, who made sure she heard it first from them so they could place sexual expression in the appropriate context of love. Prior to her relationship with Chuck, she had had only one sexual relationship, with a longtime boyfriend whom she considered marrying. Her sexual relationship with him was positive but very traditional. They made love in the dark, with him on top.

Chuck learned about sex on the streets from his friends. His father made a feeble effort to tell him about sex by leaving him a book and by inviting him to ask any questions "about men and women" he had. Chuck wasn't sure what his father was talking about and wasn't interested in pursuing it. When Chuck was older, his father advised him to "keep his pecker in his pocket." At that point his father had little credibility with Chuck. Chuck was sexually active during his late teens and early twenties. He had many different relationships, and sex was an important part of all of them.

Grace and Chuck met when they both were in their middle twenties. He was immediately attracted to her and pursued her energetically. She was flattered by his attentions but set firm boundaries about sexual contact. He respected her limits but was also challenged by them. As their relationship developed, Grace often found Chuck's intense interest in her a "turn-on" and his pursuit of sexual novelty provocative. He found excitement in the need to woo her constantly. Their differences sparked the sexual tension between them.

As time went on, his consistent sexual interest became less flattering, less exciting, and more clearly an annoyance to Grace. Her hesitancy and, at times, active resistance became less of a challenge to Chuck and more of a barrier to sexual satisfaction. Chuck's physical affection and loving attention to Grace, which had always served as an aphrodisiac to her, suffered from their sexual conflict and from the familiarity of daily contact. How could he be so attentive and loving to her when he felt so neglected sexually? To Grace, Chuck seemed less and less interested in loving her, and more interested in merely using her for sexual pleasure. How could she be sexually responsive when she felt no love from him?

What were once his loving nudges and her demure limits became, over time, insistent pressures and bald refusals. Frustration at her lack of response and anticipation of a negative reaction robbed Chuck of the gentleness and charm with which he had often pursued her. The tension of his urgent demands hardened her into resistance.

What changed in them was not only the way they dealt with their differences but the very differences themselves. His demands dampened any spontaneous interest in sex Grace might have had. Her resistance to sex and the deprivation he experienced created greater, not less, desire in him. So now he wants sex more than ever and now she wants it less than ever.

The sexual problems also created or accentuated vulnerabilities in each partner. Grace had never been completely confident of herself sexually. Now she felt even more anxiety about sexuality and, when she wasn't angry at Chuck, wondered what was wrong with her. Chuck had always taken pride in himself as a good lover. But he too, when he wasn't focused on Grace, began to wonder about himself. He certainly was not a good lover with Grace. So both became more sensitive about their own sexuality.

Grace now feels a relentless pressure from Chuck to have sex. Even if he doesn't express it directly, the way he looks at her tells her he is thinking about having sex and wondering if now is the time. Even when she agrees to sex, she feels pressure to do it in ways that make her uncomfortable. It seems as if his own desires for sex carry the day. No allowance is made for her feelings. She wonders: "How can he care about me when he pushes his own sexual agenda and shows no consideration for my feelings?"

Grace's feeling of pressure about sex is real and intense. And furthermore, that feeling is grounded in reality: Chuck does "check her out" often in the hopes of finding interest or at least concession on her part for sex. During sex he often pushes for experimentation and variety. However, Chuck hardly ignores her feelings. He scrutinizes her so intensely because he is aware of her feelings and tries to gauge her emotional state before making any sexual moves. He rarely makes a sexual advance in which he is oblivious to her mood. In fact, his sensitivity to her moods in part creates the scrutiny that adds to the pressure she feels!

With a problem this large and consuming, they each think about it a lot. She wonders if he really loves her at all. He wonders if she secretly wants to emasculate him. As they share their individual ideas about the problem, these ideas become part of the problem. They argue not just over when and how to have sex but about why they are the way they are and about possible solutions to the problem. She accuses him of using her as a sexual object. He accuses her of being frigid and compares her to other women. They generate angry and impossible solutions to the problem. He suggests that she "just do it," whether she feels like it or not. She suggests he ignore his adolescent impulses and not let them control his life. They have mixed and complex feelings about the issue. He mostly feels angry at her but is troubled by his sometimes brutish treatment of her. She is mostly angry at him for his pressure but questions her own sexuality.

How can a story like this be helpful to a couple? Their problem seems so difficult, their pattern seems so entrenched, and they each seem so stuck that no solution seems possible. But if this story accurately defines their problem and truthfully describes the defeating ways that each tries to solve the problem, the story is right. And if the couple begins to understand their problem according to this story, they may be more accepting of each other's behavior in this situation. They may ease off on the accusation, blame, and defensiveness that made the initial problem a more serious reactive problem. They may be able to find some compassion for each other among the tatters of their sexual relationship. They may feel less alone in their experience of this hurtful problem because they find a fellow victim in, of all places, their partner. They may find emotional intimacy in their struggle together. And the intimate union of those who struggle together can be a mighty force against the biggest of problems.

RECAP

The first step toward solving a problem is to define it appropriately. A good definition of a relationship problem is a story about the problem on which both partners can agree. It is a story that incorporates the kind of analysis described in Part I but for a particular couple's unique problem. Like any good story, a story about a relationship problem emphasizes certain features over others. A good story is one that emphasizes differences between partners rather than deficits in either of them, that underscores vulnerabilities in each rather than violations by either, that focuses on description rather than evaluation, that highlights the valid rather than the invalid aspects of each person's experience, that defines complex dilemmas rather than simple solutions, that accentuates conscious consequences and emotional reactions rather than unconscious intent and motives, and finally that stresses the big picture rather than the little behavior. Such a story, which is a unique "anatomy of argument" for one couple, gives each partner a rich understanding of their problem that provides a basis for both acceptance and change.

Exercise

Develop a story about an important problem in your relationship. The exercise will be most beneficial if you outline your story on paper.

- Start by identifying the incompatibilities and vulnerabilities that constitute the initial problem. If you saved any of your written answers to the exercises from Chapters 3–6, they might be helpful.
- Indicate the ways that each of you copes with this problem. Do you use any of the toxic solutions described in Chapter 7? Again, your exercise sheet from Chapter 7 could be helpful.
- Consider whether the initial problem you face leads to a more serious reactive problem. Does your struggle over the problem lead to escalation, polarization, or alienation between you? Has it led to doubts or loss of confidence for either of you?
- Look over the outline of your story now. Edit it for the features described in this chapter. For example, does it focus on differences rather than defects? Does it highlight vulnerabilities rather than violations? Is it descriptive rather than evaluative?
- If you generated a story on your own, try sharing your story with your partner. A major criterion of a good story is that both partners can agree to it. A good story about a relationship problem can be helpful to you even if you never share it with your partner. However, the story will have the greatest benefit if both of you can construct it together or agree to it once either of you has constructed it.

CHAPTER 10

Walking in Your Partner's Shoes

ACCEPTANCE THROUGH COMPASSION

Sylvia and Gerard are in constant conflict over the level of closeness in their relationship. Sylvia feels she is not a priority in Gerard's life. He seems to get more excited about a possible promotion at work or a ski weekend with his friends than about being with her. For his part, Gerard sees Sylvia as constantly dissatisfied. He can never seem to do enough for her, as if he must constantly prove to her that he cares. The struggle of it all makes him wonder at times how much he really does care.

The problem over closeness has become a chronic wedge between them. Sylvia is easily angered by signs of Gerard's lack of commitment to her. If he gets heavily involved in work, or seems too excited about recreational events that don't involve her, or shows little interest in activity with her, her anger often reveals itself in sarcasm: "I hope it's not a burden for you to go with me." Or in provocative comparison: "You seem awfully happy about going out—a lot happier than I have seen you in a while." Or in outright accusation: "You don't make me a priority in your life. I am way down on the list." Gerard typically responds by defending himself, insisting that she *is* a priority for him, that he *does* want to be with her. However, when he gets completely frustrated with her, he may counterattack: "There is no pleasing you. You are so insecure, you need constant attention." At times Sylvia gets so worn out by the conflict and feels so hopeless about getting what she needs from Gerard that she shuts down. She stops blaming, but anger pervades her silence.

Can love, caring, or compassion ever break through the cloud of anger and distance that surrounds this couple? If you and your partner are stuck in a similar vortex of anger and hurt, it may seem impossible to extricate yourselves. But when your focus shifts from the offending actions of each of you to the soft spots that are bruised by these actions, you may come to a new understanding of each other, one that cuts angry arguments short and over time brings you closer together.

This is no mean feat, of course. Anger is the most common emotion to erupt during conflict, and it tends to become a chronic state when we feel our needs are repeatedly thwarted, when we feel overwhelmed by constant demands, or when we feel slighted, discounted, or neglected day after day. Under those conditions we adopt the coping methods discussed in Chapter 7, which usually numb our compassion and blind us to what we need to stay focused on: the vulnerabilities that make us feel the way we do. Whether we opt for the familiar trio of accusation, blame, and coercion; the evasive tactics of avoidance, minimization, and denial; or a more subtle strategy of putting up defensive barriers and striking back through passive resistance, we end up not being heard and not feeling safe in a relationship that should be a sanctuary for both of us. We get trapped in an emotional bind that erodes our love for and commitment to each other. We may wish for compassion, but our loved ones seem too alienated and angry themselves to give it.

The way to break this pattern of chronic anger, withdrawal, and defensiveness is for both partners to disclose aspects of themselves that they have never or rarely mentioned or to disclose these aspects in ways that they have never voiced them before.

THE IMPORTANCE OF THE UNSAID

> What we don't say is often more important than what we do say.

Chronic conflict can leave you believing that you've already said everything there is to be said on the subject of contention—and far too often at that. In fact, though, you and your partner probably have not revealed many of your important thoughts and feelings about the conflict. You may be only dimly aware of your feelings, or you may not feel safe disclosing them. Yet it is precisely these revelations that could alter the tone of the discussion and perhaps elicit empathy between you.

The Anger Itself May Not Be Disclosed

As difficult as it may be to believe considering the tone of your voices and your mutual accusations and defenses, you and your partner may not be expressing your anger directly. One of you may be caught up in laying blame, while the other is preoccupied with self-protection, rebuttal, and counterattack. One or both of you may be distant and resentful. Neither of you says outright, "I'm really angry at you right now."

Would such a disclosure help? Possibly not. One could respond to the other's disclosure competitively: "Well, you're not as angry as I am." Or sarcastically: "Well, isn't that too bad." Or dismissively: "So?"

There is certainly no automatic benefit from this or any similar statement, so why take the risk of merely escalating the argument? Because a direct statement of anger calls attention to what is probably the most important aspect of the discussion: its emotional underpinnings. This simple disclosure can be a first step away from futile debate over the evaluation of behavior and toward a potentially fruitful discussion of each one's emotional experience.

This first step is possible, however, only if the statement is made strictly to convey information about yourself, rather than information about your partner. If you say "I am really angry at you right now" as a cover for an attack, meaning "You made me angry because of all the horrible things you do," or as a challenge, meaning "I'm angry, and you better do something about it right now," you're not shifting the discussion from blame to personal disclosure. Even if you make the statement appropriately, with all the right intentions, your partner may sense, because of his or her own defensive state, accusation, or challenge.

It will probably take more than just a simple comment, no matter how pure, to keep the focus on your emotional experience (see the accompanying diagram).

In the right boxes, Sylvia gets drawn into an argument with Gerard. In the left boxes, she avoids the temptation to attack his behavior or to defend her own. She keeps the focus on her emotional experience. Although there are no guarantees, her focus on her emotional experience may enable Gerard to listen to her and even share his own emotional experience.

SYLVIA: I'm really angry right now.

⇩

GERARD: Well, what am I supposed to do about that?

↙   ↘

SYLVIA: There may be nothing you can do. I am just upset and angry.

⇩

GERARD: You are overreacting. All I did was . . . (*Gerard defends himself.*)

⇩

SYLVIA: I am sure you have your own reasons for what you did. I am still upset and still angry.

SYLVIA: Well, you could start out by apologizing for what you have done!

GERARD: Me apologize! Why should I . . . ?

Argument

↘

SYLVIA: No, I didn't overreact. Anyone who had feelings would . . . (*Sylvia defends herself and counterattacks Gerard.*)

Argument

Genuine, Immediate Feelings May Go Unstated or Be Denied

When Sylvia is frustrated by the lack of attention from Gerard and his apparent greater interest in his work and his hobbies, she accuses him of not loving her. Gerard responds by defending himself and asserting his love for her. He recounts evidence of his love—for example, that he has been sexually faithful to her, that he hasn't tried to leave the relationship. She often replies: "You list the things you haven't done that show love. Tell me anything you have done that shows love." Gerard will then try to list times he has attended to her, like when she was hospitalized with pneumonia. She then dismisses his evidence: "That was years ago" or "That is not love—any reasonably responsible person would have helped."

In fact, Sylvia is so angry at Gerard's neglect that she is unlikely to be swayed by any factual evidence he can muster. It is as if she is saying "I don't think you love me, so I'll try to beat it out of you." And he is saying in response "I'm threatened by your upset, so I'll try to calm you with terse, dismissive recitations of fact."

If Gerard were aware of what was going on with himself emotionally at the moment and could genuinely articulate it, he would say something like "Right now I'm feeling attacked by you and want to defend myself. I'm so overwhelmed by the attack and my urge to defend myself that at this very moment, even though I know I love you, I don't feel any love."

Such a disclosure might be scary for Gerard to make. He would fear an even stronger reaction from Sylvia: "See? There—you finally admitted it. You don't love me." And he might be drawn into an even bigger defense: "I just said 'at this moment.' I didn't mean I don't love you." However, Gerard's disclosure might stop the frustrating charade they go through in which Sylvia tries to generate love through angry accusations about its absence and Gerard tries to prove his love with defensive lists of facts.

If Sylvia were aware of what was going on with her emotionally at the moment and could genuinely articulate it, she would say something like "I'm so angry at you right now that I'm not open to hearing you. I just want to attack you." Such a message would be difficult for Sylvia to make because Gerard could easily use it against her. "See, you admitted it. You don't care about whether I love you or not—you just want to attack me." However, her disclosure would prevent his fruitless efforts to prove himself to her. And it might make him listen to her.

These kinds of communications are certainly difficult, sometimes even impossible, during conflict. But they can take you another small step away from your vicious cycle of argument because you are saying what you feel like doing (such as attacking or defending), rather than actually doing it. They express the urge in place of the action.

Crucial Background Information May Be Left Out

Arguments can become so habitual and reactions so immediate that partners play their parts with little knowledge of what set them off. They may not even notice important conditions that set off a particular discussion and make it different from previous ones. Or if they do notice, they may be hesitant to disclose those conditions.

For example, Sylvia is concerned about some lumps she has felt in her breast. She tried to get Gerard to feel them, but he made only a half-hearted attempt, saying "I'm no doctor." He told her to see her doctor, which he often says in response to her (admittedly) many physical complaints. At this point, his message to "see your doctor" seems dismissive, a cover for "Don't bother me about it."

Sylvia's concern is great enough that she does make an appointment with her doctor. She lets Gerard know of the appointment in advance—to which he responds with an unconvincing "That's good." Angry that Gerard shows so little interest in her concerns, Sylvia is dimly aware that her notification of the appointment is in part a test: Will he remember her appointment and comment on it?

Sylvia has a fitful night's sleep before her appointment. That morning she awakes worried, she feels her breast, and she detects what clearly seems to be a lump. She goes into the kitchen and finds Gerard, as usual, with his head in the newspaper, eating his breakfast. He barely acknowledges her entry into the kitchen.

Her fear over her appointment turns to anger at Gerard. She sarcastically voices the observation: "That must be a fascinating article in the paper."

He replies defensively: "I said hello."

"Oh, was that hello? I thought it was some bodily noise."

Gerard assumes that this is the same old conflict: "Come off it, Sylvia. Can't a guy read the paper in peace?"

Sylvia has an urge to blurt out something about her appointment but doesn't, for fear he will dismiss her concerns. Then if her "lumps" prove to be nonsignificant, he would gloat about being right and lecture her again about not getting so worked up. The angry part of her hopes that the doctor will find something serious, so she can use it against his dismissal and lack of concern for her.

Gerard leaves Sylvia that day irritated by what he labels her "weird moodiness." He wonders in passing if she is premenstrual. She leaves that day in a mix of anger at Gerard and fear about what the doctor might find.

The crucial piece of information that would have made the morning understandable—her worry about her upcoming visit to the doctor—was never a point of discussion. Gerard forgot it. Sylvia never brought it up, partly for fear of his likely dismissal of her concerns and partly in anger, to save as a later weapon against him.

Even if Sylvia did mention her appointment, she might have done it in such a blaming way that Gerard would get caught up in defending himself rather than in hearing her concerns. Even if she were not blaming, Gerard might have been defensive rather than responsive to her. Yet her mentioning that day's appointment and her feelings about it might have served to refocus their discussion. It could have led to some genuine support from Gerard. Not mentioning it at all robbed them of that opportunity.

Other Emotions, Especially Softer Ones, May Not Be Revealed

When things happen to us that we don't like, we experience hard emotions such as anger, irritation, impatience, resentment, frustration, and disgust. These emotions, and their accompanying hard thoughts, express a strong self that says in no uncertain terms "I'm upset with the world" and "I'm not going to take this anymore." Expression of these feelings is beneficial because it often provides release for some of the negativity we feel and because it establishes our boundaries with others. Unfortunately, it also often invites a response in kind: anger may elicit anger and resentment resentment. This not only can lead to escalation but also may actually discourage the love and compassion whose absence evoked the hard emotions in the first place.

Soft emotions, in contrast, reveal a vulnerable self experiencing inward anguish. Hurt, guilt, sadness, disappointment, and fear all signal a pain inside. They reveal a wounded self rather than an assertive self. They are often accompanied by softer thoughts that express doubt and uncertainty.

Any significant negative experience in relationships is likely to lead to both hard and soft feelings and both hard and soft thoughts. If my partner ignores me at a party, I may feel anger at the neglect but I also may feel hurt and insecure. I may wonder, "How can you treat me this way?," but I may also feel hurt that my partner didn't find me more interesting. If I end up doing most of the housework, I may feel resentment at the injustice of it all, but also feel devalued as a partner because my role is to "just do the housework." I may decide not to be manipulated into being a housekeeper but also wonder about my value.

The expression of soft emotions such as hurt and fear can often trigger caring and concern in your partner. When we see others in pain, particularly others we care about, we naturally feel compassion for them. We want to comfort and protect them. We forget about our own needs and reach out to them. Unfortunately, soft emotions and soft thoughts usually go unexpressed in conflict. Often they are attempted but sabotaged by the atmosphere of hard emotion around them. One may voice "I feel hurt by you," but the manner in which the admission is delivered and the emphasis on the "by you" at the end make it more of an accusation than an expression of pain. Even the simple expression "I felt hurt" can be said more in anger than in pain.

A genuine expression of soft emotion, a voicing that you are lonely or hurt or disappointed or feel neglected or abandoned, is difficult because it opens you up. It presents you as vulnerable and defenseless. It may feel uncomfortable to do in any circumstance and impossible to do when you are angry.

Gerard and Sylvia rarely give voice to their genuine soft feelings surrounding their conflict over closeness—for the very good reasons of self-protection. Exposure of these feelings might make them more vulnerable to each other and more open to attack. Yet exposure of these feelings might elicit compassion and caring for each other. In voicing these feelings, they might be able to listen to each other's pain without assigning responsibility for that pain. They might experience connection and closeness with each other in the joint realization of how distant they are and how much it hurts. The problem could bring them together. Paradoxically they could experience closeness from a compassionate sharing of their feelings of distance from each other.

The Other Side May Never Be Disclosed

In an enduring conflict, each partner stakes out a position, argues that position, defends that position, and becomes more and more entrenched in that position. Sylvia's position is that Gerard doesn't express enough love and affection for her. Gerard's position is that Sylvia demands more than any reasonable man could give. In their regular conflicts over this issue of closeness, neither backs off or acknowledges any validity in the other's position.

In Sylvia and Gerard's conflict, as in most conflicts between couples, there is some truth in each person's position, and there are no clear external standards for judgment. Logically, then, each must question his or her own position at times. Sylvia must wonder if she is asking too much of Gerard or if she is too needy or oversensitive. Similarly, Gerard must wonder at times if he is selfish or ungenerous or unloving. Both are reluctant to express such doubt about themselves because these disclosures of doubt could easily be used against them.

Yet expression of these doubts would acknowledge the validity in each person's position. Questioning their own position or admitting to the truth in the other's view, if made genuinely, without either false modesty or pretentious nobility, might elevate both Sylvia and Gerard from the struggle over who is right and who is wrong. Then they might be able to join one another in the realization that both are right and both are wrong. Relieved of the burden of defending themselves or attacking the other, they might be able to struggle more successfully with their difficult problem. They might even feel close together as two human beings who both have limitations.

Anticipations May Not Be Shared

Even when couples are *not* in the middle of conflict, they may anticipate future conflict. Having been through certain arguments so often in the past, they know the kind of events that provoke them. These "preliminary events" take place, and couples anticipate, often accurately, that conflict will soon follow. They may be reluctant to share their anticipations for fear that the very act of sharing will hasten the conflict. Yet, without some intervening communication, the anticipated conflict may proceed inexorably.

On their way to a skiing weekend, Sylvia gets concerned that Gerard, who is a better skier than she, will abandon her on the slopes or will devote so much attention to skiing that their relationship will get short shrift. She remembers one ski weekend a year ago when he got up early to get on the slopes before the crowds arrived, skied all day, and then made noises about going night skiing. At that point she blew up and threatened to go home by herself. He didn't go night skiing, but he might as well have; they had a horrible evening together.

If Sylvia tries to express her concerns with an irritable and challenging "I hope you don't turn this weekend into the fiasco we had last year," Gerard is likely to respond negatively. He may defend himself: "All I wanted to do was try a little night skiing, and you went ballistic." Or he might counterattack: "There you go again. We're not even in the mountains, and you're already anticipating the worst."

Even if Sylvia tries to express her concern in a nonattacking way, for example, by saying "I'm worried that we're going to get into a struggle about skiing," Gerard may hear her concern as an attack. He may respond with an irritable "You just can't leave things alone, can you? Always have to worry about things going wrong. Maybe that's what makes them go wrong."

If it were Gerard rather than Sylvia who voiced concerns about the weekend, we could easily imagine a similar scenario. He might express his concerns in an accusatory way that leads to counteraccusations by her. Or he might express his concerns more cooperatively, but she might hear them as accusations, leading to an identical outcome. With such risks involved in an anticipatory discussion, both might choose to avoid a discussion and simply hope for the best.

A history of struggle inevitably leads to emotional anticipations. If Gerard and Sylvia have had difficulty coordinating their needs on skiing trips or on vacations in general, they are going to have anticipatory thoughts and feelings about the upcoming weekend. They can avoid an open discussion of their anticipations, but they can't avoid having anticipations. If those anticipations are strong, it may even be difficult to keep them from slipping into a conversation. Sylvia's seemingly innocent comment that she wants to relax and "sleep in" may be a "trial balloon" to test whether Gerard plans to hit the slopes at first light, or it may be heard by him as such a test. Gerard's seemingly innocent comment that skiing conditions are supposed to be great this weekend may be a test of Sylvia's possible reaction to his skiing as much as possible. Even Sylvia's casual comment that she hopes they have a great weekend may carry a subtext of "You better shape up and watch it" or be heard by Gerard as such.

If Gerard and Sylvia could openly disclose their concerns about the upcoming weekend without sparking a conflict, they might feel some relief in their joint apprehension. Having their concerns validated might ease those concerns.

SYLVIA: I'm a little worried about this weekend.

GERARD: You mean about us.

SYLVIA: Yeah.

GERARD: We don't have a great record when it comes to ski weekends, do we?

SYLVIA (*laughing ruefully*): No, we don't.

A discussion about the upcoming weekend could do more than simply relieve their concerns. They might be able to discuss how to manage the weekend so both get their needs met. They could make sure they have time together as well as time apart for Gerard to challenge himself on the expert slopes. It is possible for Gerard and Sylvia to have both a close relationship and good skiing, but it might take some communication and cooperative effort. Avoidance of discussion leaves a lot to chance.

RECOVERY FROM CONFLICT

In the heat of conflict, we often feel so angry or defensive that we are unable or unwilling to disclose the kinds of information just discussed, information that offers the possibility of understanding and intimacy even in the face of conflict. Even if we are able to disclose this information, our partners may not be responsive to it. Therefore, despite our best efforts to alter the course of our conflicts, argumentative patterns are likely to be repeated at times. Progress toward intimacy can be slow despite your commitment to inject acceptance and compassion into arguments.

For this reason, learning how to recover from conflict may be just as important as putting your energy into altering the course of conflict. Barring divorce, all couples recover, to some extent, from their conflicts and resume their normal behavior toward one another. But for days after a conflict partners may withdraw from each other, they may be curt with each other, or they may avoid conversation entirely. If you can short-circuit this process, if you can learn to recover more quickly and with less emotional hangover, you can lessen the total stress of conflict. Furthermore, you are more likely to achieve understanding and intimacy after a conflict than during it.

In the recovery from conflict, as during conflict itself, compassionate understanding of each other is key, as one extended conflict between Sylvia and Gerard illustrates. One Friday morning, just as he is about to leave for work, Gerard tells Sylvia that he is going to go on a camping trip the next day with his friend Daren and will be back Sunday afternoon. She reacts angrily because she thought they were going to spend Saturday together. She asks, "Why didn't you tell me sooner?" He replies defensively that they had no plans for Saturday and that no matter when he told her of the camping trip, she would have gotten angry. He leaves for work, and she is furious. As he rushes out, she accuses him of being a coward, afraid of any confrontation with her. He accuses her of overreacting to everything in life and suggests that she is mentally unstable.

Later that day, hoping she has calmed down, Gerard phones Sylvia and tries to be friendly and chatty. He is met with cold nonresponsiveness. Frustrated, he ends the conversation. He tries again for reconciliation after work. He greets her happily and proposes dinner and a movie. She refuses unless he gives her an apology. He resists: "I won't apologize for going camping with my best friend." She replies angrily: "You don't have to apologize for going camping. What you owe me an apology for is for not letting me know until the last minute—and for being such a chicken shit, not telling me until you have to leave for work so you don't have to deal with me and my reactions." Gerard bristles at the accusa tion, and they argue unproductively, first about whether he should apologize and then about camping and when he should tell her about a planned trip. Finally they set the argument aside and go out to dinner, where their interaction is tense but civil, warming up only a little over the evening.

The next morning as she lies in bed, Gerard kisses Sylvia good-bye. She tells him to be careful but to have a good time. He hears the genuine concern in her voice and tries to reassure her by reminding her when he will be back and saying he will miss her. She doesn't really believe him— he enjoys camping and his friend too much to miss her—but she accepts the warmth with which the comment was given.

Gerard has a great time camping with his friend. The day is beautiful, and the hike is invigorating. He and Daren exchange jokes, argue politics, bring each other up to date on their lives, drink too much beer in the evening, and genuinely forget all their troubles. Saturday doesn't go as well for Sylvia. She tries to make arrangements with some friends, but they are busy. She does some housework but gets resentful because she is at home working while Gerard is out having fun. Later in the evening she tries shopping and a movie, and while both are distracting, she feels lonely. On Sunday, she makes a valiant effort to put aside her resentment and disappointment. She looks forward to Gerard's arrival and wants their reunion to go well.

On Sunday they greet each other happily with a big hug and a kiss. Gerard is relieved that she is happy to see him since he wasn't sure what kind of mood she would be in on his return. Still glowing from the pleasant trip with his friend, he launches into a description of his trip. As he goes over some of the details of the trip and his conversations with Daren, he notices her interest flagging. He asks how her weekend was. She replies, "Not that great!" He offers a perfunctory "That's too bad." Then he describes how tired he is from the trip and goes into the bedroom for a nap.

When he wakes from his nap, Sylvia is angry. He shakes his head and utters a disgusted "What is it now?"

"You just don't get it, do you?," she asks accusatorily.

"No, I don't," he says, with a clear message that he doesn't really want to get it. She storms off into their bedroom. On other occasions he would have followed her, trying to find out what is wrong. Just waking from his nap and worn out by the continuous conflict, he has no motive for that now. They spend the rest of the evening in cold distance from each other. They go to sleep without the usual goodnight kiss. The next morning and evening they begin to warm up to each other again, but the whole experience has deepened each of their negative convictions about the other. She feels more strongly validated in her view: "He just doesn't want to understand me or connect with me." He feels more convinced in his: "She is just like a baby—getting upset if she doesn't get the right kind of attention when she wants it."

Any attempt by Gerard and Sylvia to recover from this incident by talking about it with each other would be risky. They might relive the incident rather than learn from it. Discussion could easily deteriorate into the blame, defensiveness, and withdrawal that characterized the incident itself. This is particularly likely if they focus on the egregious acts by the other and treat them out of context. Gerard could talk about how she called him a "coward" and a "chicken shit"; she could mention his comment suggesting she was mentally unstable.

The Buildup before the Conflict

One area that would be productive to discuss and that might aid in their recovery from the conflict would be what went on with each prior to the conflict. Gerard had actually been thinking about a trip with Daren for some time, had discussed it with him two weeks earlier, and had finalized it on Tuesday. He had gone to some pain to pick a weekend that would not interfere with any of his and Sylvia's plans. He did not let her into any of his thinking or planning because he was apprehensive about her reaction; she often gets upset when he plans something without her. Once he had finalized the plans with Daren, he knew he had to let her know. But Tuesday night he had to work late. On Wednesday and Thursday nights they were having such a pleasant time together that he did not want to spoil it by discussing the trip with his friend. He hoped that maybe the positive experiences would buffer a negative reaction. The buildup of anticipation in him about telling her got so great that he did want an easy escape—so he told her Friday morning because he couldn't in good conscience delay any longer and because he would have to leave for work immediately. Her reaction validated his fears: no strategy of disclosure would work with her.

For her part, Sylvia had been feeling good about the relationship. They had been talking a lot, sharing their experience with each other, but being playful also. They had made love during the week—on Wednesday night—which was unusual for them. Sylvia was looking forward to the weekend because they had no plans; they could just "hang out." Maybe go out for a good dinner and a movie. Maybe play some tennis. Maybe shop together. When Gerard brought up his plans for the weekend on Friday morning, she was crushed and furious. She was upset about his camping plans and angry at the way he had handled them. Why couldn't he let her know what was going on with him? The experience validated her suspicions that he could not be trusted, that she could never know what he had up his sleeve.

A discussion of this preconflict material—the events and emotions that led up to the conflict—might bridge the emotional difficulties that separate them. As Sylvia learned more about Gerard's efforts to fit his plans into their schedule, of his apprehension about her reactions, and of his search for an opportune time to reveal his plans to her, she might empathize with his dilemma. Similarly, if Gerard learned more about Sylvia's experience—her growing closeness with him during the week, her hopes for the weekend, and then her disappointment and consequent distrust of him—he might feel compassion for her plight.

If Gerard and Sylvia could voice what they had experienced prior to the conflict and if they could empathize with each other's dilemma, they would feel closer to each other in spite of—or perhaps even because of—their conflict. Such a discussion might also be a first step toward change. Even though one productive discussion is unlikely to create dramatic change, Gerard might move a step toward greater disclosure to Sylvia the next time. And although Sylvia may never greet with joy the possibility of Gerard spending a weekend camping without her, she may be more open to hearing his ideas and plans.

Attempts at Reconciliation

A second area of potentially productive discussion after a conflict is partners' attempts to reconcile. Sometimes a discussion of recovery and reconciliation is a way to facilitate that recovery and reconciliation. In the conflict between Sylvia and Gerard, each made efforts to reconcile after their initial blowup on Friday morning. Gerard called Sylvia later in the day and tried to be friendly and chatty. Although that effort was unsuccessful, he tried again that evening, but to no avail. After coming home from the camping trip, he also tried to be friendly, and he shared with Sylvia some of the interesting details of his trip. But that too was unsuccessful. Not surprisingly, Gerard became frustrated when his repeated genuine efforts to reconcile led nowhere.

For her part, Sylvia tried to reconcile also. On Friday evening, she thought she could reconcile if Gerard would simply apologize to her for what he had done. It seemed so clear-cut that he had done something—giving her very late notice of his weekend plans—that was at the very least inconsiderate. Why couldn't he give her a genuine apology? She would not hold a grudge; she can be forgiving. But she would like some acknowledgment of what really happened: that he had failed to consider her feelings. The fact that he refused to apologize not only foiled her attempt at reconciliation but also reignited the conflict.

Although it would pose dangers of initiating a conflict itself, a discussion about these failed attempts at reconciliation could lead to important new understandings between Gerard and Sylvia. Gerard's efforts to reconcile by being friendly and chatty don't work for Sylvia because she sees them as his attempt to avoid dealing with the conflict they have just had. It comes across to her as his effort to duck responsibility for the problem. But even if he did not do something that to her seemed to be so patently wrong, she cannot suddenly switch gears from being upset to being friendly and chatty with him. She wants some acknowledgment of the conflict and her hurt feelings before moving on. In the worst of scenarios, Gerard chides her for "holding on to her feelings," which just upsets her more.

Gerard also has a difficult time responding to Sylvia's efforts at reconciliation. Her demands for an apology hardly motivate him to apologize; instead, they create resistance and counterattack. Even when he has done something that he knows was not right—not telling her earlier about the camping trip—the intense anger and demandingness in Sylvia's voice make a genuine apology impossible for him. He knows that his neglect was not because of lack of concern for her feelings; in fact, he put off telling her precisely because he was so aware of her feelings. Furthermore, he believes with some justification that whenever he announced his plans, the announcement would have led to a negative reaction.

A discussion about these efforts to reconcile and how they went awry might enable them both to see that each was taking action, however misplaced, to get past the conflict. It might enable them to empathize with the other's frustration. More important, it might help Gerard realize the futility of his efforts to reconcile by putting on a happy face or help Sylvia realize the futility of demanding apologies. Neither is likely to be able to change his or her behavior dramatically or suddenly. But Gerard may be more likely to listen to Sylvia's concerns rather than meet her unhappiness with unwanted cheer. And Sylvia may be less likely to demand apologies, which, if genuine, can only be given freely.

The Dangerous Area of Pain

A third area of potential discussion, but a very dangerous one, is injury to one or both. During an argument people often make exaggerated claims and dramatic accusations. While these are hardly pleasant, they may not really injure. When there is injury, when one person's accusation hits a sensitive spot in the other, discussion can both facilitate recovery from the conflict and promote greater closeness. For example, Sylvia's comments that Gerard is a coward and a chicken shit and Gerard's claim that Sylvia is a mental case could be just part of their repertoire of conflict, but these comments might hit a vulnerable spot for one or both. If, for example, Sylvia is sensitive about suggestions that she is not mentally stable, then Gerard's accusation deserves follow-up. If their conversation about this accusation led to some disclosure about how painful it was to her and he could find a way to genuinely apologize for his comment, she may not only recover from the conflict more easily but also experience Gerard's concern for her feelings, an issue that triggered the argument in the first place. Thus, their recovery from conflict would address the central issue of their conflict.

You and your partner need to know what jabs truly hit below the belt for each other. Often threats to leave the relationship or statements about not loving the partner are poison arrows that inflict painful wounds. Specific accusations may touch a sensitive spot. A discussion, after an argument, of these below-the-belt jabs risks generating a new conflict of its own. But if partners understand the pain they create in the other and experience some compassion for that pain, then there is hope for recovery, future restraint, and even greater closeness after a conflict.

The Positives

A final area of discussion that can aid in recovery, and which is least likely to backfire, is a focus on the positive. Even in a painful struggle, such as the one that Sylvia and Gerard had about his camping trip, each partner often takes actions that deescalate the conflict or that communicate concern or caring. The morning that Gerard left for camping, Sylvia told him to be careful and have a good time. The sincerity he felt in her comment made it easier for him to enjoy his trip without guilt about her. He tried to return her warmth, and even though she didn't literally believe what he said (that he would miss her), she accepted it with the intent with which it was given. Also, when he returned from the trip, they were happy to see each other. The hug and kiss felt good to both. Any attention that a couple can give to their positive actions, any word of acknowledgment or appreciation, may help them recover from a conflict that was too filled with negative actions.

RECAP

> When all is said, it is rarely done. It is not even all said.
>
> —VARIATION ON AN OLD ADAGE

Because arguments are repetitive, couples may assume that they have said everything relevant about a particular conflict. Thus they may feel that their partners just haven't heard them or just haven't responded to what they have said. In this chapter we have discussed many things that are left unsaid in ongoing conflicts. Partners may not disclose their genuine, immediate feelings, even their anger. They may leave out important background information about what led to their feelings. They may express only the "hard" thoughts and emotions they experience and not the softer ones. Stuck in a particular position, they may never express the other side of that position, which they may fear is true. They may not fully disclose their anticipations about future conflict.

Disclosing this unspoken information is indeed risky. The information can be conveyed in accusatory ways or heard as accusatory so that it leads to further conflict. But these disclosures offer important information about the vulnerabilities of the other. The ensuing discussion could alter the course of their argument and lead to an empathic connection between the two. It could promote compassion in each for the other, a response that each needs. It could move the couple to accept each other's different behaviors and experiences rather than battle over them. Although the stakes are high for failure, these kinds of discussions can bring couples closer together in spite of their differences.

Often couples are too angry and defensive to disclose their vulnerable side to their partner during conflict. Their arguments take their usual course. But then they are confronted with recovery from the conflict. Unless the conflicts lead to divorce, couples eventually return to their normal way of dealing with one another. How can they recover from conflict more quickly and with less emotional hangover?

After a conflict, both partners are often less angry and more open to the other's experience. Sometimes couples can recover more quickly and more fully if they can discuss the conflict without reengaging in it. It is often helpful to discuss what happened internally in each just before the conflict that set the stage for the dispute. If vulnerabilities got injured during the conflict or if genuine efforts to reconcile got rebuffed, a compassionate discussion of these hurts will help. It often helps to discuss the positive actions that each took, in spite of the conflict.

Some couples experience their moments of greatest intimacy after conflict. They heal each other's wounds with love. They demonstrate that conflicts don't just alienate; they can also unite.

Exercise

It often helps to reveal more of your emotions to your partner, to find out more about his or her emotional state, and to find points where you can empathize with your partner's emotional state.

- If you are in a situation with your partner that is likely to get argumentative, try revealing more about your hopes as well as your anticipations about the current situation. See if you can discern and understand your partner's similar hopes and anticipations.
- In an actual conflict situation with your partner, try revealing something emotional that is going on with you at the moment. This disclosure might be as simple as saying "I am feeling really angry at you right now." If you are feeling like taking a bigger risk, try revealing some of your soft feelings, such as your pain and disappointment.
- Voice what you think your partner may be feeling. If you feel especially strong at the moment, acknowledge some truth in your partner's view and acknowledge that you too wonder about yourself on that dimension.
- If you are trying to recover from a conflict with your partner and feel that conversation might aid that recovery, focus on the beginning of the conflict, when neither of you was angry or out of control and you were thus easier to understand.

- See if you can understand how either your own or your partner's efforts to reconcile did not work for the other.
- If you feel particularly brave, find out if you did or said something that was especially painful to your partner during the conflict. See if you can understand how your partner might have experienced that deed or statement as hurtful. Reveal what was done that was hurtful to you.
- Finally, focus on any positive actions that may have emerged even in the midst of conflict.

None of these suggested behaviors is foolproof. Virtually any message you deliver can carry accusation or blame, which then drowns out any positive content. Even if you offer a new and important message without blame or accusation, your partner may be too angry or too suspicious of you at the moment to hear it. So don't be surprised by failure. But if you never try anything different, you may never experience the relief that comes when you accept each other's experiences rather than battle about them. And you may miss out on the intimacy that comes when difficult and troubling feelings are met with understanding and compassion.

CHAPTER 11

Getting Some Perspective on the Conflict

ACCEPTANCE THROUGH
TOLERANT DISTANCE

Emotion recollected in tranquillity . . .
—WILLIAM WORDSWORTH,
"Letter to Lady Beaumont" (1807)

*I*f compassion is the best response to a loved one's vulnerabilities, then tolerance is the optimal attitude toward incompatibilities. When our sensitivities cause conflict, empathy may prevent an escalation of argument or foster recovery from it. We may find greater emotional closeness as we accept each other's weaknesses. But when emotional soft spots are not the issue, a little distance and objectivity can remove the barbs that make our differences sting.

When both of you remove yourselves from the fray, you become more like observers and less like combatants. Distance allows you to view your struggles from a similar vantage point, to see your conflicts more clearly, and to accept each other's role in them. This emotional distance and the acceptance that goes with it may not solve the initial problem, but it often heads off associated reactive problems.

It is easy to see why tolerant distance rather than compassion is the best way to handle incompatibilities. In a case of "pure" incompatibilities, there is nothing to be compassionate about, except the struggle that the incompatibility entails. If you and your partner can never agree on whether the house is too warm or too cold or if you differ on whether to go to bed late or early, it is unlikely that either of you feels vulnerable about your position. The incompatibility does not, by itself, raise primitive fears or threaten self-esteem. Thus there may be little or no need for empathy.

Our most important struggles, however, are *not* likely to center around pure incompatibilities. In most cases, our vulnerabilities combine with our incompatibilities to produce emotional volatility. In these cases, the approaches discussed in the previous chapter are appropriate. However, the ways of seeking a joint, tolerant distance, which we describe in this chapter, can be helpful for incompatibilities even when they are powered by vulnerabilities. It can be helpful to achieve a kind of unified detachment from the problem even when the problem taps deep and sensitive emotions.

Eleanor is more emotionally expressive than Terry; when she feels upset about something or happy about something, she lets everyone know it. Terry, on the other hand, is more comfortable with understatement than exaggeration. He often finds Eleanor's expressive style irritating; in public he is frequently embarrassed by the attention her expression provokes. In extreme cases, he is overwhelmed by what he sees as her unnecessary hysteria. Eleanor is frustrated since, as she sees it, her own husband won't listen with concern to her troubles; instead he discounts them. Their incompatibility about emotional expression is fueled by Eleanor's sensitivity about being heard and Terry's about being "put upon" emotionally.

To get emotional distance from a problem about strong emotion, and to be united in their distance, will be a challenge for Terry and Eleanor. But such distance, like compassion, can prevent conflict or facilitate recovery from conflict and foster acceptance of the characteristics that lead to conflict.

TREATING THE PROBLEM AS AN "IT" RATHER THAN A "YOU"

Partners often experience their problems as "things *you* do to me" rather than as "difficulties *we* have." To move from this first position, seeing problems as a "you," to the second position, seeing problems as an "it" or a "them," is a major leap forward. It transfers the fault from one or the other to outside of both. How can couples make this experiential leap?

Broadening the Context

Because our partners' differences hurt and annoy us, it seems as if that is their intent. Terry believes Eleanor's emotional expression is intended to get his attention or upset him just because that is the effect her expression has on him. Eleanor believes Terry is trying to exclude her from his inner life because his lack of emotional expression does have that result. Neither can see that the other's behavior is her or his style of emotional expression because they are too close to the immediate conflict.

Of course, there is a little truth in each one's views of the other. Anticipating that Terry may discount her feelings, Eleanor exaggerates her feelings or expresses them more stridently than she otherwise would. And Terry does sometimes avoid telling Eleanor about his feelings because he's concerned about how she might react to them. These behaviors confirm their mutual suspicions of deliberate intent, so they hold fast to their views.

When you are too close to a conflict, a partial truth may obscure the larger truth. In the case of Eleanor and Terry, the larger truth is that their different manners of emotional expression come naturally to each of them. Eleanor's style of emotional expression is primarily Eleanor, rather than a manipulative means of provoking Terry into responsiveness. And Terry's limited expression of emotion is primarily Terry, rather than a conscious attempt to exclude Eleanor from his inner life.

By putting their differences in a larger context, couples are better able to see the larger truth that much of their behavior toward each other is not a deliberate offense but a product of many factors over which they have little control, including their genetic heritage and their upbringing. If Terry viewed Eleanor's greater emotional expressiveness as typical of women and Eleanor viewed Terry's emphasis on action over emotion as typical of men, neither would view the other's behavior as personal. Books on gender differences sell in great numbers because they make it easier for men and women to understand and accept behavior that they often find baffling in each other. If Terry were much older than Eleanor, their differences in emotional expression could be viewed as a product of the social mores of the times in which they grew up. If they came from different cultural backgrounds that put different emphases on emotional expression, they could attribute their differences to their cultural heritage.

Perhaps the most effective way to gain emotional distance from differences is to view them in their historical context. If partners have a sense of how the other was raised or what role the other played in their family of origin, they may view their differences more charitably. For whatever reason, Eleanor's family was emotionally expressive. During one of his first visits with her family, Terry observed an argument among Eleanor and her mother and father that both amused and frightened him. He worried that her family was hanging precariously together even as he was amused at the intensity of their strong feelings about what to him was nothing. In contrast, Eleanor finds Terry's family nice and polite but surprising in their careful avoidance of controversy. She wonders why they don't "engage their issues." If Terry and Eleanor viewed their own differences in the light of their divergent family experiences, their differences would make perfect sense.

Seeing your differences in the context of gender, age, culture, or personal history takes away some of the blame and fault finding. You are not "bad" or "wrong" for being the way you are. You are simply the natural product of your gender, your age, your culture, and your personal history. Without blame and fault finding, your problems are less likely to escalate or polarize or lead to alienation. In short, they are more acceptable.

Observing Rather Than Participating

Trying to discuss your problems puts you in danger of reliving them. Rather than probing your difficulties, you end up reproducing them. When Eleanor and Terry try to discuss their differences in emotional expression, Eleanor is liable to get emotional and Terry is liable to discount her concerns. They reveal the same pattern in their discussion of the problem as they do in the problem itself.

Even if you don't re-create the problem, you may create another problem. If you were trying to talk with your partner about the fact that the two of you have not made love in a while, your discussion could easily deteriorate into blame and defense. Now, in addition to the sexual neglect and deprivation you feel, you also have a problem of argument and anger.

If you can step back and observe your own interactions, you can describe what goes on between you rather than each championing a particular position. You can identify the pattern that occurs between the two of you rather than perpetuate that pattern. You can describe your problems rather than reenact them.

Observation requires distance. You and your partner must step back emotionally or physically if you are to focus on what is occurring. If a soldier is asked to report on a battle, he must temporarily stop shooting, move to a different vantage point, and focus not on aiming at a particular target but on looking more broadly at the field of conflict. A soldier cannot be a good warrior and a good observer at the same time. The demands of battle preclude observation, and the demands of observation preclude attack.

What should you be observing once you're able to step back from your conflict? You can scrutinize your coping processes. How does each of you deal with whatever incompatibility or vulnerability was triggered? You can look at the sequence of communication as you try to solve the initial problem.

For Terry and Eleanor, the conflictual sequence typically starts with an event that upsets Eleanor, such as a problem at work or an interaction with a friend. She voices her concerns to Terry, who responds by minimizing them. These comments upset Eleanor, who then expresses her concerns more vociferously. Then Terry, upset at the way Eleanor handles her concerns, remarks on Eleanor's emotional reactivity. These comments, which Eleanor feels are unsupportive at best and critical at worst, further upset Eleanor. An argument ensues, with both eventually withdrawing in anger. After some time during which they maintain emotional distance, they gradually get together again.

This bare-bones analysis could be fleshed out with a description of the triggers for each person's emotional reaction and a description of the emotional reactions themselves. The initial trigger for Eleanor is a disappointing or frustrating event that takes place in her world apart from Terry. Of course, she can also be disappointed or frustrated by Terry, but when a problem starts with her and Terry the dance is somewhat different. She talks to Terry about her problems with the world because he is the one to whom she feels closest. The emotional trigger for Terry is seeing Eleanor upset: he gets upset by her upset. In his view, she frets about every little thing that happens to her. He responds by trying to show Eleanor that she has no basis for being upset. His comments serve as a second emotional trigger for her: not only does she have to deal with the event in the real world that upset her, but now she also has to deal with Terry's dismissal of her feelings and his not-so-subtle criticism that she is too reactive to her world. Now Eleanor has to face both the issue in the outside world that originally upset her and an interpersonal struggle with Terry. Of course, Eleanor's increased upset feelings serve as a second emotional trigger for Terry. So now the two are off and running. The initial problem that bothered Eleanor has been replaced by a far more serious reactive problem between Eleanor and Terry.

One way to detach yourself from your emotions is to examine them logically, almost like a scientist would study them. Even the simple act of rating your emotional intensity on a 10-point scale, in which 1 refers to no emotional arousal and 10 refers to the greatest emotional arousal you have ever experienced, can help you get some valuable perspective on a conflict because it requires you to back away from the emotion you are feeling now and look at it in comparison to other emotional experiences. This "backing away" helps you to distance yourself from the emotion and the ratings may shed light on it. For example, Eleanor's level of emotion in response to daily upsets is usually about a 4 or 5. Of course, there are those rare occasions when she gets really upset by something, but mostly her emotional reactions to daily disappointments are in the middle of her emotional range. However, Terry's emotional reaction to Eleanor's emotional reaction is usually higher in his range, about 5 or 6. If the event to which Eleanor originally responded happened to him, he would respond with only a 1 or 2. So he can handle daily frustrations with less emotion than Eleanor, but he can't handle Eleanor's emotion about those daily events without getting emotional himself. When Terry reacts to Eleanor with a 5 or 6, she reacts to him with a 7 or 8. This in turn leads to about a 7 or 8 emotional reaction in him. So the emotional intensity goes from 4 to 8 in short order. Their interaction has amplified the emotional intensity caused by whatever event Eleanor originally experienced.

Creating a Name to Blame

There is often value in naming a problem in relationships. The name creates some emotional distance, suggesting that the problem is an "it out there" rather than "a you/me in here." Thus you can talk about the problem, the "thing" you two get into, rather than creating a problem through your analysis of it.

Try naming both the role you each play in the conflict and your communication together. A possible name for Eleanor is "volcano" since her emotional eruptions strike Terry as unpredictable and disruptive. At times they feel that way to Eleanor too. A good name for Terry would be "muffler," since his efforts are aimed at muffling the emotional intensity that Eleanor both feels and expresses. Although these mixed metaphors might not fit the canons of ideal English expression, they express the futility of their positions. There is no effective muffler for a volcano.

Be aware, though, that selecting names for the roles you each play can backfire. If names are chosen to ridicule or blame one or the other, then the names will not distance you from the conflict but instead further it. A safer route is to name only the communication process that generates toxic solutions. Since our language doesn't provide many names that describe a process between two people, simply generating a name will require creativity. But a name that describes a process cannot be used as easily against the other. Eleanor and Terry originally chose "emotional amplification and escalation," or "EAE," to describe the way their emotions built during communication, but they eventually settled on "MAD" for "mutual amplification and destruction" because it was more creative, it acknowledged the contributions of each, and they liked the irony of its similarity to the cold war policy "mutual assured destruction."

Having a name for your conflicts can enable you to talk about them without reliving them because it describes your dance without condemning either of you. You can use these names to avoid or limit the enactment of your conflicts. When Terry says to Eleanor, "I feel a MAD coming on," he often deters or lessens their conflict. When Eleanor asks Terry, "Are we fully into MAD yet?," she sometimes facilitates an exit from their conflict.

Laughing at Ourselves

Humor can create emotional distance by providing comic relief and facilitating a quick change of perspective. Exaggeration, self-deprecation, and gentle sarcasm can short-circuit automatic retorts and give you both a chance to handle the situation better than you might have without the humor. Eleanor might say, "I am really upset about this—and I know you will want to hear all about it." Or Terry might comment, "Oh, tell me all about it—you know how I love to hear the ins and outs of your emotional upheaval." These comments might work as long as they are not made with such sarcasm that they could be interpreted as criticism.

Conflict in couples has provided rich material for comics and cartoonists because intimate arguments are often filled with paradox, contradiction, and absurdity. If you catch a revealing glimpse of this absurdity, even if you never share it or laugh at it together, the intensity of your conflict may edge down. If Terry notices the contradiction in his getting upset about Eleanor's getting upset or if Eleanor observes the absurdity in their efforts to quell each other's emotional arousal by getting more aroused themselves, both may find themselves a bit removed from the conflict.

Anyone who has ever tried to relay a funny story or joke knows the difficulty of importing humor. It is even more difficult to offer any advice about humor in the context of conflict. But when partners can laugh—or even smile — at their predicament, they have achieved some healing distance from their conflict. Even a sense that "We'll laugh at this someday" can dampen the passion of the moment.

REALITY CHECK 1:
WHEN IS DISTANCE ACHIEVABLE?

Achieving the kind of intellectual distance and detachment we have been discussing is rarely possible in the heat of battle. There may be times when you can momentarily take an observer's stance during conflict. Like our soldier mentioned above, you may put down your weapon temporarily to get a better view of the battle. Even these brief attempts to observe rather than participate can dampen the current conflagration. However, it's unrealistic to expect ourselves to talk about an "it" when we have just been stung by a "you." The ability to create emotional distance and the benefit from it usually comes well before the battle or well after it.

If we see an argument coming enough in advance, our ability to anticipate its sequence can sometimes lessen the pain it causes even if it can't prevent the argument entirely. For example, Eleanor might worry aloud that she will get only a small bonus at work this year and remark, "And if I don't get a decent bonus, after all my work, I will probably have an emotional meltdown—which I am sure you will enjoy." Or if Eleanor is worrying about her bonus, Terry might comment, "Well, even if you don't get a decent bonus, I'll be able to share in your pain!" Such comments might bring a rueful smile to one or both and protect against a blowup if Eleanor does not get what she wants.

Even the act of describing an oncoming pattern of conflict may prevent or alter its occurrence. The husband in the cartoon below describes a potential sequence of argument with his wife rather than engaging in that argument. His pithy description may minimize their conflict.

Perhaps the biggest benefit of emotional distance accrues after a conflict. Establishing some distance is another way to facilitate the recovery from conflict that we discussed in Chapter 10. Let's assume that Eleanor does get a meager bonus, and she and Terry play out their usual pattern of emotional escalation. After they have calmed somewhat, humor might help them recover. Terry might poke fun at himself: "I have been considering a career change. Maybe I should become a therapist—since I'm so good at handling other people's emotional problems." Or Eleanor might acknowledge their predicament: "I think you got smothered in the ash of my volcano." With these comments Terry and Eleanor make fun of themselves and acknowledge, with humor, their role in their struggle. These comments then aid in their recovery from that struggle.

"I'm late, you're angry—we quarrel."

REALITY CHECK 2:
IS DISTANCE ALWAYS DESIRABLE?

For most of us, getting some distance from our conflicts through a broader perspective, observation, objectivity, labeling, or humor is helpful. We may take our conflicts less personally, deal with them more reasonably, and recover from them more rapidly.

However, for some couples, emotional distance may be part of the problem and therefore not a solution to the problem. For example, a husband may use his excellent sense of humor to avoid dealing with difficult issues. His strategy may be to distract his wife from her concerns with him. If it is hard for her to articulate her concerns in the first place, his efforts may be successful. As another example, both members of a couple may be adept at objectivity, observation, and analysis, but use these skills to avoid taking a stand on issues. Afraid to confront each other with their different needs and desires, they keep such a distance from the issues that they are unable to resolve them. In neither of these cases would we want to encourage emotional distance.

The "story of your problem," if it accurately captures the difficulties you face, your struggle over these difficulties, and the emotional consequences of that struggle, offers guidance as to the appropriate antidote for your difficulties. It can help you sort out what may resolve your conflicts and what will merely further them. We will discuss this notion more fully in Part III of this book.

FINDING THE BLESSING IN THE CURSE

In Chapter 5 we discussed confusing incompatibilities, those complex differences with our partners that arouse mixed feelings. Sometimes we want our partners to be different; at other times we like and support the way they are. In the heat of conflict, the negative characteristics of our partners may stand out so dramatically and may be broadcast so powerfully that we fail to see the larger context in which they appear. However, if we are able to distance ourselves from the conflict, we may get some perspective on our partners' characteristics. We may see the positive features and the attractive pull of our partners' negative characteristics. This "understanding from a distance" may help us recover more quickly from conflict and perhaps even avoid some future conflict.

Terry is often so focused on Eleanor's negative emotional reactivity that he is not aware of the pull of her emotions for him. Early in their relationship he found her broad emotional range exciting. It added color to his life. Her energy, excitement, and enthusiasm appealed to him. Even her negative emotional reactions were often engaging for him; he felt good when he could comfort her in her upset state.

For her part, Eleanor found Terry's emotional stability comforting. He was so logical and organized and reasonable that he could help her with many of the problems she faced. There was a synergy between their characteristics. Her emotionality added excitement to his life, and his stability provided an anchor for hers. Despite their conflict, they have learned from each other. His connection with her has added emotional depth to him; her connection with him has provided much needed structure in her life. Typically, their struggles over her emotional reactivity eclipse the positive characteristics that each brings to the battle. However, when either becomes evenly dimly aware of the complex exchange they have made—a measure of emotion for an equal measure of stability—they may shake their heads with a mixture of frustration and appreciation. And they may feel greater acceptance of the differences between them and struggle less over those differences.

Even when the negative characteristics of our partners don't have an obvious attractive side, they may force us to confront some of our own negative characteristics. Because Terry was not used to strong emotion and was somewhat intimidated by it, he often avoided confrontation with others. He chose to evade rather than to risk a showdown; he opted for the white lie rather than the bald truth. With Eleanor, however, his strategy of avoidance didn't work. Her "in your face" emotional reactions forced confrontation. The struggle with her drove Terry to take a stand on issues. Although Terry will never relish open confrontation, now he is less intimidated by strong emotion. And he has Eleanor to thank for it.

Eleanor's emotional reactivity seemed to have only two positions: on and off. There seemed to be surprisingly few degrees of intensity to her emotional reactions. Some trivial negative event could arouse almost as much feeling as a truly important event. In her struggles with Terry, he derided her for getting "upset over nothing." He sometimes refused to listen to her emotions. Although his actions provoked additional distress in her at the time, their cumulative impact was not all bad. Eleanor learned to choose what she needed to tell Terry and what she didn't need to tell him. Although she is disappointed that she cannot share more of her emotional life with Terry, she has learned to define what is and what is not important. Eleanor will always have something of an all-or-nothing emotional system, but she has learned to handle her emotions when they are "on" and to make some choices about what she wishes to share. Terry has been her reluctant teacher, and she his resistant student.

The grudging respect that each has gained for what the other brings to the relationship has taken some of the edge off the struggles that Terry and Eleanor have over emotionality. They still get into their arguments, but these arguments are somewhat lighter, less painful, and easier to recover from.

IT'S NOT AS BAD AS IT SEEMS

Couples conflict consists largely of significant reactions to trivial events. Although there are high crimes in relationships, most of the struggles are over misdemeanors. Some of us may betray or deceive or otherwise violate our partners, but usually the struggle is over lesser matters.

To an outsider, it may seem unreasonable that such trivial events raise such strong emotions. An objective observer might view Eleanor's emotional reaction to her frustrations at work as excessive, Terry's reaction to Eleanor's attempt to tell him about it as an overreaction, Eleanor's subsequent response as exaggerated, and Terry's subsequent response as almost hysterical.

An objective observer of Terry and Eleanor's interaction might try to explain to them the unreasonableness of their reactions. He or she might try to use logic to convince both that their emotional responses are inflated. Reason, however, is impotent in the face of strong emotion. Someone who is phobic about flying will be unaffected by statistics on the safety of airline travel. Someone who lives in terror of snakes won't make distinctions between those that are poisonous and those that are not.

Psychologists have developed powerful ways to desensitize strong emotions, particularly fear. They gradually expose the person to the feared object but in a safe and supportive environment. As people experience their feared object at a comfortable distance, they may be able to tolerate closer and closer contact until their fear eventually subsides. Likewise, we can gradually expose our partners to pieces of our behavior that cause emotional distress in them. If we know the triggers that set them off, we can create a situation in which those triggers are less likely to get activated. For example, Eleanor might approach Terry with the comment "I want to share some emotional stress in my life. Are you in an okay position to listen?" With this remark, Eleanor shows that she understands what triggers emotional reactions in Terry, she warns him of what she wants to do, and in so doing, she may enable him to handle her emotional distress without himself getting so distressed. Of course, a comment like this requires some perspective by Eleanor. If she is too distraught, she will just unload on Terry without any warning. Also, Terry may not be in a position to listen to her even if she does approach him with sensitivity to his possible reactions. She may have to accept no for an answer sometimes.

For his part, Terry could warn Eleanor of a potential trigger for her if he voiced his intent before his action. For example, he might say, "I have this urge to talk to you about your reaction and explain to you that the problem is not a big one, but I don't know if you are open to that. I don't want you to feel discounted or criticized." Such a comment would indicate considerable awareness and restraint by Terry. Depending on his own emotional state, he might simply be unable to say something like this, mean it, and accept the possibility that Eleanor might not be open to hearing him. However, on those occasions when he could make such a comment, it might enable Eleanor to listen to him.

Sometimes we can desensitize our partners and increase our own understanding of them if we stage those behaviors that upset them. A battle with fake bullets is a good training ground for real combat. For example, Eleanor might warn Terry that she is going to fake a strong emotional reaction sometime soon and try to tell him about it. She could explain that she is going to do this with two goals in mind: to increase her understanding of the role her emotions play with him and to give them both a chance to deal more effectively with emotional distress. Soon after, she could make up the event or merely exaggerate an actual event and run to tell Terry about it. Given that she is not really upset, she will be in a better position to observe what happens with Terry and between her and Terry. Her goal is to observe the scenario and interrupt it by "coming clean" with Terry if the interaction shows signs of getting out of control. Since she has warned Terry of her actions, he knows that she may be faking an emotional reaction. He can only guess which of her emotional reactions are real and which are fraudulent. This suspicion may brake his usual, instantaneous reaction to her. He too can observe what goes on between them, whether it be a fraud or the true thing.

Faking problems can often be fun for couples. Just as calmness cannot be produced on command, neither can emotional upset. Couples cannot reproduce the intensity of their emotional problems when they deliberately stage them. Their efforts to do so often strike them as funny. The humor can help create the necessary emotional distance for tolerance to develop.

To do such exercises, a couple must understand their arguments. They must know the triggers that set each other off. They must have achieved a fair amount of detachment from their conflict even to attempt these exercises. If they aren't able to distance themselves from their struggle, one could experience a faked event as an effort to show the other up or to ridicule him or her.

ON YOUR OWN—BUT WITH A LITTLE HELP FROM YOUR FRIENDS

Intellectually, we can probably all endorse the notion that our partners cannot meet all of our needs or fulfill all of our desires. We know that there are incompatibilities for which accommodation or compromise is no solution. For some of our needs and desires, we don't expect or seek fulfillment from our partners. Particularly if our partners have never met our needs in a particular area, we may have no difficulty going elsewhere. Or if our desires seem like a "male thing" or a "female thing," we may find it easy to get satisfaction apart from our relationship, with a friend of our own gender.

If a need or desire is intense and personal, however, it may not be easy to fulfill outside of the relationship. Also, if the need has historically been satisfied inside the relationship, a partner may understandably expect continued satisfaction at home. Early in their relationship Terry was happy to comfort Eleanor when she got upset, but the frequency and intensity of her emotional reactions have since discouraged Terry's responsiveness. Eleanor still believes that in marriage you should be able to share your troubles, no matter what they are, with your partner. Terry also endorsed that ideal once upon a time.

Eleanor does have several friends who serve as emotional supports for her. Often they are better help for her than Terry. But if Eleanor has to go to them too often, she gets upset at Terry for not being there for her. And she feels more distant from him because he is not part of her emotional life. Yet the reality is that Terry is not able to listen to her distress as much as she would like him to. At times, she will be distressed, and he will be unavailable. She will be alone in her upset. For Eleanor to seek comfort from her friends can be a partial solution, but only a partial solution, for their incompatibility.

Although friends offer solutions to some incompatibilities, seeking their help and counsel has risks. It's very easy to try to turn friends into allies against our partners, which only hurts our own relationship. Friends help most when they can meet some of our needs without joining in the conflict we have with our partner over those needs. Then these friends enable us to accept our partners and their limited ability to meet all of our needs.

RECAP

Because their conflicts are so painful, couples would like to exorcise them from their lives. They want to obliterate the repetitious quarreling and make it go away, right now. Certainly Terry and Eleanor would like to surgically remove their repeated trauma of Eleanor's upset, Terry's reaction at her upset, and Eleanor's further upset.

In this chapter we have provided no remedies to exorcise conflict. Rather, we have shown ways to tame conflict, to domesticate it rather than demolish it. We have shown that it is possible for couples to accept conflict and live with it.

In dealing with any problem, the first step is to identify it properly. When partners identify the problem as being one or the other, their efforts to solve the problem will often make it worse. If couples can treat the problem as an "it" that they both face, they may be able to view their differences in a more dispassionate way. They may see their differences in the larger context of their gender, their age, their culture, or their personal history. They may be able to observe the sequence of what happens between them and discuss that sequence from a mutual vantage point. They may be able to identify the roles that each plays and to see their struggle in a larger, even at times humorous, perspective. Thanks to this larger perspective, they may see the blessing in the curse: the advantages as well as the disadvantages their partners' characteristics provide them. They may be able to tolerate the negative side of those characteristics, with perhaps a little help from their friends.

It is almost impossible to maintain this larger perspective in the heat of the battle. During an actual argument each member will experience the problem as a "you," not an "it." However, after the battle, taking this larger perspective may facilitate a quicker and easier recovery from conflict.

If couples cannot exorcise their demons, maybe they can tame them.

Exercise

Think of an important conflict that you have with your partner, focusing on your incompatibilities and your ways of coping with them.

- Describe the differences between you and your partner in a larger context, such as your separate personal histories, your varying life situations, your different cultures, or your contrasting genders.
- Identify a positive feature of those differences, a valuable aspect of a negative characteristic of your partner.
- Describe the dance (or dances) that you and your partner go through when you struggle over your major differences. Give a name to that dance. What are the contradictory, paradoxical, absurd, and humorous elements in your struggle?
- Try to identify someone, other than your partner, who might meet some of your needs without causing additional stress to your relationship.

It is best if you can do these exercises together with your partner. Even done alone, however, these exercises can help you get some distance from your struggles.

At this point you may want to look at the "story" you constructed about your problems in Chapter 9. See if you want to elaborate or revise your story based on information from this chapter and the last chapter. In the next section, you will refer back to the "story" and use it for making deliberate changes in your relationship. You want to be sure it captures your difficulties accurately.

PART III

Deliberate Change through Acceptance

CHAPTER 12

The Dilemmas
of Deliberate Change

There is nothing permanent except change.
—HERACLITUS

If we want things to stay as they are, things will
have to change.
—GIUSEPPE DI LAMPEDUSA,
The Leopard (1957)

As many old sayings tell us, there is nothing as certain as change. It is
not a question of whether we and our relationships *will* change but of
how they will change. In fact, keeping things the way they are often
takes considerably more effort than changing them. If you doubt this, try
keeping your new car or new house in the same condition it is when you
buy it.

One kind of change is the slow, imperceptible modification that
comes inevitably with time. In relationships, such changes can be either
good or bad. Time and experience may mellow us. Issues that seemed
very important to us early in the relationship may seem less so later. But
sometimes our experience hardens us. We become more sensitive and
irritated by our partners. We become less tolerant. We become better
and better at being worse and worse.

The other kind of change that can occur in relationships is deliberate change. We want our partners to change in specific ways. We want
them to act and to be different so that our relationships can be different.
Sometimes we want these deliberate changes from the very beginning of

the relationship when we notice something aversive in our partner. More often, the inevitable changes that time and circumstance bring to our partners and our relationships make us seek deliberate change.

FROM ACCEPTANCE TO CHANGE

Part II of this book focused on acceptance as an alternative to change. We mentioned briefly that when you give up the effort to change your partner and instead accept him and his behavior toward you, he often makes spontaneous changes in the direction that you originally wanted. Relieved of the pressure to defend himself but with an experience of the emotional impact of his behavior on you, he may make accommodations for you on his own. Similarly, when you experience acceptance from him, you may make spontaneous changes in the direction that he desires. In the best of cases, these mutual changes promote further accommodation to each other.

This process makes sense, but it is not easy to accomplish. For acceptance, which seems the very opposite of change, to foster change, we need to develop an adequate story about our problem. Then, as we described in Chapter 9, we can understand our problem in a new way. When we see the dilemma that our problem creates for both of us, we may be moved to alter our behavior and lessen our dilemma. If, as we described in Chapter 10, we develop compassion for the pain that we cause each other, we may shift our behavior in subtle or dramatic ways that lessen that pain. And finally, if we get some perspective on our conflict, as we described in Chapter 11, we may see our problems with greater objectivity, possibly even some humor, and naturally respond in different ways that alleviate the problem.

These kinds of changes, spawned by acceptance, happen naturally and effortlessly. They are unforced. We don't have to remind ourselves or each other to make them. As a result, they often are more durable than planned and structured change. We get some of the things that we want without a struggle—because we gave up the struggle to achieve them.

Arlo was frustrated because Gabriella seemed to be uninterested in his work. She rarely asked him about it. When he volunteered information, she showed little interest and often changed the subject. For her part, she dreaded discussions about his work. She feared he would go on and on about technical details that held no interest for her. Also, she felt unmotivated to listen to him when he showed so little interest in her life.

If Arlo and Gabriella were able to develop an objective story about this problem, if they were able to discuss the isolation they feel when they cannot find a willing ear to listen to things that are important to them, if they could share a perspective on the problem—seeing it as a mutual reluctance to give because neither has felt given to—they might be more accepting of each other's behavior. However, they might also change in small but important ways. Gabriella might show more interest in Arlo's work and he in things important to her. Arlo might learn to spare her the technical details of his work. These changes might be all the more durable because they were not forced.

Acceptance can bring more than just spontaneous changes in what we seek from our partners. Acceptance can also foster a greater intimacy that may be more important than the particular changes each individual sought. For example, the discussions in which Arlo and Gabriella talk about how they each feel neglected by the other can foster a greater intimacy between them. They can feel closer to each other even if very little change actually occurs when Arlo brings up a work topic. Sometimes talking about how distant you feel from each other is a first step toward getting closer to each other.

This depiction is somewhat idealized. Acceptance doesn't always lead to spontaneous changes. Nor does it always lead to greater intimacy. Even when it does, these changes may not be enough. Sometimes we want and need deliberate change.

Our first impulse is usually to seek immediate and dramatic change.

THE SHOWDOWN:
IMMEDIATE AND DRAMATIC CHANGE

> It is only in romances that people undergo a
> sudden metamorphosis.
> —ISADORA DUNCAN, *My Life* (1942)

We may fantasize about a transformation in our partners. We may wish for a single confrontation, where we drop any pretense that all is well, where we no longer spare our partners' feelings. Instead, we point out bluntly and forcefully how their misguided actions and neglectful inactions have caused not only our suffering but their own suffering as well. We point out their limitations and their inadequacies. We provide elaborate and detailed examples, which have been preserved carefully in our memory, that illustrate their deficiencies. They may battle our logic, but it is a battle of the defeated. Inside, they know the validity of our claims.

They soon abandon any defense and acknowledge the truth in what we are saying. They summon the strength and courage to make the changes we enumerated. The next day, all is different in the relationship. A transformation has occurred. There is a sea change in their behavior and attitude. We are happier, and they are happier too. Ultimately, they are grateful to us for making change happen.

As we saw in Part I of this book, most of our efforts toward change in our partners and thus in our relationships are driven by this fantasy. And most of these efforts are unsuccessful. Yet we often persist in this tack. And when repeated confrontation brings no change, we may threaten our partners, implicitly or overtly, with negative consequences. At one extreme are destructive threats, which not only destroy mutual trust and respect but may end in violence (which is never acceptable and is discussed in more depth in Part IV). At the other extreme are empty threats. We may warn of infidelity, unforgiving anger, unbridgeable distance, or even separation and divorce. Because these threats are never carried out, our partners eventually recognize them as false cries of wolf and conclude that we are incapable of carrying out any such action.

Most threats are ineffectual at best, destructive at worst. But the most powerful threat—the *ultimatum*—has the potential to alter the course of a relationship dramatically and positively—as long as it meets certain demanding criteria. When these criteria are not met, the ultimatum's potential for inflicting damage is as great as its potential for evoking change.

Betsy and Frank had dated for a year before they started seriously discussing marriage. In those early discussions Frank professed his love for Betsy but insisted that he was not ready for the binding commitment of marriage. In his eyes, marriage was a prelude to having children, and he knew he wasn't ready for children yet. Betsy expressed some urgency to "get on with their relationship." She was not ready for children either, but at age thirty-one she wanted the assurance of a commitment to marriage and the goal of children in the future. Over the next six months they had a series of discussions about marriage that frustrated both of them. Betsy grew more and more doubtful about Frank's attachment to her and his willingness or ability to commit to marriage. Frank grew more and more uncomfortable with the increasing pressure he felt. Betsy began indicating to Frank, at first indirectly and then directly, that she would break up with him if he was unwilling to marry her. At first, Frank advised her not to give him an ultimatum. When pressured, he called her bluff. Betsy left, vowing never to see him again.

Because they missed each other terribly, they got together again, but it wasn't long before the old problem arose once more. Betsy insisted again that they either marry or break up; Frank tried to talk her out of her ultimatum. She ended the relationship a second time, but this time with greater conviction, knowing that a reconciliation without marriage would only prolong her pain. Although she talked to Frank on occasion, she refused to see him. Her actions thrust Frank into a major reevaluation of his life. He feared the loss of someone who had become the central figure in his life. He ultimately decided to marry Betsy.

Betsy insisted on a marriage in the near future, to which Frank at that point agreed. Despite some conflict about the marriage ceremony itself and some adjustment after the marriage, Frank and Betsy got along well. Because their relationship was essentially a good one, and because they cared about each other so deeply, their marriage was a solid connection between the two. Years later, they looked back with amusement at Betsy's ultimatum. Frank appreciated the strength Betsy had shown in insisting that their relationship move on. Betsy appreciated the fact that when push came to shove, Frank had been there for her.

Frank and Betsy's experience represents the best-case scenario for ultimatums. Their outcome was positive because Betsy's ultimatum met five crucial conditions.

First, Betsy's threat was real. As much as she loved Frank, she had made a decision to break up with him if he didn't marry her. He realized she was serious. Second, Betsy's ultimatum centered on a single decision: that Frank marry her. Her ultimatum did not demand unspecified changes or some indeterminate amount of change. Instead the ultimatum forced him to make a crucial choice. Third, Betsy's ultimatum demanded the change within a short time frame. She insisted they set a date immediately and that the date be within nine months. She did not demand repeated actions over some undetermined but long period of time. Fourth, Frank did not "lose face" by acquiescing to her ultimatum. Because of the nature of their relationship and the way she made the ultimatum, Frank knew that Betsy's ultimatum was no simple power move to exert control over him. He knew her decision to give him an ultimatum was a tortured one for her and that she made that move in part out of desperation. Even though he didn't want to, part of him also believed that it was time for them to make a choice about marriage. Finally, the decision that the ultimatum demanded was something that put into motion a whole series of additional positive changes. By getting married, Betsy and Frank changed their status with friends and family, had greater daily contact, and were legally entwined, among other things. For the most part, the two experienced these changes as positive.

When these five conditions don't exist, ultimatums usually fail. If you're not serious in your ultimatum, you will communicate ambivalence and probably not get an answer. If you demand something nonspecific and vague, it will be impossible to tell whether the demand is met. If Betsy had insisted that Frank show her more consideration or more respect or more love, Frank would not know exactly what he was supposed to do and when he had done it. Likewise, requiring change in an indeterminate time frame makes it impossible to tell when the demand has been met. Even if the other four conditions are met, loss of face or the experience of being controlled can make an ultimatum fail. Complying with an ultimatum means giving up something and giving in to someone. Frank could have rejected Betsy's ultimatum because he couldn't stand her telling him what to do even if he would have eventually chosen on his own to marry her. Even if Frank had succumbed to Betsy's ultimatum, the resentment he might have felt after being forced to marry her might have contaminated their marriage from its beginning.

Finally, if compliance doesn't have the prospect of creating additional positive changes, it is probably wrong. Betsy made the astute judgment that Frank's doubts indicated real but temporary anxiety on his part but did not reflect serious inadequacies in Frank or in their relationship. She believed that after marriage his doubts would fade as they enjoyed their life together. Frank eventually came to the same conclusion. Fortunately their judgments were right. If they had been wrong, then they would have married only to face the difficulties for which Frank's reluctance had been a warning sign.

Even if you meet these five conditions, your partner may refuse to comply, or the decision to acquiesce may not have the anticipated positive effects. Ultimatums are high-risk ventures and should be your last-ditch effort at change. Yet many couples owe their satisfaction, even their very relationships, to a well-placed ultimatum to have a child, to enter couple therapy, to get married, to seek treatment for alcohol abuse—or else. However, for many more couples, failed ultimatums litter the battlegrounds of their marriage.

Fortunately, ultimatums are usually considered—by all but the most histrionic—only when major relationship violations, major decisions, or major personal problems are the issue. Most of the change we seek in our relationships, and most of the change we will get in our relationships, is gradual change in everyday behavior.

EVERYDAY CHANGE

The changes we want often seem simple and direct to us: Do more of the housework. Spend more time with the kids. Don't be so critical. Pay more attention when I talk to you. Be more ambitious at work. Put more energy into our relationship.

Sometimes these deliberate changes come easily. Our partners do what we want; we do what they want. At other times the changes are much more difficult. Why?

When Change Is Easy

Specific versus General Changes

A specific change can be made more easily than a general change. If Caitlin requests that Luke "put more energy into the relationship," and he is motivated to comply, he may make heroic efforts but fail to give her what she wants because he isn't sure what that is. If what she wants is for him to do more things like plan their recreational events, she'll have more success if she specifically asks him to do just that.

Turning a general request into a specific request is complicated because any single request, however accurate, may not be sufficient to satisfy the general request. Caitlin would feel better if Luke did more of the planning of their recreational events, but that alone might not be sufficient to satisfy her desire that he put "more energy into the relationship," because there are many other ways in which he still seems unenergetic. Furthermore, if he invested more energy in general into the relationship, then the fact that he never made the plans for their Saturday nights would not bother her. Thus, there are a variety of ways that Luke could put more energy into their relationship; several changes are needed to satisfy Caitlin, but no particular change is mandatory.

Despite this complexity, Caitlin will be more successful in getting Luke to change if she lists the specific things that she wants him to do. If he knows concretely what she wants, he is more likely to act on at least some of her requests.

Taking Action versus Restraining Action

It is easier to change by doing something positive than to change by not doing something negative. It is normally easier to do more of something good than to do less of something bad. Therefore, when possible, a change should be phrased in terms of what you want rather than in terms of what you don't want. It is easier to "vacuum every Saturday" than to "stop waiting until I tell you it's time to vacuum." It is easier to "initiate sex with me occasionally" than to "stop being so passive in sex." In each case, the listener will hear a positive request for action rather than a combination of criticism and a request to stop some action.

Although this admonition to phrase requests in a positive way is useful, it can sometimes miss the boat. Luke complains that Caitlin is "too negative," and he would feel better if she were not so critical of him. She could change more easily by doing something active for Luke, such as being more complimentary of him, than by holding back her criticism. Yet this would not satisfy Luke. Yes, he could always use a few more compliments, but she is generous with her praise already. What bothers him is her criticism, and it would still bother him even if she gave a stronger dose of praise. So even though it is easier for Caitlin to increase a behavior than to decrease it, the change that Luke really wants from Caitlin is less criticism.

However, most often the changes we want from our partners are specific, positive actions on their part. In our frustration with them, we may focus on what they shouldn't do. But what we really want is for them to take some concrete actions. For example, Caitlin may chide Luke for being lazy and urge him to stop "pampering himself." However, what she may really want is for him to do specific things like getting up with the kids on a weekend and giving her a chance to sleep in. He is more likely to do what she wants if she makes the direct request for the action she wants rather than requesting the actions that she doesn't want.

Changing How You Are with Me versus Changing How You Are with the World

There are two kinds of changes we can seek in our partners: a change in how they treat us or communicate with us and a change in how they are with the rest of the world. An example of the first is Caitlin's request that Luke "pay more attention to me," while an example of the second is her request that he "be more ambitious at work." Certainly, some requests for change, such as "be more open and communicative," can cover how our partners are with us *and* with the rest of the world. However, this distinction is important for at least two reasons. First, we have more legitimacy when we request changes in how our partners treat us. When our concerns are directed at how our partners talk to us or play with us or work with us, it is clearly "our business." Caitlin certainly has a right to discuss, for example, whether Luke is attentive to her or not. However, if we want our partners to behave differently at work or with their friends or with their family, they can argue that these areas are "none of our business." Although we have joint control with our partners over what happens when we are together, they have primary control over what they do with their lives apart from us. If Caitlin wants Luke to be more ambitious at work, he can insist that it is his job, not hers.

Not only do we have more legitimacy but we also have more power to create changes in our partners when the changes concern their behavior toward us. We can observe their actions and directly influence them by what we say and do. Caitlin can usually tell, for example, whether Luke is paying attention to her or not, and then she can say something about it. However, when we request changes in how our partners deal with the rest of the world, we are not a party to the actions that concern us. We cannot observe their actions or directly influence them. Caitlin cannot, for example, directly observe how ambitious Luke is at work; nor can she intervene directly to encourage him to be more ambitious. Because of this important distinction, we should try to separate our requests for change into those that have to do with our partners' behavior toward us and those that have to do with our partners' behavior toward the rest of the world. If we want our partners to be more open and communicative in general, we might separate our request to be more open and communicative with us from our request that they be more open and communicative with the world. And we might deal with the request that they be open and communicative with us first.

Change Supported by Circumstances versus Change through Sheer Willpower

One of the easiest ways to foster change is to shift the circumstances in ways that may facilitate change. For example, Caitlin feels that she can never get a break from her kids when she is at home with them. Even though Luke is "officially" responsible for them on Saturday mornings, they still come to her with their problems rather than go to him. Indeed, knowing that she is always there as his "backup," Luke tends to slack off on his supervision. Thus Caitlin has difficulty being "off duty" even when Luke is supposedly "on duty." The quickest and easiest solution to this problem is to change the circumstances. If he takes the kids out, then she truly is free at home; similarly, if she leaves the house, then she is also truly free. In each of these cases, the kids must bring their problems to and seek attention from Luke, and he must supervise them. The circumstances allow no other option.

Similarly a husband who wants his wife to join him in an activity that she really doesn't enjoy may be more successful if he orchestrates social circumstances that would support the activity. A bike ride, for example, may be more appealing to his nonathletic wife if it included his wife's good friend or ended at a destination that she wanted to visit.

Studies of couples have consistently shown that wives do more housework and childcare than husbands even when both work full time outside the home. But when husbands and wives work different shifts, and the husbands are home with their kids while their wives are at work, husbands do much more childcare and housework. Circumstances encourage—in fact literally force—the changes the wives may have desired when they worked the same shifts as their husbands.

When Change Is Difficult

Most of us find that making deliberate changes is difficult even when we ourselves want those changes. At the beginning of each year, millions of Americans make a decision to lose weight and get more exercise. Some of those millions actually sign up for programs to help them reach these goals. All too often, however, a few weeks or months later the desire for change has vanished and old habits return in full force. Appealing food and soft couches are formidable, attractive alternatives to diet and exercise, so it's easy to understand why we often fail to make the weight and exercise changes we desire. With relationships, we have to deal not only with attractive alternatives to change but also with conflicting desires about change. It is often our partners, not ourselves, who are invested in our changing. Furthermore, there are other complexities about the nature of interpersonal change that complicate our efforts.

Why Does Change for Me Have to Be Such a Big Deal for You?

Perhaps the most important reason that change is difficult in interpersonal relationships is that it touches on incompatibilities between partners or on vulnerabilities in one or both of them. To make a change may threaten a fundamental characteristic of the other. For example, Luke wishes that Caitlin would take life easier, not worry about so many things, and just "go with the flow." His mantra to her is "Don't sweat the small stuff." And although at times Caitlin agrees that she should take life easier, she has a difficult time doing so. She is not by nature easygoing. And, for her part, she wants Luke to take life more seriously and to be more ambitious. In fact, they are fundamentally different in their approach to life, and their requests for change in each other run up against these basic differences.

Vulnerabilities can also get in the way of change. Luke wants to spend more time together with Caitlin. He likes to hang around with her, even when she is working on a project at home. But Caitlin often feels uncomfortable, even irritated, with Luke's hovering presence. Her sense of freedom and independence is abridged when he is around her all the time. She feels trapped by his presence. He cannot understand why she does not want to be around her husband more. She cannot understand why he invades her space so much.

Requests for change will often center on incompatibilities and vulnerabilities. These are the areas that create pain for each individual, so these are the areas in which partners will often make their change requests. If one partner is vulnerable about issues of approval, he or she may request that the other be more complimentary and less critical, while the other may respond with requests to be "less sensitive" or more "thick skinned." These will not be easy changes to make.

I Want You to Want To

With many changes we seek in our partners, such as wanting them to do more of the housework or wanting them to take the kids to soccer practice, there is little concern with how they feel when they are doing what we want. Of course, we would prefer them to feel happy with what they are doing. And it would create a problem if they felt resentful. But our concern is with their behavior, not with their emotional state. Our message is: Just do it!

There are other times when the changes we seek in our partners prove more complex. We want behavior change, but we also want attitude change. We are concerned not just with what they do but also with their motives for doing it and their emotional state while they are doing it. Luke may want Caitlin to be more verbally demonstrative with him. He would like it if she complimented him more often and if she expressed her love to him more frequently and more fervently. Certainly, it is within Caitlin's power to perform more of these affectionate acts. But if she forced herself to perform them, it would not be satisfying either for her or for Luke. He might accuse her of "just going through the motions." Although Luke would like more verbal affection, he also wants the motivation and attitude that usually accompany it. He wants her *to want* to do it.

Caitlin would like Luke to earn more money at his job. But apart from this concrete change, she would like him to be more ambitious in general. She wants him to be more achievement-oriented. Although he can and does listen to her dreams for a better financial future, what she really wants is for him to share her passion for that future. She wants him to get ahead, but, more than that, she wants him *to want* to get ahead.

Requests for change such as these present a difficult dilemma for couples. Making changes in behavior is quite challenging in and of itself. The one from whom change is desired must hear the request for change, respect it, endorse it, remember it, and support it. If we ask for a change in attitude, motivation, or emotion in addition to a request for behavior change, our partners are faced with a much more difficult task. Not only must they change something that is under their control—their behavior—but they must change something that is not directly under their control: their desires and emotions. They can control what they do but not what they *want* to do.

Handle Your Emotional Distress Differently

We often want our partners to act differently when they are experiencing strong emotions. We may want them to refrain from offensive actions or engage in desirable actions when they are upset. Luke wants Caitlin to stop being so critical, because he believes she searches for someone to blame every time she is upset. Caitlin wants Luke to be more expressive, because she thinks he goes off into a corner when he is upset and reveals little of what is troubling him.

The difficulties we have in making deliberate changes while emotionally at ease are magnified when we are emotionally aroused. When emotions are high, we repeat well-worn behavior patterns and are less flexible. Even if we can see alternatives to our old patterns, we may be unable to alter our behavior.

Often we want our partners to do more than change the way they act when upset; sometimes we really want them not to be so upset. Our message, stripped of any euphemistic and self-justifying wrapping, is simply "Don't be so emotional." Their emotions upset ours, so we insist that they throttle theirs. Of course, telling your partner that the circumstances at hand are not worth getting upset over only makes him or her feel invalidated and thus upsets your partner even more.

I Won't Allow the Changes I Need

> Don't call a man honest just because he never had the chance to steal.
>
> —YIDDISH PROVERB

Ernie does not trust Jade for good reason. Early in their relationship, Ernie discovered that Jade was still seeing her old boyfriend secretly. He knows Jade's style with men is to be flirtatious and provocative, and he also knows that she doesn't exactly proclaim to the world that she is married. Ernie has dealt with this problem by keeping a watchful eye over Jade. In fact, he is convinced that it is his vigilance that keeps Jade faithful. If he let up, she might also. In fact, the only way he could be assured that she is trustworthy would be for him to relax his vigilance and discover that she remains faithful to him. But he is afraid, with some justification, to engage in the actions that could lead to a trusting relationship.

Similarly, Gayle worries that Leo is not careful enough with their active, adventuresome toddler, Donny. Because Leo is not nearly as worried or as vigilant as she is, Gayle is hesitant to turn over responsibility for Donny to Leo. Even when Leo is supposedly "in charge" of Donny, Gayle keeps a cocked ear and a watchful eye. She overrules Leo when he is watching their son, and she may criticize Leo for his lack of concern. Except for occasional angry efforts to show Gayle he is responsible, Leo is actually becoming less watchful of Donny *because* Gayle is always there to back him up. And even though Gayle needs Leo to take charge sometimes so she can have a break from Donny, she fears allowing Leo full responsibility because she doesn't want to risk an accident. So Gayle wants Leo to be in charge but won't allow it. But Leo won't insist on truly being in charge either.

WHY YOU SHOULD CHANGE

When the change we've requested is difficult, our partners may question why they should change, or they may ignore or resist our requests. Even if they acknowledge the validity of our requests, they may not follow through with change. In response, we may try to justify our requests by proving why they *ought* to change.

Others Do It

One way we can justify the need for change is to point to other husbands or other wives who do what we want our partners to do: "Ben takes a lot of responsibility for their kids." "Most of the other wives go to this party." This strategy can easily degenerate into arguments about whether in fact the other spouse in question does what is claimed. "I don't think Ben does that much with his kids. He makes a show of it in the presence of others, but . . . " Or our partners can provide counterexamples: "But look at Joey and Mike. They are so busy with work they hardly know who their kids are." Or other features of the comparison spouse can be called into question. "So you really want to be married to a nerd like Ben?" What began as an effort to justify a request for change can become a fruitless argument about friends and acquaintances.

Social psychologists write about two kinds of comparisons: upward social comparisons, in which we compare ourselves to people who are better than we are by some criterion, and downward social comparisons, in which we compare ourselves to people who are worse than we are by some criterion. With most characteristics, it is possible to make either upward or downward social comparisons. So if you try to justify your demand that your partner do more by saying "You don't do as much as Joe," he can easily counter with "But I do more than Harry." And both kinds of comparisons are complicated by the fact that we rarely know exactly how much either Joe or Harry actually does. Again, the attempt to justify the original request is futile and may end in a whole new argument.

I Do It for You!

We can make a more compelling case for change through appeals to fairness or equality. "I do it for you, so why can't you do it for me?" Or "I don't treat you like that, so you shouldn't treat me like that."

During the difficult days of the Constitutional Convention in this country, Benjamin Franklin served as an excellent moderator, using his

humor and wisdom to help resolve disputes. At one point during a struggle between representatives from large and small states, he told a story
of how a rooster was trying to negotiate barnyard rules with a horse.
The rooster proposed what seemed to him a reasonable plan: if the horse
would not step on his feet, then he would not step on the horse's feet!
The horse failed to see the wisdom in the rooster's proposal, since it
didn't bother the horse how much the rooster stepped on his feet.

Similarly, proposals for change based on fairness and equality fail
to consider the fact that partners are different and that the same act
involves different levels of "psychic energy" or "psychic pain" when it is
done by two different people. It is fundamentally a more difficult task
for Caitlin to express her love for Luke than for Luke to express his love
for Caitlin. Similarly, it is much easier for Caitlin to get up early on a
Saturday morning and accomplish some household task than it is for
Luke.

When we don't accept the truth that the same act is different when
done by different people, we can create a new conflict on top of the original one.

Look at All I've Done for You!

In this case we justify our requests by pointing out that we've
tried to make our partners happy by changing in ways that they seemed
to want; now it is our turn to get the changes we want. In this justification for change, there is an implicit assumption of inequality and debt.
We have given more than they, so they owe us something.

Although it may be believed fervently, this assumption is often false.
Psychologists have discovered an "egocentric bias" when two people in
a relationship are asked to estimate their own contribution to some joint
activity: their individual, reported percentages add up to more than 100
percent because they both give themselves more relative credit than the
other does. A husband and wife may both agree that she does more child
care than he does, but he estimates that he does 40 percent while she
estimates that she does 70 percent! Psychologists theorize that this bias
occurs because each of us has more information about our own contributions than we have about our partners' contributions, so we give more
weight to our own contributions.

With or without egocentric bias, there are bound to be real inequal-
ities in your relationship. But the fact that inequality exists does not necessarily justify your demanding that it be rectified. Your partner can

rightfully argue that he or she was unaware of any reciprocal agreement for change. If a husband proposes that his wife should meet his social needs because he has adapted so much to her desires to live near her parents, she may reply: "I didn't remember agreeing to a trade-off here! You drew up a plan without getting my consent to it." So, whether there is a skewed perception of inequity in your relationship or actual inequity, you're unlikely to encourage change in your partner by trying to prove you are a victim of your partner's unfairness.

I Really Want You to Change

The simplest and in some ways the most compelling justification for change is based on our own desire: "I want you to change" or "It is important to me that you change." There is little room for argument with this honest approach because we know what we want and what is important to us. Such a message does not ensure change, but it clarifies the reason for it: the change would please me.

However, some of us don't feel entitled to request change from our partners. "Just because it would please me" doesn't seem like a sufficient justification. So we may add weight to our requests by amplifying an "I want" into an "I need." Needs sound more urgent than wants. Satisfying needs ensures survival, while satisfying wants only ensures pleasure or contentment. Therefore, if we phrase our requests as needs, we communicate that somehow our survival depends on our partners changing.

We may also buttress our request for change with an appeal to our partners' love for us. "If you really loved me, you would make the changes I seek." "If you really care, you would do this." But this tactic can easily backfire. Our partners may respond: "If you really loved me, you would accept me as I am." Or they may in turn appeal to our love to push for the changes *they* desire.

Whatever methods we use to justify the changes we request—appeals to love, to fairness, to equity—these justifications often lead to a struggle over change. Our partners experience our efforts as pressure for them to change, and paradoxically, the greater the pressure they feel to change, the more they may resist change. We may demand of them: You must change. I cannot survive without change. You owe me change, and if you loved me, you would change. In response, they may defend themselves, counter with demands of their own, or ultimately refuse to discuss our requests further.

In this dilemma, the first and most important change would be a change in the way we discuss change. We need a change in the struggle for change, a change in our communication about change.

THE MOST IMPORTANT THING TO CHANGE: COMMUNICATION

Communication is the primary means with which we pursue deliberate change. When we want our partners to change, we often begin by requesting, directly or indirectly, that change. We may negotiate or bargain with them about this change. We may struggle about change until we reach a compromise.

Communication can be the object of change requests as well as a vehicle for making change. Often what we want from our partners is that they communicate with us differently. We may want them to listen more attentively or share more completely. We may want them to consult with us and seek our opinion before taking action. We may want them to talk to us more affectionately or more respectfully. We may even want them not to talk to us so much at all.

Communication plays a role not only in change but also in acceptance. It is through our communication with our partners that we may come to experience them differently, to appreciate their positions, and to ease our demands for change. By talking to them, we come to know their softer feelings and view them with empathy rather than with antipathy. By our communication with them, we can come to view our problems from a similar vantage point, not as something they did to us, nor as something we did to them, but as something we created jointly that makes both of us part villain and part victim.

Finally, it is through our communication that we can achieve a balance of acceptance and change. Through our conversation, we can support the changes that each is able to make but foster acceptance for the inevitable limitations in what we each can genuinely change.

Because of communication's pivotal role in acceptance and change, the rest of Part III addresses changes in "how we talk."

RECAP

Change is an inexorable force. Inevitably, we change, our partners change, and our relationships change. But these changes do not necessarily move in the direction we want. What we want is deliberate change in specific areas of concern. Sometimes we want big changes immediately and end up in a confrontation, a showdown, to get what we want. On rare occasions, dramatic, positive change is possible from a showdown, but only when specific conditions exist. Most often these conditions, such as a decision point around an important event like marriage, do not exist. Furthermore, what we often want is not a single decision or a single action but ordinary, everyday changes in what our partner does or says to us.

Sometimes everyday change is easy. We ask our partners to take some specific actions in our relationship, and events conspire to support those actions. However, most often the changes we request are not easy for our partners to make. Our requests strike at the core of incompatibilities or vulnerabilities that divide us. Changes in these areas are always complicated. Furthermore, we may request change not only in our partners' behavior but also in their emotional state. We may want them to feel more passion for us or want them not to be upset when they get upset. Although they have control over their behavior, they have little direct control over how they feel. Therefore, compliance with our requests is difficult.

If our partners don't make the everyday changes we seek, we may try to justify those changes to them. We may point to how other spouses are, we may appeal to fairness or to love, or we may tout our extensive change on their behalf to justify our requests and inspire compliance. These efforts often backfire. Rather than prove the need for them to change, our efforts only generate a struggle about change. We press for the changes, and they resist them.

What is needed is change in our communication. Some of our requests are for changes in the way our partners talk or listen to us. But more important, communication is the vehicle for bringing about both change and acceptance in relationships and for modulating a balance between the two. Better communication can circumvent the struggle over change that often is the biggest barrier to change. The remaining chapters on change focus on change in communication.

Exercise

Are there any easy changes that your partner can make that would please you or that you can make that would please your partner? Is there something you would like from your partner or that your partner would like from you that does not involve complicated incompatibilities or vulnerabilities?

- Try asking your partner directly and specifically for those changes and try to alter circumstances to support those changes.
- Try to comply with the easy changes your partner asks of you.

If there are few or no easy changes, consider the more difficult changes.

- What changes do you want from your partner or does your partner want from you that invoke incompatibilities and vulnerabilities?
- What changes are you seeking or is your partner seeking that request a change in emotion and attitude as well as a change in behavior?
- Describe any struggle that ensues between the two of you about these changes.

CHAPTER 13

How Good Advice Can Be Bad for Your Relationship

ACCEPTING THE FOIBLES OF RULES

> What we have here is a failure to communicate.
> —FROM THE MOVIE *Cool Hand Luke*

What is it about enduring love that makes communication between partners so difficult?

As we've seen, love makes us especially vulnerable to hurt and anger. The stakes are high in close relationships. The lack of interest or disagreement that we view philosophically from a friend or coworker cannot be sloughed off so easily when it involves our partners in life. When our incompatibilities and vulnerabilities are triggered, our emotional reactions often impede productive communication between us. We can be too angry to communicate constructively. Even then, however, communication usually does not break down completely: we can still talk to our partners about content other than the conflict. Sometimes, however, a conflict may gradually spread until even everyday communication becomes difficult.

The legions of advice givers for couples—those mental health professionals or clergy or matchmakers or bartenders or friends who claim some special knowledge about love—are well aware that communication is at the heart of many of our problems. So they have formulated a wealth of advice for expressing our complaints, airing our feelings, and eliciting the changes we want in our loved ones and our relationships. We will now examine some of those rules, with the goal not only of promoting them but also of exposing their limits and inadequacies. Knowing the "rules of good communication" can be instructive, especially when you know why they often don't work.

"APPLE PIE" ADVICE

In the musical *Camelot*, King Arthur asks the magician Merlin for advice on how to handle a woman. He is told to "simply love her." Although this sentiment makes for a great song, it is not particularly useful advice for lovers in conflict. How can you "simply love her" if you feel hurt and angry with her?

Much of what passes for advice about communication and love is a bit like politicians' support of motherhood and apple pie. You wouldn't argue with the admonition to love your partner any more than you'd claim that motherhood and apple pie are un-American. You wouldn't disagree in theory with the advice to honor, respect, cherish, support, or love your partner for what he or she is. But these nice sentiments don't get you closer to the transformed relationship you desire any more than espousing the wholesomeness of Mom and apple pie tells voters what a politician will do once she or he is elected to office.

Advice that encourages some general, admirable state such as love or respect is well intended but oversimplified in the extreme. When our relationships are going well, it may be easy to be respectful or supportive or loving. When the relationship is not going well, we may not have a clue as to how to achieve those states.

Even advice that is more specific can be impossible to follow. The common suggestion to say something nice to your partner every day tells you exactly what to do—say you love your partner or give your partner a compliment daily—but discounts the role of your feelings in this communication. It's no problem to say "I love you" when you feel loving or to say "You look gorgeous" when you feel attracted to your partner, but what about the times you don't feel that way? Is it really a good idea to say something to your partner that you don't mean?

Another common kind of advice explicitly addresses feelings but assumes they are completely under our control. Consider the oft-repeated advice not to go to bed angry with each other, not to be angry at the same time, or to be optimistic and cheerful with your partner. When you are feeling angry or pessimistic, it may not be possible to cut off your anger on command, much less transform it into optimism and good cheer.

Our society generally recognizes the distinction between feelings and thoughts on the one hand, and behavior on the other, so it seems odd that those giving advice on interpersonal relationships often don't. For several good reasons, our customs and laws hold us responsible for what we do but not for what we think or feel. Our feelings and thoughts are private, they are not harmful to others, and, most important of all, we can't control them as easily as we can control our behavior. We can use distraction or reason to alter our feelings somewhat, especially if those feelings are not intense, and we can try to prevent certain feelings by avoiding their predictable triggers, but generally our feelings and thoughts (especially our feelings) come unbidden.

Advice that exhorts us to have certain feelings fails to consider the elementary distinction between what we do and what we think and feel.

WHEN GOOD ADVICE IS BAD
FOR YOUR RELATIONSHIP

Obviously, lots of good advice doesn't fall into either of the traps just discussed. The advice to "apologize when you make a mistake that affects your partner" is certainly specific and is directed at behavior rather than at emotions. It is also good advice. Relationships would do better overall if partners were more willing to apologize for their mistakes.

However, even good advice can be bad when it ignores the emotional context. Jamal may be angry with Letitia and demand an apology, which she gives knowing that she made an error but still feeling resentful at Jamal's angry demand. Her ungracious apology leaves them both dissatisfied. Even if Letitia was able to provide a genuine apology, Jamal might be too angry to accept it, might continue to rail against her, and might anger her in turn.

Good advice can also fail because it ignores the larger relationship context in which behavior, even "good" behavior, occurs. Evan generally uses apologies as part of an appeasement strategy, apologizing quickly to avoid Cara's anger. His evasive intent doesn't escape Cara, and she only ends up annoyed by his frequent apologies. For Jamal and Letitia as well as Evan and Cara, what sounds like "good advice" is actually bad for them and leads to a toxic solution.

We are often attracted to "good advice" that is bad for us. Advice that fits in with what we normally do is likely to appeal to us. Evan likes the advice to apologize because that is his normal tendency. And he pushes that "good advice" on Cara. But often, as with Evan, the advice we heed is not the advice we need.

When you understand your "story," you can discriminate what is good advice from what is bad advice for your particular problem. If Cara and Evan understood that blame on her part and appeasement on his, including his apologies, were part of their toxic solutions, they would know that this otherwise good advice would simply further their problem.

WHEN BAD ADVICE IS GOOD
FOR YOUR RELATIONSHIP

It was often said of Johnny Carson that his great skill as a comedian was due in part to his ability to recover from bad jokes. When a joke bombed, he would make a comment about himself, his writers, or the audience that would turn the failed joke into an opportunity for an even bigger laugh. He transformed his failures into his biggest successes.

It is possible to make a similar transformation when you try to elicit change in your relationship. When you can accept the reality that your partner won't respond to your efforts as you would like, even when your efforts are driven by good intentions and informed by expert advice, you may find that your failures provide new opportunities to adjust to each other. Somewhat analogous to the way Carson transformed bad jokes into better humor, you may transform even bad advice into something good for the relationship.

After an unpleasant discussion about their plans for the weekend, Oliver and Suzanne go to their separate corners and busy themselves with their Saturday morning tasks. Oliver hates the tense silence that comes after any argument with Suzanne and tries to follow what normally might be good advice: "Reach out to your partner after an argument." But when he proposes kissing and making up and suggests that they have the whole weekend ahead of them and can still enjoy most of it, Suzanne only feels annoyed. The fact is, Suzanne takes longer to recover from conflict than Oliver, and right now she has no interest in making up.

At this point, both are in danger of creating a reactive problem that is more serious than the initial problem of their disagreement about the weekend. If they follow their usual form, Suzanne will rebuff Oliver's overture with a dismissive wave of her hand, Oliver will get angry again and criticize Suzanne's unresponsiveness to his "positive gesture," she will question the honesty of his gesture, and they will end up arguing about the way they recover from arguments more vehemently than they disagreed initially about their weekend plans.

However, they don't follow their usual form. Both are aware of the "story" of their conflicts and have come to accept their pattern of recovery from conflict. Suzanne quells her impulse to reject his overture without a word of explanation. Instead, she says honestly and directly, "I'm not there yet, Oliver."

Even though she didn't "kiss and make up" as he wanted, Suzanne's comment explains her action. For Oliver, it is worlds different from simply waving him off. The "there yet" also implies that she will get to a place of reconciliation in due time. Therefore, her comment plus his own realization that his well-meaning overture could lead them deeper into conflict helped him to back off. He said, "I know. We each have our own pace." Then he let Suzanne be.

With the pressure to make up removed, Suzanne actually recovered more quickly from her distress than she otherwise would have. She later joined Oliver in the kitchen and helped him with the dishes. He made no demand for a kiss to mark their reconciliation but accepted her way of easing back into a connection with him. They ended up having a good weekend together.

The "bad advice" for their conflict that Oliver followed was turned into something good for their relationship because the couple had a solid knowledge and acceptance of their pattern of conflict. Suzanne has come to understand that Oliver gets anxious when there is emotional distance between them, tries to bridge that distance with efforts to make up, and then gets furious if these overtures are rejected. Her acceptance of Oliver's way of handling conflict enabled her to tell him "I'm not there yet" rather than wordlessly dismiss his attempt.

Similarly, Oliver has come to accept that his efforts at reconciliation only put pressure on Suzanne and make it more difficult for her to reconnect with him. This acceptance enables him to back off from her, to let her come back to him at her own pace and in her own way. Their combined approach, their mutual understanding and acceptance about how they handle conflict differently, enables them not only to salvage a weekend but also to begin to change the destructive way they recover from conflict.

Despite the boundless availability of good advice about communication and relationships, there are no tricks to generate a particular desired response in your partner. Inevitably we will be frustrated in our efforts to change our partners or the relationship. In fact, when we use otherwise "good advice" to try to force a response from our partners, we are liable to make the problem worse. We may create a bigger reactive problem as we use "good advice" to solve a smaller, initial problem. Our frustration with our failure to create change will generate bigger barriers to change. Therefore, the best way to implement any good advice, or any change, for that matter, is to do so with full acceptance of the fact that the effort may fail for good reason. When we approach change within this context of acceptance, we are less likely to be frustrated with our efforts and may experience failure not as a reason to denigrate our partners or ourselves but as an opportunity to learn more about each other. We will avoid the creation of a reactive problem. Rather than "try harder" to implement the same old ineffective solution, we will "try smarter" to alter our approach based on our understanding and acceptance of how we each respond. This is exactly what Oliver and Suzanne did.

The rest of this chapter will review common advice for achieving good communication that you may be tempted to try in your efforts to elicit change. Knowing the benefits, the risks, and the difficulties of implementing particular advice will enable you to approach change in the context of acceptance. It will enable you to understand that any advice may backfire, even if it is implemented correctly, and prepare you to accept and learn from those situations in which it does backfire. Sometimes we learn more from failure than from success.

EXPRESS YOUR FEELINGS

Perhaps the most common advice from popular psychology is to "express your feelings." Pop psychology tells us not only that this is a good thing to do, but also that if we don't express our feelings, particularly our negative feelings, something bad may happen to us. This advice is based on a "balloon model" of negative feelings: if we push them down in one spot, they will pop up in another. Unexpressed, our feelings may "build up" inside and then "come out" physically as ulcers, headaches, high blood pressure, and the like. Or, worse, "pent-up" feelings may affect our immune system and contribute to illnesses as diverse as colds and cancer. Psychologically, our unexpressed feelings may eventually "come out" in impulsive reactions such as emotional outbursts or rash decisions. There seems to be nothing good about holding in our negative feelings.

Not surprisingly, the scientific evidence for these notions suggests much more complexity than the balloon model would indicate. The impact of "expressing feelings" depends on what the feelings are, how they are expressed, and to whom they are expressed. Sometimes the expression of feelings can prolong or amplify those feelings. Yet, despite these caveats, appropriate expression of feelings is probably good for one's physical and mental health. A venting of feelings, particularly if those feelings are intense and have not been disclosed before, can bring great psychological relief and, according to some recent evidence, may provide physical benefits.

In addition to whatever personal benefits may come from expressing our feelings, there can be positive effects on our relationship. Appropriate expression of feelings can lead to greater intimacy and influence. Confiding deeply held feelings to our partners is one way to let them know more about us. By confiding, we may feel emotionally closer to them. And by listening to us, they may feel emotionally closer to us. In addition, as they learn about our feelings, they may take our feelings into account when they deal with us. They may alter their behavior out of consideration for our feelings.

Despite all the potential good that can come from communicating our feelings to our partners, many problems arise when we try to express our negative feelings to them, especially when those feelings concern them. Certainly, it will not be pleasant for them to hear the negative reactions we have to them. They may have trouble listening; they may interject their own negative feelings about us. But apart from their reactivity to what we say, it may be difficult for us to express our feelings honestly.

First, we may simply not know exactly what we feel. Take fear as an example. Psychologists measure fear in three different ways: by looking at behavior (people display fear by avoiding or escaping from a feared object), by assessing physiological arousal (people have faster heart rates, higher blood pressure, and sweat more when they are afraid), and by asking about subjective feelings (people can report feeling afraid). Psychologists have found that these three measures of fear are consistently high when fear is great. If people who are afraid of snakes are confronted with a large snake in a glass cage, they will try to distance themselves from the snake, they will have increased physical arousal such as faster heart rate, and they will report feeling afraid.

However, if fear is low—if those afraid of snakes are merely shown pictures of snakes—they will often not show consistency across these three measures. For example, they may show some slight avoidance behavior (turning away from the picture more rapidly than people not afraid of snakes), they may have a small increase in heart rate, but they may report no feelings of fear. They are not lying to us; they genuinely don't label their internal state as fear. In this example, we could say that they are not aware of their feelings of fear.

This example of snake phobia is simple in that only one emotion was aroused. When more than one emotion is aroused but all at a low level, being "aware of your feelings" becomes more complicated. For example, assume that a husband and wife are out to dinner with friends. His contributions to the conversation aren't particularly interesting or amusing, but hers are. Encouraged by the attention and interest she commands, she interrupts him a couple of times and tends to dominate the conversation. She does nothing rude or dramatic, but she slights his contributions and assumes control of the discussion. If we could inspect his feelings with a magnifying glass, we might see that he feels competitive with his wife, that he is jealous of her ability to entertain others, and that he is annoyed at the interruptions. Yet because the things that she did were subtle and because his feelings of competition, jealousy, and annoyance are at such a low intensity, he may not be able to articulate them. He may only experience some vague sense of dissatisfaction. On the way home from their dinner, she may express her pleasure with the fun evening they had, while he seems in a bad mood.

Another reason we have difficulty expressing our feelings honestly is that we may not be comfortable with certain feelings and may not want to experience them. The husband above not only has trouble detecting his true feelings because they are at a low intensity, he does not *want* to identify these true feelings within himself. Either he is not comfortable feeling competitive with or envious of his wife, or he believes these feelings are not justified in this instance and is therefore embarrassed by them.

When we can't or won't express our feelings honestly, we often resort to acting on them instead of voicing them. When you walk out of the room and refuse to discuss a matter with your partner, you are acting on your feelings of anger, not voicing them. If you take off your wedding ring, you are acting on your distress with the marriage, not articulating that distress. When you withdraw and sulk, you are acting on your hurt rather than verbalizing it. Even when you talk to your partner, you may be acting on your feelings rather than voicing them. As we explained in Chapter 10, our words may be stimulated by our feelings, but those words may make no mention of our feelings. When you call your partner a jerk or yell "Don't you ever do that to me again," you may think your feelings are perfectly clear, but you're really adopting the diversionary tactic of focusing on the other person's faults instead of your own emotions.

When I ask partners in couple therapy to express how they feel about an issue of concern to them, I am asking questions about one person, but I often get a reply about the other. Here's a typical response from a husband asked about his feelings about their marital communication: "She doesn't know how to communicate very well. She either blurts out her feelings no matter what—whether the situation is appropriate or not—or she just clams up. She just cannot have a simple, straightforward discussion about any disagreement without it getting all tense. I think she is afraid that she will lose out if she tries to deal with a problem rationally." Notice that the husband never mentioned anything about his feelings or even about himself.

Don't be surprised if you catch yourself "expressing your feelings" in this way. You may end up feeling hurt and frustrated that your partner has not heard your feelings. But you may never have voiced them.

Use "I" Statements

A common piece of advice designed to help couples express feelings rather than judgments prescribes messages that begin with "I feel" rather than "You." A statement that begins this way is more likely to be about one's own feelings and less likely to be a judgment, an accusation, or a blameful comment. In contrast, a "you" statement is about the other and will often be accusatory. The comment "You blew it again" could easily communicate judgment and blame and invites argument. In contrast, "I feel angry when you do that" focuses on the speaker's feelings and is less subject to debate. It's a lot tougher to argue about whether someone has had a certain emotional reaction than about whether certain behavior was appropriate, so therapists and other advice givers advocate the "I statement" formula to filter out blame and judgment from communication.

If you hope to promote change and intimacy in your relationship with the help of this advice, however, beware of the ease with which this formula can be sabotaged. Partners in conflict often preface unadulterated judgments with an "I feel," as in "I feel you are shirking your responsibility" or "I feel you are being selfish." In fact, partners may try to sanitize their most accusatory or demeaning statements by putting them under the guise of expression of feelings: "I feel you are a jerk." "I feel you don't have the capacity to love." "I feel you are worthless as a spouse."

More specific advice about using I statements suggests that the "I feel" be followed by an emotion word. Messages such as "I feel angry" or "I feel disappointed" or "I feel hurt" clearly communicate feelings rather than judgments. But, of course, there's a way around this for the person bent on blaming and name calling: "I feel angry that you are being so selfish." "I feel disappointed when you are so cruel." "I feel hurt that you are being such a jerk about this." The listener is likely to hear the accusation—selfish, cruel, jerk—more than any expression of feelings.

There's an answer to this twist too: exclude all references to the other person. Instead of "I feel angry *that you* are being so selfish" or "I feel disappointed *when you* are so cruel," try "I feel angry about this whole incident" or "I feel very disappointed."

Yes, of course, there's another loophole. Depending on the context, voice tone, and facial expression, a statement like "I feel angry about this whole incident" can communicate "You know exactly why I am angry, you did the dastardly thing that made me angry, and you are going to pay for it." When anger is intense, it may be impossible not to communicate some sense of judgment and blame, no matter what the word choice. The expression of anger may then lead to defensiveness and counterattack in a partner, a situation that the focus on the speaker's feelings was designed to avoid.

If you are to approach change in the context of acceptance, you need to be aware of these misuses of "I" statements. Nevertheless, a pure statement of feelings, without any reference to the partner, is often a good place to start a discussion. The only problem with comments such as "I am really disappointed" or "I am really angry" is that they may be too cryptic. The confused listener could very well reply: "What are you angry about?" or "What made you disappointed?" That brings us to the next section: how we can talk about our partners without attacking them.

Talk about Your Partner's Specific Behavior Rather Than His or Her Personality Characteristics

To avoid the accusation inherent in a statement such as "I feel angry that you are so selfish" and to avoid the lack of reference in a statement such as "I feel angry," one common piece of advice is to express your feelings in reaction to your partner's specific behavior: "I feel angry when you come home late and don't call" or "I am disappointed that you forgot I had a doctor's appointment today." With this kind of message, we express our feelings and we indicate what we are reacting to, yet we don't attack our partners' character or call into question their personality and put them on the defensive. Contrast "I feel angry that you are so selfish" with "I felt ignored when you didn't ask me about my day." Although a partner may not like to hear either comment, the first invites defensiveness and argument ("I'm not selfish. You're the one who's selfish."), the second invites understanding.

Just like "I" statements, specific comments can be sabotaged, however. Adrianna could get specific about Malcolm's behavior of paying attention to other women by saying "I get angry when you leer at other women" or "when you gawk at other women." While these statements contain no personality descriptions, each one contains some negative evaluation that could lead to defensiveness and argument: "I was not leering."

A more constructive approach would be for Adrianna to avoid loaded words such as "gawk" or "leer" and instead describe his behavior more neutrally. For example, she might say "I didn't like it when you glanced at Susan's cleavage" or "I got angry when you did a top-to-bottom checkout of Esther." With messages like these, she will communicate in clear and detailed language her exact feelings and exactly what behavior of his led to those feelings.

Will this approach be easy for Adrianna to take? Maybe not. She might find it phony to use such toothless language that does not accurately express her experience. Or if Malcolm's behavior was subtle, she might not be sure exactly what caused her feelings, the same way the husband who ended up feeling competitive with and envious of his wife following a party was unable to pinpoint the source of his bad mood. Or she might be wrong about what caused her feelings. Adrianna may attribute her unhappiness to her dislike of Susan or Esther and their provocative clothing, for she is only dimly aware that it was Malcolm's actions more than their manner of dress that upset her. Finally, focusing on the specific behavior may be ill advised for Adrianna because it could obscure a larger issue of concern, such as Malcolm's commitment to their relationship. Without addressing this, he could forswear ever looking at women's cleavage again, but the commitment problem would remain.

Despite these difficulties, a focus on specific behavior will be more constructive than a focus on broad personality traits. When we know the difficulties of such a focus, we may accept some struggle and confusion and persist until we discover the things that really bother each other.

LISTEN TO WHAT YOUR PARTNER IS SAYING

Listening is one of the first casualties of couples' conflict. As disagreements between partners escalate, they each make their points and produce their evidence, which fall on deaf ears. Active interruption by each makes it impossible to maintain even a pretense of listening. If partners do allow each other an uninterrupted turn at speaking, they use their silence to prepare for their turn rather than to hear what the other says.

Therapists and other advice givers have gone beyond simple exhortations to listen and devised a way to ensure that partners not only attend to what the other is saying but also truly understand it. The strategy is called "active listening," and it requires that partners alternate between speaker and listener roles. The listener must paraphrase or summarize what the speaker has said, to the speaker's satisfaction, before the listener gets a chance to say his or her piece. The listener does not have to agree with the speaker's position but must demonstrate his or her understanding of that position. Here is an example in which Tony tries to listen to a concern of his wife, Rose.

ROSE: I am bothered by all our arguments over the kids. I think they are unnecessary—we shouldn't have to have them—and they upset the kids.

TONY: So you don't like the arguments and you don't think the kids do either.

ROSE: Yes, but it is more than that. I think we should be able to discuss our differences without arguments. And I think the arguments may be harmful to the kids.

TONY: You think the arguments are harmful to the kids' mental health?

ROSE: Yes. I think it makes them feel insecure. Maybe they wonder if we are going to stay together.

TONY: So you think we ought to be able to discuss our differences without getting upset, and if we did, you think that would be better for the kids. They would feel more secure.

ROSE: Yes, that's right.

In this example, Rose got her message across to Tony. Whether he agrees or not, he genuinely understood what she had to say. Communication took place. There was nothing particularly complicated about Rose's message, but it would be easy for even this simple communication to go awry. If she stated the message accusatorily, Tony would have a hard time hearing it. Rose could have said: "I don't know why you always argue with me about the kids. It really hurts them." In this message she puts the blame on Tony (it is "you argue," not "we argue"), and she uses the inflammatory word "always." So Rose communicates that Tony is culpable and that he always does this blameworthy behavior. Tony would probably react strongly to such a message. Even if he didn't defend himself and counterattack, he might turn off to Rose and distance himself from her. Most likely he would not be receptive to hearing anything further from her.

Even if Rose did not openly attack Tony and conveyed the messages as in the example, Tony could still feel defensive and respond in ways that distorted the message and derailed the discussion.

ROSE: I am bothered by all our arguments over the kids. I think they are unnecessary—we shouldn't have to have them—and they upset the kids.

TONY: So you can't take the simple arguments we have.

Here Tony subtly twists Rose's statement, interpreting her revelation that "I am bothered by all our arguments" as a weakness in her: "you can't take" the arguments. Calling the conflicts "simple arguments" implies that she cannot take what any other ordinary person could take. See where this might lead.

ROSE: I didn't say I couldn't take it; I said I was bothered by it.

TONY: Well, you seem to be so bothered that I think you can't take it.

ROSE: It is not an issue of whether I can take it; I have taken it for far too long. It is an issue of whether it is good or appropriate for the kids.

Now they are off on an argument about their arguments over the kids.
A listener can make an even more subtle perversion of the speaker's
message by restating the speaker's words precisely but adding a *seemingly* innocent word or two.

> ROSE: I am bothered by all our arguments over the kids. I think
> they are unnecessary—we shouldn't have to have them—and
> they upset the kids.
>
> TONY: So you want to feel bothered by all our arguments over the
> kids.

By throwing in the "you want to feel," Tony accuses Rose of intentionally getting upset. He implies that her distress is her own fault. Let's
see where this could go:

> ROSE: I didn't say I want to get bothered. I said I was bothered.
>
> TONY: But you have some control over your emotions, don't you?
> You are not a victim of your emotions, are you?
>
> ROSE: Of course I am not a victim of my emotions.
>
> TONY: So if you feel bad, you must want to feel bad.

So now the two are off on an argument that may seem to plumb
philosophical and psychological issues about control of emotional reactions, but it is really an argument over who is to blame for the conflict.
Tony feels accused for the arguments over the children and thus tries to
blame Rose for being upset about those arguments.

Attempts to summarize the speaker's words can include much more
obvious distortions than those in the preceding examples. The listener
can editorialize about the speaker's message or ridicule that message in
his or her supposed summaries of the speaker's message.

> ROSE: I am bothered by all our arguments over the kids. I think they
> are unnecessary—we shouldn't have to have them—and they upset
> the kids.
>
> TONY: You think we have too many arguments about the kids.
> More than the ideal couple who never have conflict and are
> always sweet and agreeable.

Here Tony editorializes about what might be going on in Rose's mind—namely, that she is comparing their arguments to some ideal. However, Tony's message really serves to invalidate Rose's statement. In so many words, he is saying: Your feelings are not justified because you are comparing our normal arguments to your unrealistic ideal.

Let's look at a final example in which the listener, under the auspices of summarizing the speaker's message, ridicules that message.

ROSE: I think we should be able to discuss our differences without arguments. And I think the arguments may be harmful to the kids.

TONY: So you think our little tiffs are going to make the kids go crazy!

Here Tony minimizes the arguments ("little tiffs") and exaggerates the possible impact ("make the kids go crazy") in a message that is far from capturing Rose's concerns, but rather invalidates those concerns by ridiculing them.

So far we have focused only on the verbal content of the listener's message. The way the listener communicates nonverbally—the posture, the voice tone, and the facial expression—can overshadow that message. For example, Tony might make a verbally accurate comment such as "You are really worried that our arguments are going to make the kids feel insecure" but say it with a tone of voice and manner that communicate understanding and sympathy. Or he could say it in a voice tone and manner that communicate "That's the craziest idea I've ever heard."

Why is it that listeners have such a difficult time with the simple request to summarize what the partner is saying? The difficulties usually arise when the listener feels blamed or challenged by the speaker's message. The listener then makes a statement that may attempt to capture the speaker's concerns but at the same time invalidates those concerns.

The complication for couples is that any conversation over a common problem is likely to include some implication of blame. When the focus is on something that one is upset about in the relationship, it is impossible to communicate that without also communicating some accusation. For one last time, let's consider the speaker's initial message:

ROSE: I am bothered by all our arguments over the kids. I think they are unnecessary—we shouldn't have to have them—and they upset the kids.

Even if Rose matched these nonblaming words with a nonaccusatory style of speech, there is a clear message of culpability. She is suggesting that Tony should not be doing what he is doing to contribute to the arguments. Certainly, she is not shifting all the blame onto him. But Tony, knowing Rose far better than we do, might accurately see that the nice message is a cover for the real underlying message that "you are the cause of our arguments that upset me and the kids." Or Tony may be so defensive that he responds to even an implication of shared blame with defensiveness.

These difficulties in listening to our partners and demonstrating to them that we have understood their message does not mean that we should give up the effort. Quite the contrary. Often we may be able to hear their message and they may be able to hear ours, even when discussing a relationship problem. However, knowing the difficulties of really listening may enable us to be more accepting of our partners when they fall short of understanding. We may also realize our limitations in understanding them.

NEGOTIATE REASONABLE COMPROMISES TO YOUR PROBLEMS

Better bend than break.
—SCOTTISH PROVERB

A compromise is a settlement by which each side gets what neither side wanted.
—EVAN ESAR,
20,000 Quips and Quotes (1968)

The man who says he is willing to meet you halfway is usually a poor judge of distance.
—EVAN ESAR,
20,000 Quips and Quotes (1968)

The idea that marriage involves compromise is probably as old as marriage itself. What is more recent is the emphasis on the process of problem solving, in which partners negotiate and compromise as a means of dealing with their differences. The influence of business and law, in which people hammer out detailed agreements with others, has been influential on marriage. Many have noted that getting married and raising a family is in part a business and is governed in part by law. The sheer frequency of divorce has alerted most of us to the possibility that our marriage may not last forever and has encouraged a pragmatic view of self-protection in the face of that possibility. Young love has been forced into an uncomfortable relationship with prenuptial agreements and estate planning.

Some approaches to couple therapy and many self-help books have advocated rational problem solving in marriage. Partners should sit down, in a businesslike manner, and discuss their differences, negotiate and bargain to fashion compromises, write down their agreements, and let these guide their behavior almost as if they were legal contracts. Sometimes couples are encouraged to engage in this process early in their relationships so that expectations can be clarified and problems averted. Let's look at some of the specific advice commonly offered to couples.

Set the Stage for Problem Solving

Often couples try to solve problems when they are most upset by them. At those points the problems seem dramatic, and they have the energy to focus on them. But they may also be too angry to compromise or too upset to evaluate possible solutions. So they are advised to engage in problem solving only when they are calm and unhurried. The only problem with this advice is that couples often don't want to focus on controversial issues when they are relaxed and feeling good about each other. So this advice may often lead couples to avoid the issues of concern altogether.

Focus on Only One Specific Problem at a Time

Discussions of problems often escalate in intensity and expand in content, both horizontally and vertically. Horizontally, the content includes more and more specific topics; vertically, content may expand from specific topics to broad categories. Rose and Tony may start out with a discussion of their arguments in front of the children but end with a discussion of their abilities as parents and how much each really loves the children. The advice to focus on one specific topic at a time is meant to counter this tendency.

However, it may be important for couples to explore broader

themes as well as specific problems. For example, Rose may have a more important point to make to Tony than just that they shouldn't argue in front of the kids. She may be concerned that they as a couple and Tony as a father do not attend to the impact of their actions and words on the kids. Not observing the impact of their arguments on the children may be just one example. She may also be concerned that he doesn't seem to notice the impact of his moods on the children. The challenge for Rose and Tony is to be able to discuss this broad theme, and maybe even Tony's related theme about Rose overprotecting the children, without the discussion escalating into a confusing and distressing confrontation that brings in "the kitchen sink." Thus, our challenge is to narrow our focus on a particular problem but without limiting a full and broad exploration of that problem.

Separate Problem Definition from Problem Solution

Often one or both members of a couple will generate solutions before the problem has been clearly defined and agreed on. As we saw in Chapter 9, this tendency leads to oversimplified solutions that are toxic. So it makes sense to first take a systematic, logical approach to defining the problem.

But human thought and emotion rarely follow the lock-step sequence that logic might dictate. Sometimes consideration of possible solutions helps define the true problem. Let's assume that Rose raised the problem of arguments in front of the kids and that Tony, ignoring our advice, proposed that he would be willing to move their arguments into a private setting away from the kids if she would simply request it at the time. Although this solution would solve the problem as Rose initially defined it, she was not satisfied with the solution. In her consideration of this solution and her discussion with Tony about it, she came to realize two important facets of the problem: (1) In addition to whatever direct impact they had on the kids, the arguments upset her and made her less able to deal with the kids. Merely keeping the kids away from their arguments would therefore deal with only the direct impact of their arguments on the kids. It would not deal with the indirect impact: how the arguments upset her and made her less capable as a mother. (2) She was in part concerned that Tony was not tuned in to the kids. She wanted him to notice the impact of arguments as well as the impact of his own behavior on the kids. If she had to notify him when the kids were affected, it would not solve her concern.

Generate Solutions and Negotiate an Agreement

Once a problem has been defined so that both members agree on exactly what it is, they can move to the solution stage, where they generate, evaluate, and negotiate ideas to resolve the problem. A common piece of advice is to "brainstorm" solutions, that is, to generate as many ideas as possible without evaluating their quality. To focus on evaluating solutions may thwart creativity in generating them. Often an enthusiastic partner proposes a possible solution only to be deflated with the reaction of the partner who says in so many words "That will never work."

After all possible solutions have been generated, couples are advised to go though their list and systematically evaluate them, looking for the pros and cons of each. This evaluation process becomes a negotiation over possible solutions, in which couples give and take until they reach a compromise on a solution or set of solutions to implement. At this point couples are encouraged to write down the solution; the mere act of putting it on paper will make it more concrete to them. They are then advised to implement the solution and see if it is helpful. They can later sit down and discuss how the solution worked and perhaps modify it accordingly.

In Tony and Rose's evaluation of possible solutions, Rose might push for delaying their arguments until later. Tony would be reluctant to accept that plan because he knows Rose would push "later" back later and later. He might agree to a delay in their disagreement if they agreed to set a specific time period to resume the discussion that is sooner rather than later. Even if they could work out some agreement on this solution, Rose would be concerned, based on her experience with Tony, that he might push for the last word before they delayed their discussion. It would be hard for her to return her attention to the children if she were still fuming over Tony's ending remark. Thus, even apparently simple, concrete solutions, such as agreeing to delay discussion of a conflict, require discussion and negotiation before agreement is possible.

Problem solving can be a difficult and tedious process, but if it results in new behavior that solves an old problem it is well worth the effort. Problem solving is most likely to be successful when it addresses actions in which emotions play little or no role. Couples can use rational problem-solving strategies to handle conflicts over household chores, work schedules, and childcare more easily than they can use these strategies to solve conflicts about how they argue or how they express anger. Tony and Rose can negotiate about who does the laundry more easily than they can negotiate about their arguments in front of the kids. Especially difficult are negotiations about behaviors that normally require positive emotions. Being "in the mood" is largely irrelevant for complying with an agreement to vacuum the house or pick up the kids on Tuesday. However, it is hardly irrelevant for an agreement about being more affectionate or sexual or attentive. You can easily follow through with the former, even if you don't feel like it. Not so with the latter.

Even when the strategy of rational problem solving works—when partners address a problem that lends itself to the strategy, when partners are able to follow a logical sequence, and when partners can agree on a workable solution—the outcome is often surprising. Partners may come to an agreeable solution but never implement it! Rose and Tony struggled with the issue of their arguments in front of the children. After considerable effort they worked out a plan in which they would delay their discussions until later; they would agree on a particular time for the later discussion; Tony would not level a zinger at Rose before the delay; and Rose would stop what she was doing and talk at the agreed-upon time. In the weeks that followed the agreement on this plan, Rose called for a delay only once. Tony agreed, but both forgot to return to the topic later. On a number of occasions neither Tony nor Rose initiated the solution when they got into a disagreement about the kids in front of the kids. This failure to implement the agreement was due in part to the fact that their disagreements in front of the children were not as intense as they were before. In reflecting on the problem, it was clear to Rose that she just wanted her concerns to be heard and taken seriously by Tony. The process of problem solving accomplished that. Afterward they both were more careful about how they dealt with disagreement in front of the kids. So their "solution" became irrelevant almost as soon as it was created. Yet their problem solving had been successful.

RECAP

In this chapter, we reviewed some of the most common rules of communication. We dismissed the "apple pie" advice that simply exhorts people to maintain a particular attitude or emotional state without any information about how to achieve that state. Then we focused on three broad categories of advice that give behavioral prescriptions about what to do: express your feelings, listen to your partner, and negotiate reasonable compromises. All of this advice can be useful, especially if you understand and accept its limitations and are prepared for failure.

Exercise

Although some of the rules discussed in this chapter are useful for everyday conversation, they are applicable primarily for discussions about relationship problems. It is these discussions that are most likely to deteriorate into accusation, defensiveness, counterattack, and withdrawal. Therefore, it is these discussions that need the structure that rules can provide.

Try using some of these rules in discussions with your partner about relationship problems.

- Express your feelings to your partner by using "I statements" and by focusing on the specific behavior that bothered you.
- Listen to what your partner is saying and demonstrate that you have heard him or her by summarizing your partner's message to you.
- Try to negotiate reasonable compromises to your difficulties: start problem solving when both of you are in an appropriate mood for it; focus on one specific problem at a time; separate problem definition from problem solution; generate solutions and negotiate an agreement.

As we have amply illustrated in this chapter, there will be times when mood and emotion prevent either you or your partner from using these rules appropriately. Sometimes these good rules will be bad advice for your relationship. However, your understanding and acceptance of the inevitable difficulties you will face in trying to communicate with your partner, no matter what rules you use, can create an opportunity out of your failure. As we will see in the next chapter, you can create genuine change rather than simply repeat "the same old thing."

CHAPTER 14

Why a New Approach Can Lead to the Same Old Thing

USING YOUR OWN STORY
TO MAKE GENUINE CHANGE

Sal and Hava were locked in a pattern of distance and criticism. Distressed at what she felt was Sal's abdication of any responsibility in the family—he rarely helped with childcare or housework—Hava criticized him relentlessly. From Sal's point of view, nothing he could do would please Hava. So why bother to do anything, except tune her out?

In my initial work with this couple, I established some reasonable, positive goals for therapy, to which both agreed: Sal would become more involved in the household and Hava would provide more acknowledgment and appreciation for Sal's efforts. As my first intervention with them, I asked Hava to keep track of her daily expressions of acknowledgment or appreciation for Sal's efforts and Sal to keep track of his daily efforts to participate more in the household.

At the beginning of the next session, I asked for their records. Hava had hers ready at the top of her purse and produced it proudly. She had carefully made a calendar of the days of the week and faithfully recorded every instance of Sal's actions on behalf of the family and her corresponding communication of appreciation or acknowledgment. Sal, it turned out, had forgotten to do the assignment until late in the week and then only when Hava reminded him. He tried to keep track mentally of what he had done and later to write it down. Hava noted that he had not written it down until they were in the waiting room before the appointment.

As I read over the very sketchy and hurried notes that Sal had made, Hava looked at me with the confidence of a prosecuting attorney who has just handed the jury the smoking gun. Then she launched into her husband: he could not even do therapy right. His behavior in here was a perfect example of his behavior at home: too little, too late. Sal shook his head and tuned her out.

My therapeutic effort to change their behavior had simply given them a new occasion to exhibit the same old behavior. My assignment had given Sal a new opportunity to fail and Hava a new opportunity to criticize him. They were using my assignment to engage in exactly the same pattern that my assignment had tried to end!

The kind of experience I had with Hava and Sal is just one way my therapeutic efforts sometimes backfire. Sometimes couples use the positive action I suggest to justify their existing behavior. Let's say that, as one positive step toward resolving conflicts between a critical husband and a withdrawn wife, I urge the couple to express their feelings to each other. The following week the husband harangues his wife over some misdeed of hers. In the next session, he justifies his criticism of her by saying, "I was just expressing my feelings, like you said."

Sometimes I offer partners a crutch to help them communicate, and they end up hitting each other over the head with it instead. The critical husband may use my suggestion to express feelings as another opportunity to attack his wife: "You never express your feelings! How can you expect me to respond to you when you don't even do a simple thing like that, which the doctor here recommends?"

My predicament as a therapist bears some odd resemblance to an amazing historical incident in nineteenth-century France. In 1815, Napoleon sailed back to France from exile with about 1,000 of his followers. Arriving in Cannes, he marched toward Paris, gathering supporters along the way. In Paris, King Louis XVIII sent troops out to meet and arrest Napoleon, but when they saw their old leader, they joined him and declared him emperor. As a therapist, I sometimes feel like Louis XVIII. The interventions I've sent out to "arrest" the enemy instead join the other side.

Attempts at change, I have learned, often lead instead to more of the same. As a therapist I've allowed this to happen by failing to anticipate the interplay between my intervention and the vicious cycles of interaction in which the couple is stuck. You can avoid the same trap by looking honestly at the steps you're taking to try to elicit change and anticipating, based on your story, how your own partner is likely to react.

WHEN OLD PATTERNS COME DRESSED IN NEW CLOTHING

Chan has a stronger sex drive than Gwen and has pushed for more frequent and diverse sexual contact. In response to Gwen's resistance, Chan makes vague threats about the viability of their marriage and hints about "looking elsewhere." Although disturbed by these threats, Gwen often challenges them: "If you think threats are a sexual turn-on, you have a lot to learn about women."

Chan doesn't really want to leave Gwen or to threaten their relationship further by having an affair, so he decides to try to make some positive changes on his own. Knowing how pressured Gwen feels by him, he decides to pull back, to give her "more room sexually," as she has often requested. That would certainly be a change, and a difficult one for him to make. Maybe it would help.

Chan tells Gwen: "Look, I'm not going to push you sexually anymore. If there is going to be any sex, you'll have to initiate it. I'll just wait and see how this works."

Although his actions may have seemed like a major change to Chan, their impact on Gwen was the same as that of his old behavior. "I'll just wait and see how this works" felt like another form of pressure to her, and the comment came with a veiled but vague threat that he might take more drastic measures if Gwen didn't start initiating sex right away. His comment that "If there is going to be any sex, you'll have to initiate it" was made with resentment and anger. Despite Chan's genuine efforts to do something constructive, his actions were merely variations on his theme of pressure and threat.

To an outsider, a couple's efforts to change can be amusing because they are so transparently "more of the same." A husband who wants more say in his marriage pleads with his wife to let him make more of the decisions. A wife who realizes the truth in her husband's complaints that he takes most of the responsibility for housework asks him to remind her when things need to be done. They, however, are so mired in their vicious cycles of interaction that they don't see any irony in their efforts.

Realistically, of course, the husband who wants more power may need his wife's assistance in becoming more assertive and the non-domestic wife may need some gentle reminding as she takes on more responsibility for the housework. If they can recognize the irony in their requests, convey this irony to their partners, and their partners can hear these requests with accepting compassion, the changes they desire are more likely to occur.

WHEN "MORE OF THE SAME" BECOMES "WORSE OF THE SAME"

When a tolerant understanding of each other is missing, efforts to change can exacerbate an existing conflict by escalating a negative pattern of communication. The couple gets better and better at being worse and worse.

When Allie feels that Ogden has set himself up as her superior and evaluated her performance as both wife and mother, she withdraws from him verbally and emotionally, which upsets Ogden. After one particularly painful incident where Ogden critiqued her behavior toward their daughter, Allie withdrew in hurt and anger and started brooding over how unfair it was that Ogden criticized her but never turned his forever pointed finger at himself. She decided to teach him a lesson and refused to talk to Ogden at all. In that she had never before *completely* refused to talk to him, Allie's response to Ogden was new and different, but it was hardly a change in the pattern. Instead it was an intensification of the old pattern.

There is a mythical Danish village whose people are known for their goodness and tenacity on the one hand and their ignorance and stupidity on the other. Many wonderful stories are told about this group. In one particularly relevant story, some members of the group dig a well so they can have easily accessible fresh water. Although the well is successful, the well-digging project leaves behind an ugly pile of dirt. Wanting their project to be aesthetically pleasing as well as functionally successful, the villagers decide to get rid of the pile of dirt. They dig an appropriately sized hole and put the dirt from the well in the hole. Of course, what remains is the new dirt that was left over from digging the new hole. They dig another hole for that dirt but are again faced with the same problem. Once more they repeat their efforts but to no avail. How can they get rid of the remaining ugly pile of dirt? They consult their wise leader, who listens to their story carefully. He goes to the site of the dirt and studies the situation. Then he spends valuable time alone thinking about the problem. Finally, he announces the solution, which the whole village agrees is brilliant. The village will dig a huge hole, which is big enough to hold all the dirt!

DELIBERATE CHANGE STARTS WITH AWARENESS

To enact genuine change in your relationship, you must be aware of what is going on in your relationship. Chapter 13 showed how rules that ignore the importance of emotional context are doomed to failure. If you don't know your own story—the vulnerabilities and incompatibilities that have contributed to your conflicts and how the two of you have developed certain patterns, even vicious cycles of interaction, in a vain effort to solve your problem—you can simply make things worse rather than change your relationship for the better. You can fool yourself into thinking that you are doing something positive when you are not.

In-the-Moment Awareness

In Chapter 9 we taught you how to develop a true and workable story about your problem. The construction of that story should have helped you develop an awareness of your problem, which could enlighten your efforts to solve it. However, a broad awareness of your story may not be enough to help you make change. Unless you understand how your general story plays itself out in particular incidents, you will not see how your efforts at change are likely to be, and produce, more of the same. Awareness of the here and now, a sense of what is going on emotionally right now in this particular discussion with your partner, can foster genuine change.

One Saturday morning as Norman is putting away the breakfast dishes, Cheri asks in a nice voice, "Do you know when you'll be done with the garage?" Norman replies with annoyance, "I'll be done when I'm done." Cheri walks away without a word. About fifteen minutes later, Cheri approaches Norman again and asks politely, "Want to do our run now?" Norman looks at her incredulously and replies, "Not really." Cheri says sarcastically, "You're certainly in a great mood today," and she storms out of the room. Norman follows her and tries to apologize: "Don't get so upset. I just didn't feel like a run. Maybe we can do it later." Cheri locks the bedroom door from the inside. Norman yells in at her, "Damn it, I hate it when you do this."

To become more aware of what went on emotionally in this brief encounter, let's first consider the "general story" of this problem for Cheri and Norman. Cheri is far more invested than Norman in organization and order. She feels most comfortable when things are put away in their proper place. Although Norman has no objection to order in their household and even finds it helpful, disorder doesn't bother him as long as he can "kick back" in his easy chair and read. For him, rarely is the goal of a well-organized closet or shelves or drawers—or even an organized counter—worth the effort required to achieve it. So Norman's motivation for order is rarely enough to spur him into action. In contrast, Cheri often will put forth energy to keep the counter neat, to see to it clothes are in their right place, and so on. Yet she doesn't feel like she should have to do all the work while Norman sits and reads. What particularly upsets her is getting stuck with sorting and organizing his stuff. So Cheri resorts to encouragement, reminders, and prompts as a way of getting Norman more involved in keeping the house in order. Norman has grown sensitive to these gentle suggestions. He doesn't want to be the henpecked husband; nor does Cheri want to be the nagging wife. Yet without some intervention on her part, Norman won't take much action. Like with the garage, which he promised he would clean up.

To see how this general story plays out in this particular incident of the garage, we have to take a look not only at the words and actions of Cheri and Norman but also at the emotional communication that was part of those words and actions.

Words Spoken or Actions Taken	*Emotional Message*
CHERI (*nicely*): Do you know when you'll be done with the garage?	I want to remind you to work on the garage, but I don't want to cause an argument, so I am asking nicely.
NORMAN: I'll be done when I'm done.	I don't like to be nagged, even when you try to camouflage it with a nice exterior.
(*Cheri walks away.*)	Gosh, I try to be nice to you and you get irritated.

CHERI (*politely*): Want to do our run now?	I don't want us to fight today. I am trying to be conciliatory by suggesting that we do something we both enjoy. But my patience has its limits.
NORMAN (*incredulously*): Not really.	You nag me, which I hate, and then come in and act like nothing has gone on and we should just go on a run together. I don't get it.
CHERI (*sarcastically*): You're certainly in a great mood today. (*She storms out.*)	I try to be nice to you, and it just doesn't work. I'm angry. I'm done with you.
NORMAN (*follows her*): Don't get so upset. I just didn't feel like a run. Maybe we can do it later.	Oops! Now she's really upset. I hate that. I'll take back what I said. I'll do anything to appease her if she just won't go off in such an anger.
(*Cheri locks the bedroom door from the inside.*)	I'm really angry. This is over for me.
NORMAN (*yelling in at her*): Damn it, I hate it when you do this.	The day is ruined. There is no way I can pull her back. I'm angry and upset.

When you are aware of the emotional messages in a conversation, you have the option of openly expressing these messages. For example, Cheri might have opened the discussion by saying, "I don't want to be a nag or create an unpleasant scene between us, but I'm eager to have the garage cleaned." Or Norman might have said, no matter how Cheri started the discussion, "It bothers me when you remind me about something I've agreed to do." Because these comments are more direct and open, they have a better chance of success.

Awareness of emotional messages also allows each of you to acknowledge the other's reactions. Instead of proposing a run, Cheri might have said, "I bet you're annoyed that I mentioned the garage." If Cheri had proposed a run, as in the original exchange, Norman might have said, "I know you're trying to be nice and smooth over any tension between us by suggesting a run, but I just don't feel like it." This acknowledgment of what the other is experiencing can often prevent emotional escalation.

Third, awareness allows for the possibility of positive actions by either party. Knowing that Cheri was concerned about the garage yet not wanting to fuel an argument, Norman might have offered her a time line for completion. With the knowledge that Norman was upset about her mention of the garage, Cheri might have delayed her request for a run. Either of these actions might have prevented the emotional distress that followed.

The same benefits of in-the-moment awareness can be seen in a conversation that took place between Chan and Gwen one Saturday evening when they had no plans.

Chan looks through the cable TV guide and suggests a movie to watch. He reads the short description and notes, "I've heard it's supposed to be kind of sexy."

There is a long pause from Gwen. "It doesn't sound that interesting."

Chan replies with some disappointment in his voice, "Well, there's nothing much else on."

Gwen says, "You can watch it. I have reading I'd like to do."

"I was hoping we could do something together," Chan replies.

"We'll both be in the family room. Maybe I'll see if it's interesting."

Chan says "Great" sarcastically and leaves the room.

Gwen calls after him, "So if we can't do exactly what you want, then you're not happy?" Chan doesn't bother to reply.

We already know the general story of Chan and Gwen's issue with sex. Let's see how this conversation sent emotional messages that both failed to hear.

Words Spoken or Actions Taken	Emotional Message
CHAN (*reading the description of the movie*): I've heard it's supposed to be kind of sexy.	I hope this movie will put you in a sexy mood and we can make love.
GWEN: It doesn't sound that interesting to me.	I'm feeling pressure to have sex. I don't want you to get your hopes up.
CHAN (*with disappointment*): Well, there's nothing much else on.	I am disappointed. I wasn't insisting on sex, just hoping it might happen.

GWEN: You can watch it. I have reading I'd like to do.

I don't want you to be disappointed, but I don't want to feel pressured.

CHAN: I was hoping we could do something together.

I can't believe you won't even allow us the possibility of sexual intimacy.

GWEN: We'll both be in the family room. Maybe I'll see if it's interesting.

Okay. I'll allow for that possibility. But it's just a possibility.

CHAN (*sarcastically*): Great.

I'm getting upset. Let's forget the whole thing.

GWEN: So if we can't do exactly what you want, then you're not happy?

I'm angry. I offer you the possibility, and you reject it.

If Chan and Gwen were more aware of what was going on between them, they might be more open with their own emotional messages. For example, Chan might have opened the discussion by saying, "The movie is supposed to be sexy. Maybe it can put us in the mood for making love." Even if Chan had opened the conversation as he did, Gwen might have said, "When you describe a movie as sexy, I feel you're telling me you want us to make love afterward, and then I feel pressure and I start resisting that pressure."

Awareness would also enable them to acknowledge the other's reactions. At some point in the conversation, Chan might acknowledge that "I bet you feel pressure for sex when I propose a sexy movie." Or Gwen might acknowledge, "I think you're disappointed that I may be rejecting any possibility of sex tonight."

Awareness also opens the possibility for positive actions. Chan might decide not to comment on the movie's sexiness, knowing the effect that might have on Gwen. Or Gwen might make a humorous comment: "I'll watch the movie with you, but I'm going to keep my chastity belt handy."

Thus awareness of emotions makes it possible for *either* partner to acknowledge his or her own feelings *or* the other's feelings *or* to take actions that can change the course of their discussion. None of these alternative actions are foolproof ways of avoiding an ugly conflict, yet they often promote more constructive communication.

All of our examples of alternative actions that could avert conflict focused on the early stages of the discussion. Once emotions run high, partners may be too upset to be aware of the struggle going on between them. Or, even if aware, they may be too angry to take any constructive action. Once Cheri had locked herself in the bedroom, both she and Norman were too upset to be aware of what had led to their struggle, to be aware of what positive actions could lead them out of it, or even to be receptive to any positive actions by the other. They simply needed distance from each other to calm down.

To be fully aware, moment to moment, of what is going on emotionally during a discussion with your partner, even during the early stages of such a discussion, is an ideal goal. Typically, people have only limited awareness of their own emotions and even less awareness of their partners' emotions. Tension and conflict may further block awareness. We on the outside may see the emotional interplay between Cheri and Norman and the unspoken sexual dialogue between Chan and Gwen, but it is much more difficult for them to see it as it is happening. Any increment in their awareness of their "general story" and how it plays out in a particular incident provides them with more options to alter their usual pattern. But there are serious limits on their moment-to-moment awareness, as well as on our own.

Hindsight Awareness

Fortunately, awareness does not have to occur "in the moment" to be helpful. A retrospective awareness can aid us as well. Hindsight awareness may not be able to prevent a conflict from happening or even interrupt its course, but it can enable you to accept the conflict and recover from it more quickly. To illustrate, let's pick up Cheri and Norman's conflict where we left off.

Cheri is now locked in the bedroom, angry, and replaying in her head the scene she has just had with Norman. "I have no impact on him," she thinks. "I try to be nice to him, I approach him kindly and ask him a simple question about the garage, and he rejects me. Like a fool, I hang in there, try to be nice, invite him for a run, and he rejects me again. When am I going to learn? He has *no* consideration of my feelings. The only effect I can have with him is when I really blow up; then that gets his attention. So I have to be furious to get a response from my husband. Is this any kind of marriage?"

Norman also fumes over the conflict they have just had. "What's with her?," he wonders. "She nags me again, and then she can't stand it that I'm annoyed. I turn her down for a run, and she acts like I've committed murder. Now she's the one who acts hurt and angry. But she started it all!"

Thoughts and feelings like these will make it difficult for Norman and Cheri to recover from this conflict. Any discussion based on these internal experiences will further inflame their argument. If at some point after the conflict they became aware, even in hindsight, of what really happened between them, they might recover more easily and quickly. For example, if Norman realized that his procrastination created a problem for Cheri, or that her manner of asking and her proposal of a run were genuine efforts to be positive, or that he was being overly sensitive to reminders, then he might be more accepting of her behavior and of his own. Similarly, if Cheri realized that her reminders presented a problem for Norman, even when masked in kindness, or that she had difficulty tolerating rejection from him, or that he had difficulty with her emotional distress, she also might be more accepting of him and of herself. An awareness of any of these features of the conflict might have eased a return to normalcy by them both. Cheri might get over her anger and come out of the bedroom sooner with this hindsight awareness. Similarly, Norman might get over his anger sooner and initiate some reconciliation between them.

A few specific guidelines might help in achieving hindsight awareness. First, we (and our partners) are probably more blaming than we (or they) realize. During arguments, even during the most civil arguments, we may say things that reflect negatively on the other. Without ever calling each other names or engaging in character assassination or even raising our voices, we can manage to convey plenty of accusation and blame. Consider a conflict between a husband and wife about whether to visit her parents on the weekend. During the course of the discussion the husband might say, "Do we have to visit them again?"—implying that his wife already pushes them to visit more often than is reasonable. He might further ask, "Can't you manage without seeing them one weekend?"—implying that his wife is too dependent on her parents and can hardly survive psychologically without constant contact with them. She might be stung by these remarks, yet he may be unaware of how subtly aggressive they were. Similarly, she might ask during the discussion, "Can't we do what I want to do for at least one weekend?"—implying that he selfishly determines what they do and never accommodates her needs. In addition, she might offer during the discus-

sion, "I'm sure it will require a little unselfishness on your part to go"—
implying that he is very selfish and would have difficulty being even a little selfless. As with the husband's comments, these comments by his wife
may hurt and anger him, but she may be relatively unaware of their
accusatory power.

A second guideline for hindsight awareness is to remember that our
partners have their own side of the story, their own experience in the
conflict, and *it is a legitimate one.* Most of us could agree that each person in a conflict has his or her own take on it, but how can it be a legitimate position if it is diametrically opposed to ours? And how can it be a
legitimate position on those occasions when they are clearly in the
wrong? Won't their version simply be an excuse for their failure to do
what was right?

Let's consider an example in which one person is clearly in the
wrong: Sterling did nothing for Joyce's birthday—no card, no gift, no
acknowledgment, nothing. By most of our standards for thoughtfulness,
consideration, and love between spouses, we would judge that Sterling
had done wrong. Joyce's hurt and anger are justified. In fact, she is so
hurt and angry that she really doesn't want to hear anything from him,
because any explanation he might have would seem like an excuse.

But there is a story behind Sterling's failure to acknowledge Joyce's
birthday, and it is important for Joyce to be aware of it. Consider some
possibilities:

1. Sterling makes very little of events such as birthdays, anniversa-
ries, and the like. He has never been very good at remembering them. He
doesn't get upset if others forget his birthday (he often doesn't remember
himself), and so he can't understand why Joyce makes such a big deal
about it. He is not fully aware that even though birthdays don't mean
much to him, they are important to Joyce.

2. Sterling was very aware of Joyce's birthday. Yet he is furious at
her for several things she has done to him. He deliberately avoided any
action on her birthday because he wanted to hurt her as she had hurt
him.

3. Joyce's birthdays have been controversial for a long time. Sterling feels that no matter what he does, it is not good enough for Joyce.
The card he picks is funny rather than romantic. The gift he buys is too
practical. He is not clever enough to surprise her. Nothing he does seems
good enough. Sterling was aware of her birthday, didn't feel right about
buying her a romantic gift and card, knew she would resent anything

less, and didn't know how to resolve the problem. He avoided dealing with her birthday and got caught up with work right before it and genuinely forgot about it. Maybe at some level he was saying: If you don't like what I do for you, maybe I will do nothing for you.

Each of these stories is very different. None portrays Sterling in a positive light, but they all show the human side of his error. Each makes his action understandable, if not acceptable. Both Joyce and Sterling need to be able to understand his side as well as hers, so they can deal with the problem effectively. Of course, the first challenge will be for Sterling to voice his thoughts and feelings, without seeming like he's making an excuse or transferring blame to Joyce.

A third guideline for hindsight awareness follows from the second. If our partners' message does not make sense to us, if their story seems unconvincing, then we probably have no awareness of what is really going on with them. Maybe they have not been able to articulate their position. Maybe the message became too clouded with blame and accusation or with defensiveness. But whatever the reason, we are missing a major piece in the puzzle.

Carlisle has been without work for three months, ever since his company closed down. Because he has been unable to find a job, they and their two teenage daughters have survived on Janie's income. Janie does not understand why he has not been more aggressive in pursuing a job. It seems as if she is more concerned about his getting a job than he is. Does he want to be dependent on her? Does he lack the drive to get out there and fight for a job? She has begun to lose respect for him. She just doesn't understand what is going on.

For his part, Carlisle sees Janie not as an ally in his job search but as an adversary. She seems so cold and angry with him. She tries to control him. She comes home and demands an account of his performance. She feels the TV to see if it is warm. She wants to know how many calls he has made—a tally of his activities. Now he often refuses to answer her. Why should he have to answer to her? What is going on with her?

Because neither is aware of what is going on with the other, Carlisle and Janie have distanced themselves from each other. They are struggling individually with strong emotions, but they struggle in isolation. In this difficult situation, neither has the support of the person who cares for them the most.

What would each ideally convey to the other, even if they could not completely articulate it? What does each need to be aware of in the other?

Janie's message would be: I'm frustrated that you haven't found a job. That's probably obvious to you. But more than that, I'm anxious that you won't get a job. I fear for our financial future. I'm worried that we'll have to survive on my income alone. Then there will be no way for us to all fly back east and visit my parents, no way for us to pay for college for the girls. I'm not even sure we could continue to keep the house. In the face of these powerful and realistic fears, I need to see that you are concerned. I need reassurance that you also feel some urgency about the situation. When I don't get any information about what you're considering in terms of a job and what you've done, I get suspicious. I fear that you don't care about it. That you've done nothing. And then I go into my controlling mode—checking up on you, interrogating you about what you have done. I need information to calm my fears, and I'm not getting that from you.

Carlisle's message would be: Getting laid off and trying to find a new job is the most difficult crisis I have faced in a long time. I have lost confidence in myself, and I don't think I have all the technological skills I need to make it in a new job. I have to struggle with myself every day to motivate myself to take some action. I definitely avoid action because I don't feel up to it, because I anticipate another failure. And if I can motivate myself, I must also struggle with the various employment bureaus and personnel officers and counselors. And if that's not enough, I also have to struggle with you. I hate it when you check up on me, when you interrogate me about what I've done, when I see disgust all over your face. It makes me feel worse about myself.

In the heat of their struggle, neither Carlisle nor Janie could articulate their positions as clearly as we have laid them out. Nor could they fully understand each other's position in the midst of their conflict—even if they each could articulate their positions. However, any communication that either could make that approximated their position, even if made after a struggle—a hindsight communication—would be helpful for them because it might increase their awareness of their predicament. Even without communication, each might be able to achieve some increment in hindsight awareness simply by thinking through the problem on his or her own.

Carlisle and Janie face two problems. There is the initial problem of Carlisle finding a job. But now there is the reactive problem of their struggle about this job. Because the initial problem is so difficult, they may not be able to solve it without first solving the reactive problem. In other words, Carlisle may not be able to find a job, or at least find it as quickly, if he is in a struggle with Janie. He may not be able to fight a battle on two fronts: one for a job and the other with Janie.

The advantage of any gains in hindsight awareness by either Janie or Carlisle is that it may lessen their interpersonal struggle. If Janie understood what Carlisle was experiencing, she might change in any number of ways. She might be less angry with him or less cold toward him. She might not monitor him so closely. Or she might be more positive in her dealings with him and more forgiving about his difficulty in motivating himself. She might be able to encourage or support him in ways that really did motivate him. If Carlisle understood what Janie is experiencing, he also might change in any number of ways. He might feel some strength, even be empowered, if he could assure her that her financial fears would not turn into reality. He might make a stronger, more consistent effort to find work. He might be more forgiving of her efforts to control the situation.

If we follow these three guidelines for hindsight awareness—that we may have been more blaming than we realize, that our partners have a legitimate position, and that we may not understand that position—then we may be able to accept our arguments and recover more quickly from them. We may be able to return to a discussion that erupted in argument. Our hindsight awareness can enable us both to accept the struggle we are in and to pursue a more effective path toward its resolution.

RECAP

Efforts to change a relationship, whether by an outside therapist or by ourselves, may have unintended consequences. Instead of creating change, our efforts may simply be more of the same. In fact, we can create a situation that is a worse version of the same old problem. To prevent our well-intentioned efforts from falling into these traps, we need awareness of what is going on between us. A good starting point is awareness of the story of our problem, elaborated in Chapter 9. Then we can see how the general story of our problem plays itself out in everyday interactions; we become mindful of the emotional communication in our discussions with each other. This awareness shows us options for altering the course of our conflicts, sometimes preventing them or at least minimizing their impact and facilitating recovery from them. Although such in-the-moment awareness is often difficult to achieve, a hindsight awareness of what went on between us can also help by facilitating acceptance of an argument, a quicker recovery from that argument, and motivation to pursue a more productive discussion.

Exercise

It's easier to start with hindsight awareness than with in-the-moment awareness. Look back at a recent argument. Can you see how the general story of your problem played itself out in this particular argument?

- How were each of you more blaming than you may have realized at the time?
- What were the main messages that each of you was unable to get across to the other?

Now try to achieve a greater in-the-moment awareness. When you're beginning to sense that an argument may be coming on but before things are really heated, try holding back a moment and questioning yourself.

- What is going on with me emotionally at this moment?
- What may be going on emotionally with my partner at this moment?
- Try to express directly what is going on with you.
- See if you can listen to what may be going on with your partner.

CHAPTER 15

Lost Battles
Can Win the War

HOW CHANGE AND INTIMACY
CAN EMERGE FROM DEFEAT

*D*efeat is inevitable for those seeking change—as the last three chapters have demonstrated. Good advice is bad for us because it doesn't consider the emotional context of our conflicts. Rational rules become nonsensical because they fall into the trap captured by W. C. Fields, whose advice for conquering insomnia was "Get plenty of sleep." New approaches to each other are unmasked as simply more of the same old behavior because it's so hard for us to recognize how our relationship story comes into play in every encounter between us. Even when we do everything right, our partners may have good reasons for not responding well to our efforts to change them.

Now for the good news: Being prepared to accept lack of change opens up a wealth of opportunities for transforming your relationship into the peaceful, intimate union you've wanted all along. When you accept the failure of your efforts, you head off arguments about the change you believe should have occurred. Your partner may even respond to your acceptance in ways that lessen the need for change. Finally, you may end up less discouraged and frustrated than if you had been intractable, which may open you up to pursuing other, more successful avenues of change.

In this chapter we shift our attention from anticipating failure to change to taking positive steps to prevent it or profit from it. Instead of better rules for communicating and behaving, we will offer flexible guidelines that incorporate acceptance of whatever may come and that bend to accommodate your unique circumstances.

With this forgiving, adaptable, accepting approach, you can succeed in bringing about improvement in your relationship whether any particular effort to make change succeeds or fails. You can win even when you lose.

TO CHANGE YOUR RELATIONSHIP, FIRST CHANGE YOURSELF

As you've now seen many times, most efforts to improve relationships are directed at changing our partners. A fundamental shift occurs when we focus on changes *we* can make rather than on changes *they* can make. Rather than implying that we are culpable for whatever problems exist, this shift acknowledges that we have direct control over and responsibility for our own behavior alone. Likewise, only our partners have direct control over and responsibility for their behavior. It is empowering to know that we can make a change, rather than waiting in frustration for our partners to make a change.

Gerda appreciated Nat for his many fine qualities. He was a good man: honest, generous, hard-working, and committed to the family. She knew he loved her and would never be unfaithful to her. Yet some of his difficulties in communication were frustrating to her. He often didn't listen to her, he was easily distracted when she talked to him, and he would interrupt her in midsentence.

She first tried to talk to him about the problem. At times he would acknowledge the problem; at other times he would defend himself. But nothing seemed to change, so Gerda bought him a book on communication. With some persistent prodding on her part, Gerda got him to read a few chapters. He acknowledged some valuable points in the book, but again his behavior did not seem to change. Finally, Gerda proposed they go to a communication training class that was offered through the local college extension program. But Nat put his foot down at that point. The class was not held on a good night for him. Furthermore, he was tired of her constant complaints about his "inability to communicate." She should just accept him for what and how he was.

That confrontation precipitated a minor depression for Gerda. She didn't want to break up the marriage over some seemingly simple problems in communication. Yet these problems were a daily frustration to her that dimmed the value of Nat's more positive qualities and eroded her positive feelings for him. In her despair over the problem, she withdrew from Nat. This prompted more attention and concern on his part; he really wanted her to be happy. Gerda responded to his attention, became more engaged with him, but knew their problems wouldn't go away.

At this point, a fundamental shift occurred for Gerda. In her frustration over the possibility of never effecting a change in Nat, she decided that she could stop one annoying event from happening: his habit of continuing to watch TV or trying to read the newspaper while he listened to her. In the past when she had complained about this diversion of his attention, he would argue that he could listen to her and still keep one ear turned to the TV or one eye on the newspaper. So the TV stayed on and the newspaper remained in his lap.

Mustering her courage, one evening Gerda told Nat she wanted to talk to him but wanted the TV off and the newspaper off his lap before she did. He was annoyed by the request and launched into his argument that he could easily do two things at once. He recalled a previous occasion where she had accused him of not listening but where he had proven to her that he could recall everything that she had just said even though he had been glancing at the TV. Because Gerda had carefully considered her approach to him and had already anticipated his reaction, she was prepared for this argument. She accepted his point but made her request anyway: "You may be able to listen to me and watch TV or read the newspaper, but it is uncomfortable for me. I would prefer to have your undivided attention when I have something important to say."

She had added the word *important* to justify her position, which she felt might be too extreme. However, that word served to stimulate Nat's curiosity. He argued with her a bit, but when he became convinced that she would not be swayed, he turned the TV off with annoyance and said, "All right, what is it?" Gerda persisted that he needed to put the newspaper aside also. Frustrated, he threw the newspaper on the table, but he was all attention. Intimidated by his anger, she told him of an event that had happened at work that day, trying to make it as interesting as possible. At the end of her story, he commented sarcastically, "Well, that was certainly worth turning off the TV and putting aside the newspaper." He went back to his TV. Gerda went upstairs and cried.

Because this first incident had gone so badly, Gerda almost gave up her struggle with Nat over the TV and newspaper. However, she knew that getting Nat to change his habits would not be easy, and she told herself that she was worth getting his full attention. She persisted with her plan; she would only greet him and exchange minimal information while he was involved with his TV and newspaper. She would request time to talk to him without either. Sometimes he refused or delayed any conversation. There were also frustrating times when he would turn off the TV and put away the newspaper with resentment or argue with her about her position. But gradually they established a new pattern in which he listened to her without the distractions of the TV or newspaper.

Even during these diversion-free conversation times there were problems. Sometimes Nat's attention would wander, particularly if Gerda went on and on. At times she was so needy for conversation time with Nat that, given his undivided attention, she would luxuriate in it, without thought to what he was experiencing. Also, he would often interrupt her and talk over her. In an attempt to deal with these problems, Gerda tried to curb her tendency toward monologue. She also decided to confront Nat's interruptions directly.

Gerda was so accustomed to Nat's interruptions and so used to yielding to them that she often was not aware of them at the time. Only later in the conversation, as her frustration with being unable to voice her ideas increased, did she realize that he had been interrupting her. Then sometimes she would criticize him for his interruptions, he would defend himself, and an argument would ensue. Only as she became aware of his interruptions at the moment of their occurrence was she able to intervene in ways that allowed her to prevent the interruption but without creating an argument. She would say, "Wait. I'm not finished yet," or "Excuse me. You interrupted me. I am not done." These comments would often allow her to continue her communication to Nat.

Needless to say, Nat was not particularly pleased with these comments. They were interrupting his interruptions. Even though they did not necessarily create an argument, he was frustrated by her efforts. He would let her continue with what she had to say, but he was often irritated at her comments. Although Gerda wavered at times in her efforts, wondering if she had a right to be so insistent, questioning if it was worth dealing with Nat's negative reactions, feeling guilty for upsetting the status quo between them, she persisted. She counseled herself: Of course he is going to react negatively, I am upsetting his usual style. But I have a right to be fully heard by him.

A turning point came, paradoxically, when she was so frustrated with the tension her efforts created that she was ready to give up. She burst out to Nat: "I really don't want to create tension between us, but I am in such a bind. I can let you interrupt me and keep peace, but then I feel bad about myself, that my ideas are not worth your attention. Or I can stop your interruptions and complete my thoughts, but then I create tension between us. Neither way seems to work."

Because her emotions and words rang so true, Nat heard her message. He was sympathetic to her position. Surprisingly, he encouraged her in her efforts, and he tried to interrupt her less often.

Dealing with his interruptions in public created different challenges for Gerda than dealing with them in private. She feared creating a scene; she didn't want their friends to detect tension between them. But after achieving some success in stopping his interruptions in private, she went public with her efforts. At first she intervened cautiously, almost apologetically, when he interrupted her in public. The tension that her action created was painful for her. What she had not anticipated and what was even more difficult for her was seeing the hurt look on his face when she stopped him.

Over time, Gerda's efforts paid off. Nat would not only attend to her without TV and a newspaper as distractions, he would also interrupt her less. Occasionally he surprised her by stopping himself in mid-interruption and letting her finish her comments. Although he would never make it to the "Listeners' Hall of Fame," he did listen to her more attentively. He changed in some very clear and concrete ways—but only because Gerda had changed first.

Although Gerda was not blameless—she had a tendency to ramble in her conversation—most of this problem was clearly in Nat's corner. It would have been easy for Gerda to persist in trying to get him to change his inconsiderate ways. In changing her own behavior, Gerda not only had to get over her self-righteousness, she had to face her own doubts, fears, and frustrations; she had to deal with Nat's negative reactions; and finally she had to deal with the repeated failure of her efforts. At first it seemed unfair that the burden for change fell on her, the one who was in the right, but toward the end, as she started to see Nat changing gradually, the experience was empowering for her. She did not have to wait—impatiently—until he changed. She could take matters into her own hands.

Perhaps more important than the specific changes Nat made, though, were the changes that occurred in their relationship. Because a frequent source of his resentment diminished, Gerda felt more positive about Nat, she was able to be lighter with him, and he responded in kind. Also, because Nat was now more attentive to Gerda—she had insisted that he be so—he adapted more to her feelings and opinions. Thus Gerda felt more important to Nat and he in turn became more important to her. The "little" changes that Gerda had made created "little" changes in Nat, but in combination they had large ripple effects on their relationship, enhancing their intimacy with each other.

DO LESS OF THE SAME—AND MORE OF THE DIFFERENT

There is always the danger that change, even a change in ourselves, will turn out to be more of the same—that what seems new is really but a variation of the old. Awareness of what is happening in the relationship—awareness of the "story" you composed and have been using since Chapter 9—can prevent this kind of false change. With awareness of what is going on, you can then make a genuine effort to do something different.

In the previous section, we urged you to change yourself first. In this section, we urge you to change yourself by doing something truly different. In the sections that follow, we target specific areas where you can do something different.

Rather Than Complain and Criticize, Take Constructive Action

A common trap in relationships is to get caught in the pattern of complaining or criticizing your partner about a problem but doing nothing else about it, even though constructive action could change it. To paraphrase a line from Eleanor Roosevelt, some would curse the darkness rather than light a candle.

In trying to create change in communication, it was easy for Gerda to complain *after* Nat had tuned her out and turned on the TV or to complain *after* he had interrupted her. But her complaints only created arguments without ensuring the changes she wanted. What was harder for Gerda—and would be for most of us—to do was to intervene at the moment rather than complain afterward. She had to push herself to ask Nat to turn the TV off and to put the newspaper aside before she talked to him. She had to become aware of Nat's interruptions as they occurred so she could intervene at the time of an interruption and thus prevent it.

Let's consider another example of constructive action rather than complaints. Zack is upset over how controlling Samantha is. Everything has to go her way or, in Zack's words, she "throws a fit." She is adept at managing the situation so that the only reasonable alternative seems to be the action she desires. It is easy for Zack to grumble about Samantha, to say sarcastically, "I guess we should do what you want to do—because you never get your way," or to whine, "Let's do it your way again." In a calm moment, not near the scene of any relevant incident, he is even able to bring up the problem of her control as an issue to be discussed. Samantha usually ignores his sarcasm and whining. When he brings the problem up for discussion, she usually tries to justify her position.

It is hard for Zack to state his desires constructively and to push for them assertively in the moment of decision making. Samantha usually has a blueprint for their activities before Zack has thought of an alternative. Because everyday decisions are so much more important to Samantha than to Zack, she can trump his casual predilection with her decided preference.

Although any particular decision is usually not that important to Zack, his cumulative lack of influence *is* important to him. To alter this pattern, Zack will have to decide when to push his own preference and when to go along with Samantha's. On the one hand, he doesn't want to precipitate a struggle over an issue that matters little to him. On the other hand, if he just defers to Samantha because the decisions are not important to him, then he feels bad about her, because she is so controlling, and bad about himself, because he lets himself be controlled. Once he decides to push for his preferences, he has to confront her questioning and resistance. "Do you really want to do that? It's so boring." He also may have to confront realistic limitations on what he can do, limitations that are sometimes exacerbated by Samantha's careful planning. For example, one Saturday morning they were driving to visit friends a couple of hours away when Zack saw a scenic area he wanted to stop and visit briefly. Samantha explained that she had told their friends they would arrive by noon for lunch so there was no time for this detour. To take the detour he wants, Zack would have to call the friends and make a potentially disruptive, last-minute alteration of the plans Samantha had made without his input. Of course, she makes plans without him because he often shows little interest in them at the time.

To follow the guideline in this section, Zack will need increased awareness of his own desires and increased involvement in Samantha's planning so that he can see to it that he gets more of what he wants rather than complain, after the fact, about not getting his needs met. It won't be easy, but it will probably be worth the trouble. When Zack feels powerless in the relationship, he feels bad about himself and angry with Samantha. He withdraws from her, which exacerbates her own feeling that she has to go it alone in the relationship, and deprives them both of the intimacy they desire. Any movement that Zack made toward developing greater awareness and asserting his own desires would be a step toward altering their dilemma. Furthermore, if Zack could discuss his feelings about the problem, emphasizing his own sense of powerlessness rather than Samantha's controllingness, he might find her an ally rather than an adversary in their struggle.

Do Something Positive for Your Partner— with No Strings Attached

When partners are in conflict, much of the daily positive attention they normally give each other may cease. Therefore many advice givers urge us to make a point of extending to our partners the little courtesies and considerations, the tokens of appreciation and affection, that we have been denying each other out of anger and resentment. Unfortunately, this advice falls into the W. C. Fields category: If we could follow the advice, we wouldn't have the problem; if we have the problem, we can't follow the advice. As we saw in Chapter 13, our hurt and anger over our partners' offenses may make following such advice all but impossible. Either we can't give these gifts freely or we can't face the way they might be received. For this reason, positive gestures toward your partner should probably not be offered unless you can make them without requiring your partner to respond in kind—without, in fact, predicating your action on any kind of response at all. The most powerful positive act is offered in the context of acceptance—an acceptance of your partner's negative feelings, which may lead him or her to reject your positive action. When your positive gestures are made independent of your partner's reaction, they remain positive no matter what the response.

After a particularly unpleasant confrontation, Samantha says to Zack, "I know that I can be controlling and hard to deal with at times. I just want to say that I love you a lot and I am willing to work on this or any other problem." This statement acknowledges her own role in their problems, assures him of her love, and indicates her willingness to work on the problem. We could hardly imagine a more positive gesture. However, Zack may be too upset to respond in kind. He may be suspicious of her positive response and test it. He might reply angrily: "Well, you have finally acknowledged some responsibility. Now what are you going to do about it?"

If Samantha reacts to his negative reaction, they are back into another argument. If she can accept his negative reaction, perhaps because she has some compassion for his struggle with her, she may say: "I know you are angry now. Maybe we should talk later, but I want you to know that I do understand your feelings." Granted, these positive words would require considerable strength on Samantha's part. But when she offers them to Zack, she is giving the only genuine gift—one that comes without strings. If Zack takes a moment to review this interchange later, he may very well be touched by his wife's generosity and courage. In fact, it would be difficult for him not to be affected by a positive action that withstood even his own attempts to test it. Her simple unencumbered gesture toward him could in time lead to a powerful reconciliation between them. Beyond the resolution of their immediate conflict, her message communicates to Zack that she hears his. She gets it. As a result, he may have less need for protective distance from her.

Do What Your Partner Has Been Asking You to Do

One clue about what we can do that is really different, that is not more of the same, lies in our partners' complaints. What they accuse us of not doing, what they demand that we do more of, may include prescriptions for constructive action on our part.

As an example, let's consider a conflict between Enrique and Rosa about childcare and housework. She complains, with considerable justification, that he does not take his share of the responsibility for childcare and housework. He complains that she insists childcare and housework be done to her exacting standards and that she does not acknowledge his contributions. A simple, positive action that he could take would be to do what she has been asking him to do: get more involved in childcare and housework. Because of his flair for the dramatic and surprising, he decides to offer Rosa a complete Saturday off. He will take care of the children, and she can have the day to herself.

This seemingly simple, positive action could, however, be complicated for Enrique to implement. First, he has to deal with his own feelings that making such a positive gesture to her will indicate weakness, that he has given in to her and that his position has no validity. A second challenge for him is to make his offer of a Saturday off without a grudge on the one hand or martyrdom or heroism on the other. If he comes in with an attitude that smacks of "You've been complaining so much, I guess I'll finally do something to shut you up," he won't get a good reception for his offer, and his offer, contaminated by his resentment, will just lead to another argument.

Third, Enrique may also need to be prepared for skepticism and suspicion. Rosa may not know what to make of his offer, and therefore may not respond to his first effort with wild appreciation. Fourth, he may face some practical obstacles. Maybe the Saturday that he wants to "give her" doesn't work for her. Finally, Rosa may have difficulty "letting go" for a whole day, perhaps because she feels guilty about being away from the kids or feels guilty that Enrique is taking the entire burden this Saturday. Just because she genuinely wants him to take more responsibility doesn't mean that she can easily give up that responsibility herself.

Even if Enrique and Rosa meet all of these challenges, some unexpected comment by one or the other could rock their precarious boat of genuine change. Let's say he makes the offer of a free Saturday for Rosa, she takes him up on it, and he carries it off well. On her return home, he shares his experience with her. Perhaps he had some difficulty with the kids and now has a greater realization of how challenging it can be to spend a whole day with them. He recounts his difficulties and his frustration and says, "Now I know more what you mean about how hard it is to take care of them for hours on end and keep your sanity at the same time."

Rosa may feel guilty about being gone all day. She may anticipate that he will use this day against her—that he will hold it up as evidence of what he does for the kids, that this one day will invalidate all her charges of noninvolvement. As a result, she may jump on his expression of frustration. "Well, now you know how difficult it can be. Maybe from now on you will be a little more sympathetic with me and offer to help more than once in a blue moon."

If Enrique were strong, he might hold on to the positive change and not be drawn into an argument: "I know it is difficult. And I plan to get more involved. Today was just a start, but it was a genuine start." However, after a day with the kids, this might be too much to ask. He responds to her provocative comment with an angry retort: "I can't believe it. Here I spend the whole day with the kids and all you can do is jump on me."

She responds: "Well, you think one day is all you need to do. So your work with the kids is done for the year, right?" And an argument is off and running.

However, this argument need not signal the white flag of defeat; it need not destroy the positive effort to change. A couple can salvage an argument and recover the thrust of change. After this unpleasant argument, Rosa mulls over her day alone and the fight they have just had. She achieves some hindsight awareness of what has just happened. She realizes that her husband did make a genuine effort and that she, out of her own anxieties, used his expression of frustration against him. Although she still has her fears about what one day of action on his part will mean, she apologizes to him. She expresses appreciation for what he has done.

Enrique's actions show Rosa that not only has he heard her message, but that he is willing to take constructive action about her message. Her apology shows him that she is willing to admit error and to acknowledge his efforts. Those actions could do more than start them on the difficult road to changing responsibility for childcare. They are the kinds of actions, even when born out of argument, that can foster appreciation and closeness with each other.

TAKE BETTER CARE OF YOURSELF

> A handful of guilt is better than a truckload of resentment.
>
> —PROVERB

Our genuine desire to protect our partners' feelings may make us conceal our own feelings and curb our behavior that hurts their feelings. Although these loving acts of protection may ensure peace in the short term, if extensive, they may create resentment in us that, ironically, generates more distress than had we not been so protective. If we took better care of ourselves, we might have to deal with conflict in the short run, but we might increase our satisfaction over the long run.

In our sexual relationship, for example, we may forfeit potential pleasure rather than risk injury or embarrassment to our partners. To mention that something feels uncomfortable or that we need a slower pace might upset our partners or create tension in our relationship. To ask for some action that might arouse us could embarrass our partners and ourselves. Our sexual relationship could be disrupted. Our effort to improve our sex life could backfire and make things worse. So we endure discomfort or forgo pleasure to preserve what we have. We pass up opportunities to improve our own, and ultimately our partners', level of sexual satisfaction.

Although our sexual relationship is often a particularly sensitive area in which we may protect our partners' feelings, we can do so in almost any area. For example, you may be watching a TV show that interests you, but your partner interrupts you to tell you something. Not wanting to hurt your partner's feelings, you do not say honestly, "I really want to watch this show. Can you tell me later?" Instead, you give your partner half your attention, leave the other half focused on the TV, and feel vaguely resentful. Meanwhile, your partner may feel irritated at the less-than-full attention you provide.

These examples are not meant to oversimplify. Voicing your wishes may create hurt feelings, generate tension, or precipitate an argument. The distress may not be worth the freedom of expression. Because your partners' feelings do matter to you, it may be better to suppress your reactions and let the situation pass under certain circumstances. A useful guideline, like taking better care of yourself, can never substitute for good judgment.

When a problem comes up repeatedly, however, confrontation may be better than protection. Cara would like to spend more time away from Matthew. She enjoys a few hours shopping by herself and would like to go out with her friends without Matthew more often than she does. In contrast, Matthew prefers doing things with Cara and will adjust his schedule to go with her on every occasion, from social events to errands. Cara usually does not have the heart to tell him she wants to do her shopping alone or that she would prefer to go on her errand by herself. So he tags along, and she finds herself mildly irritated by his presence. Her only solution so far is to be slightly devious: she times her errands for when he is away or seems too busy to join her, or she makes up excuses for not taking Matthew along when she gets together with a friend. She feels slightly guilty about these deceptions, and then she gets angry at Matthew for putting her in this defensive position. But to take better care of herself and assert her right to independent activity would mean doing things that would hurt Matthew's feelings, which in turn would mean more guilt for Cara. It might also precipitate an argument or spur Matthew to withdraw in resentment.

There is no easy way for Cara to resolve her need for independence. But by taking the more devious avenue—carefully timing her errands or her shopping, offering half-truths about what she and her friends are going to do—she forces herself to repeat these measures every time she wants some time without Matthew. Confronting Matthew more directly about her needs would require her to handle his emotional responses and her own, but in time genuine change might take place. A new pattern of greater independence for her in their relationship could emerge.

Cara might start by discussing her concerns with Matthew. It would be important for her to focus on her desire for time apart from Matthew rather than on any presumed deficiency in him, such as his insecurity. If the conversation emphasizes his inadequacies rather than her desire for independence, it will almost surely fail. However Cara approaches the subject, Matthew will certainly be hurt by it. At some level, he will see her desire for more independence as a rejection of him. He may well try to reframe her desire for independence as lack of love, or he may withdraw and sulk in a guilt-inducing way. It will be a challenge for Cara to maintain both that she does love him *and* that she needs more independence from him. It may help for Cara to share her own vulnerabilities with him: her guilt about hurting him, the appeal his constant presence had for her early in their relationship, her fear that this issue may dampen her love for him. It is possible for them to be allies rather than adversaries in this effort.

Whether Cara starts with a "heart-to-heart" discussion or not, the real challenge for her will come in the everyday decisions about how to spend her time. She will need to tell Matthew in so many words "I want to go shopping by myself today" or "I want to spend some time alone with Candace." Undoubtedly, she will have to deal with some negative reactions on his part. At times she may decide not to push the issue; at times she may need to reassure him that greater independence is not her only goal. At other times, despite their best efforts, her actions may precipitate an argument.

If Cara persists in this struggle, she will achieve her immediate goal of more time apart from Matthew. However, she may achieve much more. Once she has more independence and feels less guilt about achieving it, she may find that she values her contact with Matthew even more. Rather than tolerating his contact with mild irritation, she may enjoy his company. Although Matthew may find the initial rejection from Cara painful, he may end up with a more loving and appreciative partner. He may decide that a smaller portion of a genuine Cara is worth a greater portion of a half-hearted Cara. Furthermore, her insistence on greater independence may force him to reevaluate his own dependence on her and his connection with other friends and family.

Genuine change threatens conflict, but it offers the potential for greater personal growth and increased intimacy.

MINIMIZE DAMAGE

Love puts us in harm's way. Although physicians try to follow the adage "First do no harm," lovers cannot. Because we care so much about our partners, who are different from us in what they want and think and feel, they will inevitably do things that disappoint, sadden, hurt, and anger us. They will, of course, also do things that excite, please, relax, and gladden us. But pain will always be part of the picture of love.

One important feature of good relationships is "pain management" and "damage control." Partners in any long-term relationship inevitably will experience tension and distress. The challenge is to contain these experiences, to prevent them from escalating out of control. An argument, a disappointment, a misunderstanding can create hurt and angry feelings that escalate into damaging statements ("I never really loved you") or intimidating threats ("I am going to leave you and this relationship"). These are the kinds of damaging words and actions we want to prevent. The following guidelines are designed to control damage.

If You Can't Get Your Message Across, Change the Medium

It may be impossible to talk constructively about some issues with your partner. A controversial topic may have such a history of conflict that neither of you can bring it up without tension. The mere mention of the topic can initiate a chain of emotional arousal that leads to an impasse.

You can change the circumstances of your discussion. You may bring up the topic when both of you are calm. You may talk about the topic when you both are at a restaurant, where neither of you would want to make a scene. You may talk on the phone since the extra distance that comes with a phone call may prevent the escalation of your emotions. All of these strategies are reasonable attempts to create a setting where constructive discussion may take place. However, if they are unsuccessful, a more dramatic change may be necessary.

You can change the medium of your message. Rather than talking in person or on the phone, you can write a note, send an e-mail, leave a voice-mail message, or make an audio or video recording. This change in the medium may catch your partner's attention, particularly if you don't normally communicate this way. Your partner may be intrigued by getting a note, an e-mail, or a tape from you. Changing the medium also allows you to say your piece without feedback or interruption. You will not be deterred by your partner's looks of annoyance, thrown off by his or her attempts to "correct" your version of events, or riled up by the rolling of her or his eyes. You can also deliver a more considered, thoughtful, and deliberate statement of your position. You can prepare what you're going to say, deleting a phrase that doesn't seem right or erasing a section of tape that may be inflammatory. If you use the written word, there will be no angry voice tones or tense facial cues to distract from your message. Finally, if your partner chooses to respond in kind, he or she will enjoy some of the same benefits: freedom of expression without feedback or interruption and the opportunity to prepare a more thoughtful response. As a result, the process of communication may be less accusatory and less defensive. The change in medium may change the message.

When Discussion Deteriorates into Argument, Focus on Emotions Rather Than Content

Listen for the melody, not the words.

Tara and Ned are discussing their summer vacation in California. Although she is not fully aware of it, Tara is feeling increasingly irritated that Ned is taking over the discussion and the planning of the trip. He mentions that they can easily drive in one day from Los Angeles to San Francisco. She strenuously objects.

TARA: No, we can't drive from LA to San Francisco in a day.

NED: Of course we can. People do it all the time in less than a day.

TARA: No they don't. Unless they're race car drivers.

NED: Look. You're no judge of distance and time. We can take the 5 freeway; it's only a few hundred miles!

TARA: Bullshit! It's more like 500 miles. And is that your idea of a vacation—driving on a freeway?

NED: My idea of a vacation is to get where you want to go as quickly as possible.

TARA: Well, I may want to take the scenic coastal route.

NED: Great, then we can spend all our vacation in the car.

In this example Tara and Ned focus on details—the distance between LA and San Francisco and whether to take the inland or the coastal route—but ignore the growing tension between them that will prevent them from ever coming to a decision. Like the story of the family who has an elephant in their living room but never discusses it, they ignore the powerful emotional interplay going on between them and focus only on the superficial details of their discussion.

In *The Talk Book*, my colleague at UCLA, Jerry Goodman, offers the following advice: "When in trouble, self-disclose on the double." Statements such as "I am beginning to feel tense" or "I dread where this conversation seems to be going" or "I think we are getting stuck" can shift a conversation away from its often superficial content to its more important emotional tone. A self-disclosure can put the emphasis on the melody in a conversation rather than the words. With this attention to emotion, it is possible to calm the discussion rather than inflame it further. Or at least postpone the discussion until a later time when emotions are calmer. Let's see how this might happen.

TARA: I'm not sure why, but I'm getting really irritated by this conversation.

NED: I can tell.

TARA: Well, you're not exactly Mister Calm.

NED: That's true. I'm frustrated too. I have this incredible urge to get an encyclopedia and prove to you that LA and San Francisco are less than 500 miles apart.

TARA (*smiling*): Please don't. Even if you were right, you'd win the battle but lose the war. Because I might refuse to go to California with you at all.

By talking about her emotional state, Tara was able to stop the escalation of emotion and inject some welcome lightness into their discussion.

Like all interpersonal advice, this advice comes with no guarantees. It is hardly a surefire solution to tension-filled talk. One danger is that we will comment on our partners rather than disclose about ourselves.

Statements such as "You're overreacting to this whole thing" and "Why are you getting so angry?" change the focus from the content of the discussion to the emotional tone of the discussion. However, rather than disclosing how we're feeling, they make a judgmental evaluation of how our partners are feeling. Furthermore, even if we make a genuine disclosure about our own emotional state, we may imply that our partners are to blame for causing those emotions. For example, the comment "I'm getting really frustrated" can be made as simply a statement of one's emotions or with an overtone of "and you are such a jerk for making me frustrated." Even when we do it right—we are getting tense in a conversation so we change the focus from the content of our discussion to the emotions we are feeling—our partners may be so distressed themselves that they ignore what we have said and barge forward with their own points.

When All Else Fails, Take a Time-Out

There comes a point in arguments when nothing good will happen. Emotions are too high. Your partner is not listening, and neither are you. The looks and words that pass between you are only angry condemnations. It's time for a "time-out," a break in the communication where you can get out of each other's presence. You may mentally rehash the argument and get more inflamed, but at least the destructive comments have stopped. And eventually you will calm down. The retreat offered by a time-out can be a victory for the relationship.

Time-out is widely advocated because it has the compelling logic of a cease-fire. The first constructive act is to stop the fighting. And implementation seems simple: Just part company. Leave the immediate scene. Don't talk to each other until you're both calmer.

Of course, nothing is that simple between lovers, and time-out is no exception. It may be overused by those who want to avoid conflict and resisted by those who prefer to push ahead at all costs. And whether time-out is effective depends to a great extent on how it's initiated. The initiation itself can contain a heavy accusation, as in "You're getting hysterical, so I'm going to take a time-out" or "I can't talk to someone who is unreasonable, so I'm going to leave until you calm down." Or time-out can be the punctuation following a telling point or a dramatic summary of our position, which is precisely the wrong timing for our partners. It leaves us with the last word and our partners recoiling from our final shot. Not surprisingly, they may not cooperate with our proposal.

We can initiate a time-out with hints that it may be more than temporary or with the overt statement or covert implication that we will refuse to talk about this topic ever again. Or we can simply leave the scene, insulting and confusing our partners with our sudden departure.

Perhaps the best way to think about time-out is as a self-protective strategy for use in cases of failed discussions. If you view time-out as a way of taking care of yourself and the relationship when you're too upset to be reasonable or constructive, you're less likely to invoke it accusatorily or to use it to get in the last word. Even if your partner is the one who is hysterical, while you are still able to be reasonable, you can use time-out as a self-protective strategy. Sometimes when your partner is very upset, you can act in ways that soothe and comfort, but when the hysteria is directed at you, engaging with your partner will only upset you too. So calling a time-out still delivers the same message: I cannot act constructively in this current situation. I want a time-out as a way of protecting myself and our relationship.

When you view time-out in this way, you may become more respectful of your partner's needs for self-protection and thus more accommodating when your partner calls a time-out. Rather than preventing your partner from leaving the room or following your partner, you will allow him or her privacy and freedom of movement.

When you use time-out appropriately, you acknowledge a mutual failure: neither of you was successful at making the conversation constructive. This acceptance of failure, however, can prevent further damaging escalation in the argument. Furthermore, it allows you to recover more quickly from the argument and renew your efforts to relate to each other. Your acceptance of failure can plant the seeds of later success.

Conflict is a window on both the best and worst of human relationships. During conflict, otherwise loving partners can relentlessly attack a vulnerable other or withdraw from a needy other, emotionally wounding the other even as they themselves are wounded. Conflict is often the tortuous road to separation and divorce. However, conflict can also spark powerful reconciliations, inspire intimacy and commitment, and invigorate relationships. It is often the occasion when partners voice, albeit in exaggerated form, what they have not been able to voice before. It can lay bare vulnerabilities and incompatibilities but in so doing stimulate efforts to address them rather than avoid them. These positive features of conflict can occur only if damage during the conflict is kept to a minimum. Thus time-out, by limiting damage, can pave the way for a more fulfilling, intimate relationship.

RECAP

Making positive, deliberate changes in our relationships is not easy, but it can be done. Although our tendency is to focus on what our partners should change, we will be more successful if we focus on what *we* can change. If we do less of what we normally do and more of what we typically don't do, we may achieve positive change. In particular, we can take constructive action instead of complaining and criticizing. We can do something positive for our partners even though there is negativity between us. We can do what our partners have asked us to do. None of these seemingly simple acts will be simple to implement. We may run up against our own resentment or a less-than-enthusiastic response from our partners.

Sometimes we can make a genuine change in our relationships by taking better care of ourselves. If we do not protect our partners so much, we may find ourselves less resentful. But we must deal with our own inhibitions and guilt about upsetting them by doing what we want to do.

At times, our disagreements with our partners may veer out of control. Our feelings and their feelings are so strong that constructive discussion becomes impossible. A positive change may simply be to minimize damage. If certain topics seem impossible to discuss constructively, we can change the circumstances or medium of those discussions. At the first signs of emotional distress, we may be able to salvage a discussion by focusing on the emotional interplay between us rather than by persisting with the particular topic that led us astray. When a discussion is not salvageable, we may need to call a time-out to cease the discussion between us and allow for a cooling-down period. A time-out represents an overt acknowledgment of the failure of our discussion, but, by preventing damaging escalation, it can facilitate reconciliation after the conflict and a quicker recovery to "normal." We get less painful conflict and sometimes, with a compassionate reconciliation, greater intimacy.

Exercise

The most fundamental and far-reaching change you can make in your relationship is to focus more on what you can do differently and less on what your partner can do differently.

- Consider some of the things you complain about. What kinds of constructive action could you take to improve those situations?
- What are some simple positive actions you could take for your partner?
- What actions could you take that would satisfy your partner's desires for change in you?
- Do you protect your partner's feelings unnecessarily, at the expense of your own resentment? What could you do to be more honest with your partner?

One important way to improve your relationship is to minimize damaging interactions.

- If you are completely unable to communicate about a particular topic constructively, try changing the circumstances or medium in which you communicate.
- If a particular discussion begins to deteriorate, focus on the emotions, not the content.
- Try using time-out as a way to protect yourself and the relationship when an argument is no longer salvageable as a constructive discussion.

WHERE ARE WE NOW AND WHERE ARE WE GOING?

At this point, we hope that reading this book and doing the exercises has helped you achieve several broad goals. First, from Part I, you should have a greater understanding of the complexity of intimate conflict. Specifically, you should understand how your differences and vulnerabilities lead to initial problems between you and your partner and how your efforts to cope with these problems can lead to more serious reactive problems. Second, from Part II, you should have taken this general knowledge of conflict and applied it to your own particular struggles with your partner and created a "story of your relationship problems." Based on this story and your reading in Part II, you should have more compassion for your partner's position in the conflict and should have been able to communicate that compassion. You should be able, at times, to see your struggle with some healing distance, as more of an "it" and less of a "you." All of this can make you more accepting of the struggles in which you find yourself. Finally, from Part III, you should have a greater understanding of the difficulty of making genuine, deliberate change, an awareness of how often efforts at change create more of the same. Hopefully, you also are empowered with the notion that genuine change, though difficult, is possible if you start with the only person you have control over: yourself. Furthermore, genuine change is worth the struggle because it not only reduces conflict but leads to greater intimacy. Ideally, the total impact of this book will lead to a softening of your position vis-à-vis your partner, and to an appreciation of your partner's human limitations and vulnerabilities as well as your own, even as you struggle to create a better, more fulfilling relationship. Perhaps you have now begun to move away from adversarial incompatibilities to reconcilable differences.

At this point, you might find it helpful to evaluate your progress. If you have not achieved some of these objectives, it might be wise to reread a chapter or section or to do some of the recommended exercises. It is also possible that some special problem—an affront by your partner, such as an affair, violence, or verbal abuse, or a serious disorder in your partner, such as depression or alcoholism—prevents the kinds of positive changes we have envisioned. It is also possible that your difficulties, whether or not they are exacerbated by special problems, require more than either of you can do. You may need professional assistance for your difficulties. In Part IV we address each of these special problems.

TEST YOUR LEVEL OF ACCEPTANCE

Log on to www.acceptancesurvey.com (active as of the date of this April 2000 printing) to complete our questionnaire on the level of acceptance in your relationship. You can obtain feedback about your relationship, and your anonymous responses will contribute to our ongoing data collection. After completing the questionnaire, your responses will be scored automatically by our site. You will then receive information on how your score compares to couples seeking therapy from our project; satisfied couples we have studied as a comparison group; and thousands of others who have visited the site on their own. We do not know how long this site will be available, so we invite you to visit it soon.

PART IV

When Acceptance Is Not Enough

CHAPTER 16

"Don't Do That to Me!"

VIOLENCE, VERBAL ABUSE,
AND INFIDELITY

*T*hroughout this book we have promoted several important ideas: There are at least two sides to every conflict. No one partner is responsible for an interpersonal problem; both members contribute to it, usually unintentionally. Interpersonal pain comes in part from the action perpetrated and in part from a vulnerability to that action. Crimes of the heart are usually misdemeanors, but our vulnerabilities make them feel like felonies.

Yet sometimes true felonies are committed in relationships. Sometimes one partner does something that is way out of line, something that is really wrong. The problem is not that we are sensitive, although we may be. The problem is that our partners have done something that we should not have to accept or even tolerate.

This chapter discusses three all-too-common categories of action in relationships that should not be accepted because they raise moral as well as interpersonal issues: violence, destruction, and physical coercion; psychological, emotional, and verbal abuse; and infidelity. These three kinds of behavior are very different and have different consequences. We don't want to equate their degree of seriousness. Clearly, violence is the only one that can literally be deadly. Also, specific acts within each category range dramatically in their severity: being pushed is very different from being beaten. Yet each of these three types of action is destructive in relationships. In each case, there are victims. The victim of all three types of action can convincingly say, "Whatever I did that was problematic in our relationship, I didn't deserve this."

VIOLENCE, DESTRUCTION,
AND PHYSICAL COERCION

It seems obvious that violence, destruction, and physical coercion should not be accepted in any relationship. Yet they are so widespread that it bears discussing in the context of acceptance and change.

We envision home as a safe haven, a place where we are protected from the struggles of the world. We may be injured daily by an uncaring outside world, but in our homes we can heal our wounds and return to the outside world refreshed. Evidence from the last twenty-five years has shown that many American homes are a stark contrast to this image. Instead of being a sanctuary of safety and support, they are dangerous sites of violence and destruction.

In 1985 Murray Straus and Richard Gelles conducted a national telephone survey of more than 3,500 households containing a currently married or cohabiting couple. These households were selected so that they would be representative of the U.S. population at large. Among other questions, the researchers asked about specific violent acts that might have occurred in the last year between husband and wife. Their results showed that violent acts, such as pushing, shoving, slapping, hitting, kicking, and beating up, occurred in 16 percent of couples. Severe violence, which they defined as kicking, biting, hitting with a fist, hitting with an object, beating up, threatening with a knife or gun, or using a knife or gun, occurred in 6 percent of couples. Because these reports were made to a stranger over the phone, they probably underestimate the true prevalence of violence in couples.

Not surprisingly, rates of physical aggression are higher in distressed couples seeking counseling than in the general population. Studies suggest that about half of all couples who seek therapy engage in at least some physical aggression. For example, in one study of 132 couples attending a marital clinic, about 50 percent of both husbands and wives reported that the husband had pushed, grabbed, or shoved his wife. About 20 percent of both spouses reported that the husband had slapped his wife. Fifteen percent of husbands and 19 percent of wives reported that the husband had kicked, bitten, or hit his wife.

In contrast to the information on violence, there is little information on the frequency of destruction and physical coercion in the population. *Destruction* occurs when one partner deliberately damages a possession of the other. *Physical coercion* occurs when one partner physically forces the other to do something, such as have sex, or physically prevents the other from doing something, such as going out with a friend. Although there is not much information on these kind of acts, they go hand-in-hand with violence.

Both men and women are violent, but men are more likely to commit severe violence, and the physical and psychological effects of violence on women tend to be more damaging than those effects are on men. Because men are generally bigger and stronger than women, they are more likely to prevail in any violent episode. In fact, women are twice as likely as men to experience physical injury from violence. Furthermore, women are more likely than men to suffer psychological consequences, such as lowered self-esteem, depression, and stress as a result of the violence. In their landmark study of battering, Neil Jacobson and John Gottman reported that men virtually never experienced or reported fear during altercations, whereas women were typically terrified before, during, and after. Also, violence seems to have a different purpose for men and women. Men are more likely to use violence as a method of control, intimidation, and subjugation, whereas women are more likely to be violent as an act of self-defense or as an ineffectual expression of anger. Finally, male violence is more likely than female violence to escalate in intensity.

Can couple therapy or the techniques advocated in this book help stop violence in a relationship?

To answer this question, we need to distinguish between battering on the one hand and low-level physical aggression on the other. In battering situations, almost always male to female, women are afraid of their partners, and there is almost always at least occasional injury. The woman gets bruised, scratched, or cut, whether intentional or not. Battering includes acts such as hitting with a closed fist, slapping, kicking, hitting with an object, throwing the other down or against a wall, biting, and beating up. Even if there are no such acts of violence, there may be intimidation. The woman may be afraid for her physical safety. She may be scared to speak her mind, lest her partner retaliate against her.

We do not do couple therapy, nor do we recommend it, for couples in which there is battering, that is, where there has been injury or where the purpose of the violence is control, intimidation, or subjugation of the woman. Therapy could be dangerous for these women. Because therapy engages both partners in discussions of conflict-laden topics, the therapy could precipitate violent episodes. For example, as therapists we could encourage a wife to explain her point of view, her husband might become furious at her for what she then says in front of us, and he could retaliate at home by beating her up. As therapists, we would have then unwittingly precipitated violence.

Furthermore, if we agree to do couple therapy where there is battering, we are treating the husband's problem as if it were a *marital* problem.
This comes in handy for the husband, who typically blames his wife for the
violence, but it is destructive for the wife. It places the therapist in the
untenable position of implicitly blaming the victim. In fact, stopping battering is the husband's responsibility and his alone. Furthermore, by treating the pair as a couple, we imply that this is a relationship worth saving.
We are endorsing the couple's staying together rather than separating. But
that is seldom the right course for a couple where there is battering.

Finally, there is little evidence to suggest that any treatment will stop
battering, including couple therapy. The evidence in favor of rehabilita-
tion of any kind is meager and suggests that batterers will be batterers as
long as they are physically able. The best solution to battering is for
women to leave, which they usually do once they have an adequate safety
plan. But the short-term risk can be to place battered women in even
greater jeopardy if they try to leave. Although many battered women
escape abusive relationships eventually, the escape is all too often followed
by more serious beatings, stalking, harassment, and even murder. *We
advise battered women interested in escaping safely to call the National
Domestic Violence Hotline: 1-800-799-7233.* This hotline refers battered
women to local low-cost help from trained advocates, who can assist battered women in their safety needs. This may be the most important phone
call that battered women ever make.

Reading this book is not going to help battered women any more
than couple therapy would. If you are in such a violent relationship, you
are reading the wrong book. We recommend *When Men Batter Women:
New Insights into Ending Abusive Relationships* (Simon & Schuster,
1998) by Neil S. Jacobson and John Gottman. Also, we recommend
Getting Free by Ginny NiCarthy (Seal Press, 1986) as an excellent guide
for battered women on how to get out of abusive relationships safely
and how to recover from them later.

What about physical aggression where there is no battering? What
can be done about those angry exchanges that lead to low-level violence,
such as pushing, grabbing, or shoving, but where there has not been
injury or intimidation?

Take Violence, Even a Push or a Shove, Seriously

One of the troubling things about violence in couples is that
neither partner may take it seriously. In the study of 132 couples who

attended a marital therapy clinic (mentioned above), husbands and wives were asked to write down the "major problems you see in your marriage." Only 6 percent of wives and 1.5 percent of husbands reported physical aggression as a major problem in their marriage, even though, when asked directly, over 50 percent of both husbands and wives reported some violence in the relationship. Even cases of what we would call serious violence were not seen as major problems by most spouses.

The tendency to ignore violence is especially likely when the level of violence is low. Why make a big deal out of an occasional push or shove? *Mild violence should always be taken seriously because it can easily escalate into more serious violence.* The shove can be reciprocated; then the shoving match can turn into kicking or hitting. What was once seemingly innocent can become dangerous. Mild violence can also cause accidental injuries—for example, a person who is shoved can trip and fall. If you have children, you have another good reason to take mild violence seriously. Any display of violence between parents is harmful to children, not only because it sets a terrible example for them but also because it triggers anxiety in the children toward their parents. They may feel scared and protective of their mother who gets shoved or pushed. It may complicate their feelings toward the two people most important in their lives.

What does it mean to take violence seriously? You need to acknowledge it openly as a problem. You need to talk about it with your partner and establish a goal of nonviolence in your relationship. You need to insist on a standard of "zero tolerance" for violence. The remaining sections will discuss steps to achieve this goal.

Establish Responsibility for Violence

A primary assumption in this book is that both partners contribute to problems between them. Unfortunately, those who have been violent, destructive, or physically coercive often use this rationale to justify their own behavior: I would not have pushed you if you had not been so insulting. I would not have torn up our wedding picture if you had not been so rejecting. I would not have kept you trapped in the kitchen had you been willing to talk to me.

There is, of course, a certain logic to these arguments. Without the insult, there might not have been the pushing incident. Without the rejection, the wedding picture may have remained intact. And with a willingness to talk, there would have been no necessity for coercion. This does not mean, however, that insults, rejection, or uncommunicativeness directly cause violence or that violent acts are of a kind with insulting words or rejecting words or refusal to talk. Freedom of speech, even insulting speech, is guaranteed for all, as is freedom of movement. Violence, destruction, and physical coercion are illegal acts, except in cases of self-defense. Therefore, the one who was violent, destructive, or physically coercive owns full and sole responsibility for these actions. Both partners are responsible for conflict and arguments, but only the perpetrator is responsible for violence, destruction, and physical coercion.

Remember That Perpetrators Can Control Violence

Violent partners may argue that they get so upset that they can't control their violence. Conflict provokes their anger so that they can't help grabbing or shoving, breaking things, or hindering the other's free movement. In fact, mildly violent partners can control themselves and are already controlling their violence. They have not crossed certain lines. Despite their anger, they have not engaged in wanton destruction or actually battered their partners. They have demonstrated repeatedly that they can and do control their impulses, proving that the insults or whatever made them angry are not direct causes of their violent reaction.

The task in these cases is to move back the line of what is acceptable, to shift that control so that any violence, any destruction, or any physical coercion is off limits. You can verbally insist on this standard of "zero tolerance." More important, you can refuse to engage in violence, destruction, or physical coercion yourself, even in retaliation. You can discourage the initiation of violence by vowing never to respond to violence with violence. Unless it is critical to your self-defense, any retaliatory act of violence may signal your partner that you find mildly violent behavior as acceptable as he does.

End Arguments before Violence

Battering may sometimes come "out of the blue." A drunken husband may strike his wife for no apparent reason except that he is mad at his boss and therefore had too much to drink when he got home. The low levels of violence that are the focus of this section, however, usually develop out of an argument. There is a buildup of conflict, an increase in intensity, until you are not listening to your partner and your partner is not listening to you. No constructive discussion is taking place. And then the shoving or grabbing or pushing begins.

This buildup may be rapid. Like a souped-up car in a drag race, you may go from a zero of calm conversation to the 100 miles per hour of intense anger and frustration in less than a minute. But it is possible to be aware of that transformation, no matter how rapidly it occurs. And it is possible to take control, to apply the brakes, before violence breaks out.

Chapter 15 discussed time-outs, stopping an argument in midstream. You and your partner can use this strategy to end arguments and postpone discussions and thus avert violence. You must become aware of the buildup, be tuned in to the shift from constructive engagement to futile argument. And then it is possible to stop the discussion before violence happens.

Even if you are not violent yourself, you can assist in this process. If your partner requests a time-out, you can honor it. You can even assist in the detection of a futile argument. You can say, even if your partner doesn't, "This argument is getting out of control. Let's take a break." It is not your responsibility to prevent your partner from being violent, only to prevent yourself from being violent. However, if you can stop an unproductive discussion, you will help your relationship. And if your partner is the violent party, you may make it easier for your partner to control his or her violence.

Seek Professional Assistance

If you are unable to end violence on your own, seek professional assistance. Even though we do *not* recommend couple therapy for battering, it may be useful for low-level violence that erupts from arguments. If one partner has a problem managing anger without resorting to low-level violence, destruction, or coercion, individual therapy may be helpful. The next chapter discusses professional assistance in more detail.

VERBAL, PSYCHOLOGICAL, AND EMOTIONAL ABUSE

> Sticks and stones may break our bones, but words
> will break our hearts.
> —ROBERT FULGHUM

Words can hurt. The carefully aimed criticism, the dismissive comment, the blunt rejection, and the taunting joke can create psychological suffering that makes physical pain seem mild in comparison. Even the absence of words can create a comparable emotional anguish. Physical withdrawal in response to affection, a bored look that greets excitement, or preoccupation that shuts down emotional expression can all break our hearts.

Although most of us know that love brings its share of pain, some words are more hurtful than should be allowed. But where does "unkind" or "troubling" or "unfair" end and "abusive" begin?

Defining Abuse

The term *verbal abuse* focuses on the actions of the abuser, the unacceptable words that the abuser uses. We often use this term to describe epithets and insults that anyone would consider unacceptably cruel. A pattern of cursing, swearing, or name calling is certainly abusive. No one should have to tolerate expressions like "You ugly bitch!" or "You worthless idiot!" or "You miserable cunt!" or "You complete loser!"

Certainly, threats of physical violence, *even if they are not carried out,* are another form of blatant verbal abuse. You should never have to hear threats such as "You say that again and I'll smash your face in" or "You do that again and I will hit you so fast you won't know what happened to you." Even if violence is not specifically threatened but only implied, it is abusive: "You wouldn't do that if you know what's good for you" or "You do that again and you're going to regret it real bad."

Other kinds of extreme threats, involving illegal or unacceptable actions, are also abusive, whether they are carried out or not. You should not have to hear threats involving the deprivation of your freedom ("I won't let you leave the house") or threats about contact with your children ("You do that again and I will take the kids and you will never see them again") or threats about access to your friends and family ("I won't let you go see them") or threats that deny you normal adult autonomy ("I won't let you have any money, and then see what you can do") or threats about the destruction of your property ("Next time I will burn your stupid little diary"). All these actions are abusive; the threat of them, whether carried out or not, is verbal abuse.

Apart from these obvious examples of verbal abuse, it is difficult to specify which actions and words are verbal abuse and which are merely undesirable. In her book *The Verbally Abusive Relationship: How to Recognize It and How to Respond,* Patricia Evans developed an extensive list of fifteen "categories of verbal abuse." Along with obvious ones such as threatening and name calling were withholding, discounting, accusing and blaming, judging and criticizing, and forgetting. Clearly, most of us would be guilty of verbal abuse by this broad and varied definition. In fact, in a study by Julian Barling and associates of 398 New York couples six months after marriage, none of whom was seeking marital therapy, 89 percent checked off the item "insulted/swore at him/her," 82 percent checked "did/said something to spite him/her," 84 percent checked "stomped out of the room/house/yard," and 97 percent checked "sulked/refused to talk about an issue." Not surprisingly, rates are higher for couples in treatment: 90 percent or more admit to each of these behaviors.

The term *abuse* refers to some action that is morally wrong, that is unacceptable human behavior, that should be condemned by all. We may be tempted to use the word to describe something that is merely negative or unpleasant for us, because it adds weight to our protest, invoking moral sanctions against our partners. Even if we use it in the desperate hope of deterring the unpleasant behavior, however, describing all negative or unpleasant actions as "abuse" is a misuse of the word. Rather than halting the unpleasant behavior, the charge of "abuse" may be another form of accusation that inflames an argument. Furthermore, it can backfire. For example, one husband's description of his wife's criticisms of him as "abusive" did not change her behavior. Instead, it gave her the opportunity to discount his objection altogether: that he would see her criticism as abusive just showed how ridiculously sensitive he was to her "constructive criticism."

How, then, do we distinguish the verbally abusive from the non-abusive? Perhaps we can find a clearer definition of abuse if we shift our focus from the abusive actions of the perpetrator to the emotional reactions of the victim. Some actions are termed *psychological abuse* or *emotional abuse* because the effect on the victim is abusive. What does it mean to feel emotionally or psychologically abused? It is much more than simply feeling hurt or upset by something, even if that hurt or upset is extensive. We can be very hurt that our partners forgot our birthday or flirted with someone else or made a critical comment about our appearance, but their behavior, in and of itself, is not abusive.

Feelings of emotional abuse involve fear and intimidation. You are emotionally abused when you feel subjugated and controlled by your partner. When you are emotionally abused, you are frightened, you feel bad about yourself, and you may blame yourself for the problems in the relationship.

Of course, it is possible to have feelings of fear, inadequacy, intimidation, and self-blame even when your partner is not being particularly abusive. These feelings can come more from yourself than from your contact with your partner. Furthermore, even if your partner is clearly abusive—yelling, swearing, and threatening you—you may not experience these bad feelings about yourself. You may fight back by yelling and swearing and threatening in return. Although the communication is clearly destructive, no one is feeling abused, just angry.

Therefore, to get a clear understanding of emotional and psychological abuse, we must consider both people in the relationship. If a woman feels intimidated and her husband is trying to dominate her: if she is feeling unworthy, and he looks at her contemptuously and tries to put her down; if she is feeling self-blame, and her partner is heaping on the accusations; or if she is feeling weak and inadequate, and her partner is trying to control her, then emotional and psychological abuse is occurring. Abuse happens only in a context of power inequities. When a man is on top and trying to take advantage of it and a woman is on the bottom and feeling scared, the situation is abusive.

Thus, words that are abusive in one relationship may not be abusive in another relationship. What is merely unpleasant for one couple may be poison to another. A wife could deride her husband with comments such as "You really blew it. You messed up royally. Can't you get it right for once?" If he found her comments annoying and simply fought back verbally ("Oh, get off my case"), this would be an argument, not abuse. However, if he said the same things to her, and his attack occurred within the context of a history of violence and intimidation, the same message would be abusive.

Battering is almost always accompanied by psychological abuse. When men batter their wives and girlfriends, their threatening words carry the reality of real violence. Their words are often used in conjunction with their fists to subjugate and control. We noted above that this book is not helpful for couples in a battering relationship. Nor is it helpful in dealing with the psychological abuse that accompanies battering.

How often does psychological abuse or emotional abuse occur in the absence of violence? It is certainly possible for someone in a relationship to be intimidated, subjugated, and controlled even without the threat or actual occurrence of violence. A powerful man might use money, along with his abusive words, to control his wife, without ever beating her or threatening to beat her. We simply don't know how often this occurs. However, this book is not appropriate for those cases of control any more than it is appropriate for cases of battering. We would recommend that someone in this kind of relationship begin with the resources we described above for battering.

Discouraging Verbal Abuse

The suggestions that follow do *not* apply to cases of battering or abusive control and subjugation. Following these suggestions could easily precipitate violence in a battering relationship or additional abuse in a psychologically or emotionally abusive relationship. These suggestions apply only to cases of cruel and unacceptable language such as cursing, name calling, and nonviolent threats. As always, your emotional or psychological reaction is the key to determining whether the behavior was abusive, warranting action. Some partners can occasionally tell the other to "go to hell," or call the other a "jerk," or threaten separation or divorce without causing serious harm. Although these are hardly laudable acts, they may be just part of the way one or both express anger. If these acts are extremely painful, a serious affront to your dignity, then they are abusive, whether they occur once or repeatedly, and you should take action.

Talk to Your Partner

It's important to talk to your partner about an abusive comment that is a painful affront to you, but only in a calm situation, not during the heat of the argument. Tell your partner the specific words or comments that offend you and focus on the impact of these words on you. Railing vaguely against "the way you talk to me" may leave your partner unsure of exactly what you find offensive and may invite defensiveness and arguments about your own sensitivity.

Consider how April tells Kerry of her feelings and resists being drawn into defending them.

APRIL: I really don't like it when you call me a "bitch" during an argument. I find that term degrading and offensive.

KERRY: Oh, I just say it when I'm angry. I don't really mean it.

APRIL: You may not mean it, but I find it offensive, and I would appreciate it if you wouldn't say it anymore.

KERRY: I think you're making a mountain out of a molehill. It's just a word.

APRIL: It is just a word, but for me it's an offensive word. And I would appreciate, out of consideration for me, that you not use that word.

Take Action in the Moment

An effective way to deal with verbal abuse is to take action that shows you will not tolerate it when it occurs. By "action" we don't mean a discussion such as just described but instead quick action to end the abuse right now. If your partner is cursing you or calling you an unacceptable name, you can simply announce, "I won't listen to you talk to me like that," and leave. Or you can leave without comment. You don't have to tolerate threats or name calling or insults. Take a time-out from the situation and leave your partner without an audience.

Ending a conversation when your partner makes an abusive comment communicates a powerful message about that comment, but it's not an easy action to take. You may be so stung by your partner's abuse that you want to attack. You don't want to leave the situation; your impulse is to stay and fight. Often this leads to more verbal abuse, perhaps on both sides. Similarly, if you are invested in the conversation or if there is some urgency to the conversation, you may not feel like ending it and waiting for a better time.

Don't Abuse Your Partner

If you want your partner to talk to you without name calling, yelling, cursing, or threatening, give your partner the same respect. Verbal abuse is often the end product of an escalating argument. Stop the escalation by avoiding verbal abuse on your own part, and you may decrease the chances that your partner will escalate into verbal abuse. You may need to invoke time-out to stop the escalation.

INFIDELITY

Most serious, committed romantic relationships endorse monogamy. In fact, the agreement to be monogamous is fundamental to most relationships. That is why having sexual relations with someone else is considered infidelity: more than being simply an act of intimacy with a third person, it means betrayal of a fundamental trust—and often a great deal of deception as well. Actually, sexual intercourse itself may not even need to be a part of infidelity.

For months Clayton met secretly with his coworker, Alicia. Although he told his wife that work demands were keeping him late at the office, it was really Alicia. He poured out his soul to her, revealing all his marital problems, including difficulties in their sex life. She became his primary confidant. Behind his closed office door, Clayton and Alicia not only talked to each other, they kissed and fondled each other. They deliberately avoided intercourse, however, because Clayton felt that intercourse would clearly be a violation of his marriage vows. Furthermore, Alicia wanted to save sex for the day when Clayton left his wife.

Although Clayton took moral reassurance from the fact that he had not actually had intercourse with Alicia, it would have provided little solace for his wife. She would have been outraged by his secrecy, lies, and misleading comments. She would have been furious that he had shared their marital secrets with another woman. She would have felt foolish for comforting him after he came home late after a long workday. The fact that his physical contact with Alicia had never crossed the line into intercourse would not have consoled her. Even if Clayton had never kissed and fondled Alicia, his wife would have viewed his relationship with Alicia as an affair of the heart that violated their marriage.

In a recent national survey of human sexual behavior, about 80 percent of women and 75 percent of men indicated that they had been sexually faithful in their marriages. A British survey with an expanded definition of infidelity that included "adulteries of the heart" found, however, that only 60 percent of their participants were faithful. And one report suggests that 60 percent of couples seeking therapy had been affected by extramarital relationships that were either completely sexual or were affairs of the heart. It seems clear that, although most couples manage to stay faithful to each other, there are many who do not.

The Impact of Affairs

The discovery of an affair may be a pivotal point, like the death of a family member, which burns itself into your memory and changes your life forever. If you have no inkling of the affair and then get an anonymous letter or catch your mate with someone else, you may feel shocked and stunned. If you are strongly attached to your mate, you may experience the event as a trauma, more severe in its emotional impact than a car accident or a robbery at gunpoint. You may experience trauma's incumbent symptoms: constant and intrusive thoughts about the affair, inability to experience the emotions you normally experience, or hyperarousal and supervigilance, such as scrutinizing your partner for further evidence of affairs.

Even when the discovery is not traumatic, it can be destructive in other ways. If you suspected your partner's infidelity, finding out the truth may give you a strange sense of relief because it shows you that your suspicions were not crazy, as your partner may have implied. Still, confirmation of your suspicions can cast a dark shadow of distrust or erect a wall of anger that affects all your contact with your partner.

Is an affair a terminal condition for a marriage? Infidelity certainly presents a crisis, and it may signal the end of the relationship. Sometimes infidelity brings an already severely deteriorated relationship to a sudden, crisis-ridden end because neither partner has the desire to put the relationship back together. But even if a relationship is capable of recovery, the experience of moral and emotional violation may be so vast that the betrayed partner is unwilling or unable to give the relationship another try. There is much good in the relationship, but the infidelity crossed a line that could not be uncrossed. Another possibility is that even though both partners want to make the relationship work, their efforts at recovery create such powerful additional problems that they eventually break up. This is a special case of the reactive problem ending up causing more trouble—the end of the relationship—than the initial problem, the affair. It is such a common trap for couples that the rest of this section is devoted to helping you steer through the difficulties of getting past infidelity.

Find Out Information about the Infidelity

You may have a strong need to know what happened. Your partner's affair may feel like community property, as much your business as your partner's. You certainly have a right to know about any risk to your physical safety. Did your partner practice safe sex? Is there a risk of sexually transmitted disease or of pregnancy? Should your partner be tested? Should you be tested?

Once questions about physical safety have been settled, you may desperately want to know details about the infidelity so you can understand what has been violated and gauge its impact. How long did the relationship last? How serious was it? Did they ever discuss marriage? Did they go to the same special, romantic places that you as a couple frequent? Did they ever have sex in your home?

Often a struggle will develop over revelations about the affair. Because your partner doesn't want to anger you further or stoke his or her own guilt, your partner may conceal details of the affair. He or she may minimize the time spent or the gifts purchased or the intensity of feelings. As you sense his or her unwillingness to disclose what really happened, you may fear the affair was a bigger deal than it actually was. You may push for details, while your partner resists. You may wonder if you will ever get the whole story. Because your thirst for information never seems satisfied, you might find yourself slipping in questions at the oddest moments. Passing a hotel in town, you may ask, "Did you ever go there with him/her?" Your partner will surely get frustrated by what seems like a never-ending stream of questions: "Can't you ever give this up?"

In couple therapy we often set up a limited period for full disclosure. We find out whether the perpetrator of the affair is willing to answer any and all questions during a limited number of therapy sessions, say, two or three. During these sessions we ask the unfaithful partner not to minimize involvement in the affair. In fact, we may ask him or her to "round up" rather than "round down." For example, if a husband saw his affair partner once or twice a week, he should say twice a week rather than once a week. In this way his wife may get a clear, unminimized picture of the affair and his involvement in it.

We ask the partner who has been violated to agree to ask questions only during these specially designated sessions. We encourage this violated partner to think of all possible questions and even to write them down before the session. The payoff for the violated partner is complete disclosure as long as the violated partner is willing to keep the questions within these specially designed therapy sessions. The payoff for the unfaithful partner is that the questions will cease if full disclosure is made as agreed.

If you are struggling with the aftermath of your partner's affair and have a strong need to know what happened, you may want to set up something similar. A few sessions of full disclosure may enable you to get the information you want without either of you enduring a constant struggle over what happened.

Close the Door on the Other Relationship

To move your relationship forward, the affair must stop. Your partner will probably understand this. He or she may have considered a termination or even attempted it before you discovered the affair. But it is a decision that affects three people, and it is important to keep that in mind. The third party is often a victim too, having been deceived by your partner in much the same way that you were. For example, Clayton misled Alicia about his intentions to divorce, one time telling her he had consulted an attorney when he had not. Even if your partner has not misled the "third party," he or she may have legitimate concerns about that person's feelings. Your partner may need to consider how best to end the relationship.

You may want your partner to terminate not just sexual relations but any relationship with his or her lover. Because of the strong feelings that were generated in this other relationship, your partner may want to maintain close ties, even if no sexual relationship. He or she may still wish to have intimate conversations. He or she may want to keep that other relationship open just in case the relationship with you fails to heal.

You will have a hard time ever trusting your partner again, but it may be impossible if your partner doesn't cut off the other relationship completely. It would be perfectly natural to worry that if a so-called platonic relationship continues, a casual conversation will turn into an intimate conversation or an intimate conversation will turn into sexual intimacy. The progress of your relationship will be hampered if your partner maintains even a warm connection with the person who once had a more intimate and intense connection with your partner than you did. Nevertheless, your partner may be unwilling or unable to cut off all ties. The other person could be a coworker, and your partner may be unwilling to make a career sacrifice. You may walk a tightrope: do you press your partner to make a sacrifice for your relationship or try to accept your partner's limited relationship with the other person?

Reviving trust may be easier if you can participate in the termination of this other relationship or at least be privy to its termination. Perhaps you and your partner can compose a letter that tells the other that the affair is over and that the two of you are going to put your relationship back together. Or perhaps you can listen in as your partner talks on the phone and tells the other that he or she wants to end the affair and work on your marriage.

What is important in this process is to shift the balance of intimacy and secrecy. During the affair, their relationship was secret from you. They talked about your marriage and its problems. You knew nothing of their relationship. Now you, the victim, have an understandable desire to know about their relationship, now past, and an equally understandable need to deny the third party any further information about your marriage as it now stands. You quite naturally want to shut the door to the person who had an affair with your partner so you can open it to your relationship.

This approach will feel right to you, who have been violated by another relationship, but it may not feel right to your partner, who still has feelings for the other man or woman. Your partner may claim, rightly, to be unable to turn off his or her feelings for this other person. But you are not asking your partner to turn off feelings, only to turn off the behavior toward this other person, behavior that your partner can control. Your partner may feel bad about hurting the other person by terminating all contact. And if the other person did care about your partner, the termination will hurt her or him. But the problem of a lover's triangle can never be solved without pain. Usually it is pain for all three. And one person must be eliminated from the triangle.

Establish Responsibility for the Affair

Your partner may blame problems in your relationship for the affair. The fact that the relationship wasn't close or that the sex wasn't great drove your partner into someone else's arms. Or your partner might take it one step further and blame you directly. Because you did not listen to your partner's concerns, or because you were so selfish, or because you were not sexually responsive, your partner sought comfort elsewhere. Thus, the affair is as much your fault as your partner's—maybe more so.

In your own thinking about the affair and in your discussions with your partner, you need to clarify and separate two points. First, there may well have been problems in your relationship or problems in your responsiveness to your partner's needs. Affairs always happen in context; they don't happen when both partners are completely satisfied with their current relationship. But the second point is even more important: affairs are not designed to solve relationship problems, and they usually make those problems worse, not better. There are many other constructive ways of responding to relationship problems that don't involve secrecy and betrayal. Although you and your partner are jointly responsible for problems in the relationship, your partner is solely responsible for choosing an affair as a bad solution to those problems.

Let Go of the Affair

Three weeks after he had confessed his affair, Joe felt there was no letup in Mary Louise's anger. It seemed that every conversation eventually turned to the affair. Her looks cast a thousand knives at him. Couldn't she realize that it had been a mistake on his part? He was hardly the first human being to make such a mistake. And he had been honest enough to admit the affair and strong enough to end it. Couldn't she focus on that?

For her part, Mary Louise found Joe's stance incredible. He seemed to want compliments for the fact that he had confessed the affair and ended it rather than criticism for the fact that he had had the affair to begin with. Why couldn't he focus on her pain and distress rather than justify his own position? Why couldn't he give her a genuine, heartfelt apology? She didn't need him to cry her a river, but she did need him to make amends.

Joe found it difficult to apologize to Mary Louise because of her intense anger. He read in her anger, "You have committed a horrible crime" or "You are less than human for doing what you did to me." An apology would feel to him like admitting to being inhuman or confessing to an unforgivable sin. Instead of offering an apology or displaying remorse, he tried to convince her that the affair was not serious and that the other woman meant little to him. But to Mary Louise, Joe's attempts to explain the affair came across as efforts to invalidate her feelings. She heard in his comments the message "You shouldn't be so upset, I didn't do anything very bad." So his efforts to explain himself made her angrier. And her anger made it more difficult for him to see her pain and respond to it.

A struggle, like that between Joe and Mary Louise, often develops over letting go of the affair. Naturally, your partner wants you to move on, to stop focusing on it. Your partner may encourage or even insist that you not dwell on the past, that you look to the future. Your partner may question why you bring it up when it only creates upset. But the affair may have so shaken your confidence or been so emotionally traumatic that you have difficulty letting go. You cannot avoid thinking about it. You are frequently reminded of the affair. You bring it up.

Even if your partner verbally acknowledges responsibility for the affair, you may not feel much relief or satisfaction. Your partner may come to that acknowledgment only reluctantly, after you pushed him or her on the point. Your partner may put more energy into justifying the affair by pointing out the inadequacy in you or in the relationship than in acknowledging his or her own personal responsibility.

If you saw that your partner understood your pain and was truly sorry for what he or she did to you, you could let go of the affair more easily. But instead you see defensiveness about the affair. Your partner's apologies may seem too cheap and easy. In response, your anger is heightened and your focus on the affair more intense.

Your partner may find it difficult to express genuine remorse. In the face of your angry accusation, he or she may resist making even a nominal apology. Your partner cannot see the suffering behind your accusations.

To break this kind of struggle requires one of three possible actions. Your partner can put aside his or her own feelings, realize that your anger masks your suffering, and respond to your suffering with genuine remorse and apology. Conversely, you can let go of some of your accusation, allow your pain and vulnerability to be more obvious, and create a context in which your partner can experience empathy for you. Either one of these actions, if taken unilaterally, is difficult and for many people impossible. A movement by both you and your partner is a more likely avenue for letting go of the struggle and ultimately of the affair.

The Ongoing Issue of Trust

You may wonder if you will ever trust your partner again. He or she betrayed you once; it could happen again. Going down a strange path is easier the second time around. How can you recapture your trust in your partner once it has been broken?

You may try to restore trust by seeking evidence of your partner's faithfulness or unfaithfulness. You may question your partner about his or her activities while not in your presence. You may carefully note the times your partner leaves home and returns from work. You may interrogate your partner if his or her behavior deviates from the usual—he comes home a little late, she is not at the office when you call, he has "errands to do" on Saturday morning.

In response, your partner may get irritated at your distrust. You also may wonder if you can ever trust again. From your seemingly inno-cent questions about his whereabouts to your interrogation of her over anything suspicious, your partner may fear that he or she will never be free again. Your partner will be boxed in by your mistrust.

Battles over trust can sometimes create as many or more problems than the infidelity itself. You get angry at your partner because he or she won't tolerate your distrust. Here you had to tolerate infidelity, but your partner is annoyed that you won't suddenly trust again. Your partner gets angry at you because of your suspicions, your questions, and your vigilance. Your partner may feel tortured by your distrust.

I once worked with a couple who was trying unsuccessfully to recover from the husband's infidelity. The wife was convinced that he was still seeing his former girlfriend or had started seeing other, new girlfriends. She called him repeatedly to check his whereabouts. Each evening she questioned him about his day.

The husband protested his innocence and expressed his dismay over her tactics. He felt as if he were a little child, answering to his mother about what he had done every day. At times he gave his wife a detailed accounting of his activities; at other times he refused to submit to her interrogation.

My work with them had little impact. Clearly, their attempts to deal with distrust were creating more problems for them than his original infidelity had. She was becoming obsessed with his infidelity; he was becoming totally turned off by her. Either she was paranoid or he was a liar.

I explained to them the notion behind the proverb "Never call a man honest who never had a chance to steal." I suggested that she needed to give him the space to be untrustworthy, so she could ulti-mately trust him. I noted that in their relationship she had become a dis-trict attorney and he had become an uncooperative suspect. She needed to release him on bail. And then she needed to shift roles from district attorney to detective. Sometime after his release, she should check up on him. Because she was a busy professional and was financially well off, I suggested she might even turn over the duties of detective to someone else. Have a private detective check up on him to assure herself of his honesty.

Although he liked the idea of being "out on bail" and being released from questioning, he was not excited about his wife or anyone else becoming a private detective. She was amused by the notion of a private detective but was not certain that she could stop her distrust or the questioning it generated. Soon after this session the couple stopped coming to see me. I assumed that I had not been able to break their cycle of distrust.

A number of months later the wife made an appointment to see me alone. She told me that she had carefully considered my advice and followed it. She had let up on her husband; she had quit her interrogation of him. She tried just to enjoy their relationship for a while. Then she hired a private detective to track him. As she talked to me, she passed me an envelope of pictures the detective had taken. They showed her husband coming out of a motel with another woman. Based on those pictures, she had initiated divorce.

She wanted to thank me for my suggestion: being a detective had been much more productive than being a district attorney. She also wanted to show me that she was not paranoid; all of her suspicious had been confirmed.

This example illustrates that gathering evidence is more productive than relentless questioning. Also, the example shows that evidence can lead to dramatic change. Based on the pictures she obtained, my client was able, despite the great difficulty involved, to leave her husband for good and start a new life of her own.

When your partner has been unfaithful, you may look for evidence that will be as convincing as the evidence was for my client. However, the problem with evidence is that it is only convincing in the negative, that is, when it points to an affair. Positive evidence is always suspect. If you find no evidence of suspicious calls on the phone bill, it may mean only that your partner used pay phones or work phones to make calls. If you find no suspicious credit card receipts, your partner may have simply torn them up or paid in cash. Even in the extreme case of hiring a private investigator, an absence of evidence could simply mean that your partner's lover was out of town or otherwise unavailable during the period of surveillance.

For building trust, what is more important than evidence about what your partner does when he or she is not with you is the experience you have with your partner when he or she is with you. You can have experiences together with your partner that build trust apart from any evidence about what your partner does when you are not present. Some of these experiences occur as part of the process of discovery of the infidelity. For example, if your partner felt so guilty about the affair that he or she stopped it and revealed it to you, even when you had little or no suspicion, you may find in that revelation a basis for trust. Your partner could not persist in the infidelity; the commitment to you and personal integrity made your partner stop. Certainly, this kind of experience, no matter how upsetting, sets more of a basis for future trust than a case in which you yourself discover the infidelity in full bloom.

Even if you discovered the infidelity, there are experiences around it that can promote trust. If you see your partner's genuine guilt and remorse, you can be reassured that your partner has strong feelings for you and an intact sense of integrity. If you experience empathy from your partner for the pain you endured, you have a reason to believe your partner won't hurt you again.

Your partner's sensitivity to your feelings can also bolster trust. He may make extra efforts to call you when he is away on business trips, so you can feel the security of contact with him. She tolerates your insecurity and your questions. He can pass up a party at which his former lover may be present.

Greater openness is a direct antidote to distrust. Secrecy and deception are a necessary part of infidelity. If your partner make efforts to be more open, so there is less that is unknown between the two of you, your partner will promote your trust. He may offer more information about what goes on with him. She may include you in her social circles at work so you know her colleagues and friends.

What ultimately will build your trust are your partner's efforts within your own relationship. If your partner addresses the problems in your marriage, you know your relationship is important to him or her. You know your partner wants to be with you.

What complicates all of these trust-building experiences is that they cannot be mounted by your partner alone. Your accusatory fury can dispel your partner's empathy. Your demands can quash his sensitivity. Your interrogation can prevent much openness. To have trust-enhancing experiences with your partner, you must give as well as receive. You may want and need your partner to make the first moves, but the process of rebuilding trust will require you both.

Seek Professional Assistance

If you are not able to deal successfully with an affair on your own, you may need professional assistance. Couple therapy could help you get past the infidelity and resolve some of your relationship problems. In the next chapter, we discuss couple therapy.

RECAP

Three common ways in which we can be mistreated in relationships are (1) through violence, destructiveness, or physical coercion; (2) through verbal, emotional, or psychological abuse; and (3) through the infidelity of our partners. These kinds of actions are very different from each other, particularly in their danger to us, but are all similar in that they are wrong. For most of this book, we have tried to get you away from moral judgments, to get you to see your problems as incompatibilities and vulnerabilities rather than as moral issues. However, some actions, even if they are common, are simply wrong. You should not have to endure violence, abuse, or betrayal from someone who loves you.

The actions encompassed by these three categories are not equally wrong. Being pushed is very different from being beaten up. Being called "an ass" is very different from having your life threatened. We made an important distinction between battering on the one hand and low-level physical aggression on the other. Battery involves injury and intimidation and is almost always committed by men against women. If you are in a battering relationship, this book is not for you. It is important that you seek help elsewhere, for example, by calling the National Domestic Violence Hotline at 1-800-799-7233. Our comments on violence, destruction, and physical coercion concerned only low levels of these acts.

Like battering, psychological and emotional abuse involves fear and intimidation. They often go hand-in-hand with battering, and women in these kind of relationships should consult the resources we provided for battering. Our comments focused more narrowly on verbal abuse, such as name calling and cursing.

Finally, we discussed infidelity, the betrayal of a vow of monogamy. Unless a partner reveals his or her actions immediately, infidelity also involves deception. Infidelity almost always creates a crisis for a relationship, challenging a core assumption that partners have made about the relationship and raising an enduring question about whether the restoration of trust is possible.

Although coping with each of these threats to the relationship has its own special requirements, there was one similarity across these issues. Our partners may believe that we contributed to their infidelity or their verbal abuse or their violence by what we did in the relationship. Even though they were the perpetrators, our actions led them to do what they did. We too may believe that we bear responsibility for our mistreatment at their hands. Maybe we deserved it.

It is important that we and our partners establish responsibility for the infidelity, the verbal abuse, and the violence, destructiveness, and coercion. Yes, we bear our share of the responsibility, along with our partners, for problems in the relationship. But our partners bear the *full responsibility* for reacting to those problems by being unfaithful, verbally abusive, violent, destructive, or physically coercive. No relationship problems force individuals to resort to these kinds of actions. No one deserves to be treated with lies or with abuse. These actions do not mean our partners are monsters or inhuman, but they do mean they were wrong.

Recovery from infidelity, verbal abuse, and low levels of violence, destructiveness, and physical coercion is possible, particularly when appropriate responsibility for these acts is first established.

CHAPTER 17

Call in the Professionals!

COUPLE AND INDIVIDUAL THEAPY

Sometimes self-help is not enough to solve problems that plague relationships. If you've been quite unhappy in your relationship for several months or more, and your constructive efforts to talk to your partner, to implement the suggestions in this book, and to make positive changes in yourself have failed to improve your relationship substantially, you may want to seek professional help. You will not be alone because relationship problems are one of the most common issues that send people to mental health professionals. The first half of this chapter explains who might benefit, what kinds of help are available, and how to find the best person to assist you.

Self-help is particularly likely to fall short when your partner has individual problems that are affecting the relationship. Throughout this book we have tried to steer you away from laying blame for intimate conflict on your partner. But sometimes one of you does have a behavioral or emotional problem, and this problem clearly does play an important role in marital struggles and in recovery from them. Research has indicated that the quality of intimate relationships is associated with anxiety, depression, substance abuse and dependence, and sexual dysfunction—the behavioral and emotional problems for which people most commonly seek help. A poor relationship can contribute to your partner's depression or anxiety or substance abuse or sexual difficulties, but these problems can also contribute to a poor relationship, in a kind of vicious cycle.

You may have an important role to play not only in getting your partner to seek professional help but also in assisting him or her with his or her individual problem. The second half of this chapter will explain how.

WE NEED HELP!

It's not hard to understand why so many people seek couple therapy. About half of all first marriages end in divorce, and the prospects are even dimmer for second marriages. Many couples stay together only because financial or religious barriers prevent them from separating or because they believe staying together will be best for their children. If your relationship has ceased to be a positive factor in your life, a pleasure or a support for you, and is instead an emotional burden, couple counseling may help. Even if you are extremely dissatisfied with the relationship—either because of a preponderance of negative emotions like anger, resentment, guilt, and disappointment or because there is little emotion of any kind, positive or negative—you are a good candidate for couple therapy if you are still committed to the relationship. There are no clear-cut answers to how unhappy you must be to try couples therapy or how committed you must be to ensure its success, but unless you sincerely want the relationship to succeed and are willing to do your fair share to make it work, couple therapy is doomed to fail.

"The work being done on your marriage—are you having it done, or are you doing it yourselves?"

What Is Couple Therapy Like?

Asking what couple therapy is like is a little like asking what treatment for cancer is like. Just as the treatment that one patient receives for cancer will depend on the type of cancer, the variety of treatment options available, the philosophy of the doctor, and the receptiveness of the patient, your experience in couple therapy will vary depending on your specific problem, the treatment approach chosen, the type of therapist you consult, and what the two of you are willing to do.

Couple therapy is usually done conjointly. Although the therapist may want to see each of you alone at times, both of you will be present during most of the sessions. It is possible to undergo couple therapy without your partner, but the willingness of both partners to come to treatment will certainly increase its effectiveness.

You should also be aware that therapists normally take a neutral position about the conflicts that divide couples. Many couples come to therapy seeking specific advice on how to solve a particular conflict, but therapists usually will not say how a conflict ought to be resolved or how they would solve the same problem in their own relationship. Although they may make suggestions, therapists serve primarily as mediators who assist couples in understanding their problems and coming up with their own solutions for them.

People who seek couple therapy sometimes want not advice, but affirmation of their own righteousness. Many clients mentally rehearse the "evidence" against their partners before the first session. Others come fearing that the therapist will find fault with how they have behaved in the relationship. Because there is usually an excess of fault finding in couples who seek therapy, the therapist will work toward helping partners communicate better and find common ground rather than at directing blame.

This does not mean, however, that the therapist is passive. Those who have not experienced therapy before often hold a stereotypical image in mind of a patient lying on a couch, complaining about his or her problems, while the therapist sits nearby, quietly taking notes. This image is truer of psychoanalysis than of psychotherapy. Most individual therapy today would not proceed this way, and certainly couple therapy would not. Typically, partners in a couple sit so that they can speak directly to the therapist as well as to each other. Furthermore, the therapist is an active participant in the communication, rather than a note-taking observer. Because a couple in therapy can easily get into arguments, the therapist often serves as an active mediator in their conflicts.

What Types of Couple Therapy Are Available?

In a very real sense, there are as many types of therapies as there are couples in therapy. Each therapist develops his or her own way of working with couples and adapts that strategy to each individual couple. However, there are several broad approaches to working with couples that have influenced therapists.

One broad distinction is between those approaches that focus on the past and those that focus on the present. A substantial portion of therapists, who call themselves psychodynamically oriented or psychoanalytically oriented, look to the past for answers to the puzzles of the present. They believe, for example, that spouses' marital difficulties stem from their past relationships with their mother and father. Therefore, these therapists will be interested in the childhood histories of the spouses and will be on the lookout for connections between the present marital relationship and patterns in the past. For example, maybe the husband had a critical mother and learned to deal with her by withdrawing inward and avoiding direct communication with her. Now, when his wife is critical of him, he feels like he did with his mother and copes in the same way, by withdrawing. Or a wife may have gotten generous praise and admiration from her father when she was a girl. If her father was not forthcoming with adoration, she may have pouted and sulked. Perhaps she behaves similarly with her husband, seeking his praise but pouting if she doesn't get what she feels is an appropriate response from him. Therapists who focus on the past believe that when people achieve insight into the childhood origins of their own behavior and their partners' behavior, they will learn new and more constructive strategies for dealing with each other.

Therapists who focus on the present don't deny that the past is influential. But they don't believe it is necessary to attend to the past to solve the problems of the present. Furthermore, they wonder about the accuracy of people's recall of their childhood histories. In any event, they examine couples' present behavior, emotional reactions, and thought processes to help them approach their problems more constructively.

One major approach, called *behavioral couple therapy*, focuses couples on positive actions each could take to solve their problems and promote a better relationship. These therapists have partners generate lists of actions they could take that would make the other more satisfied, they encourage partners to engage in behaviors from these lists, and they debrief any actions that are taken to be sure that partners are acknowledging each other's efforts. This strategy of focusing on positive changes is also a mainstay of clinicians who call themselves *solution-focused therapists*.

In addition to this focus on positive actions, behavioral therapists teach partners communication and problem-solving skills, such as those discussed in Chapter 14. Similar to how coaches teach athletic skills, therapists may have couples practice the skills in session, give them feedback about their performance, and then assign them exercises to do at home to enhance their communication skills.

A group of clinicians who call themselves *cognitive behavior therapists* may use all the strategies just described, but they add an emphasis on the interpretation of behavior. Will interprets Claire's lack of interest in physical affection one evening as her punishing him by withdrawing affection. In fact, her intention may not at all be to punish him; she is simply not interested in being affectionate. In this case, a cognitive behavior therapist would analyze Will's interpretations of Claire's behavior in an effort to help him understand her better and respond to her more appropriately.

Other therapists focus on the present but attend more to emotions than to cognitive interpretations. A group of clinicians who call themselves *emotionally focused couple therapists* look at the primary emotions that partners arouse in each other. For example, partners may get so distressed with each other because they feel hurt by the other or fear abandonment by the other. These therapists help partners express these primary emotions of fear and hurt rather than engaging in verbal attack of the other or withdrawal from the other. The expression of these primary emotions will often generate a positive, sympathetic response in the other that can lead to closeness and intimacy.

Researchers have studied the effectiveness of each of these approaches in couple therapy. More research has been conducted on behavioral couple therapy than on any other approach. In fact, studies conducted in the United States, Canada, Europe, Australia, and South America have consistently shown that this form of therapy helps a majority of couples, at least in the short run. Research conducted by one of us (N.J.) suggests that some couples relapse one to two years following treatment, so that only about half of the couples treated experience long-term improvement. Although less research has been done on the other approaches to couple therapy, evidence from several studies shows that cognitive behavior therapy and emotion-focused therapy also help couples.

We have developed an approach called *integrative couple therapy* that utilizes strategies similar to a number of the therapies already discussed, as well as new strategies, but focuses on emotional acceptance in relationships. This book is a description of that approach but written for couples themselves. Some preliminary research we have done, and two small studies that others have conducted, suggest that integrative couple therapy is an effective treatment, perhaps more effective than behavioral couple therapy, the most studied therapy to date. Because of our research, the National Institute of Mental Health has funded a large study of this type of therapy that we are conducting in Los Angeles and Seattle. This five-year study should provide conclusive evidence about the effectiveness of our treatment.

Who Does Couple Counseling?

There is no such thing as a couple counseling profession. Several different professions with different kinds of state licenses or certification engage in couple counseling. State licensing laws mandate what kind of professional practice a person holding the license can engage in. State certification laws mandate who can use a specific professional title.

Psychiatrists

Psychiatrists are first of all physicians. Just like their colleagues who will later become surgeons or radiologists or specialists in some other area of medicine, they go through four years of medical school, complete an internship or residency, and must pass a state licensing exam to practice medicine. Specialty training in psychiatry comes primarily during a residency in psychiatry, which happens after receiving an MD and lasts three or more years. Typically, this residency focuses on medical treatments, such as the use of drugs and hospitalization, to treat serious mental disorders such as depression and schizophrenia. Psychiatrists also learn how to consult with other physicians about patients with physical disorders that may be complicated by psychological factors. Couple therapy is usually not an important focus of their training.

Clinical Psychologists

Clinical psychologists have a PhD or PsyD (doctor of psychology) rather than an MD (doctor of medicine) degree. They go through four or more years of graduate school in psychology, where they study the assessment and treatment of psychological disorders. Their training also includes a year's internship, often in a hospital or mental health clinic, before they receive their doctorate. Prior to licensing or certification as psychologists, they must complete an additional year or more of postdoctoral training in assessment and treatment. Some exposure to couple therapy is usually a part of training, although only a small number of psychologists, such as the authors, specialize in it.

Social Workers

Social workers attend a two-year graduate program before obtaining a master's degree in social work, an MSW degree. Before becoming licensed or certified as a clinical social worker, they need two additional years of supervised training. Those social workers who specialize in psychiatric social work will learn about mental disorders and individual, group, couple, and family therapies.

Counselors

Most states have licensing or certification laws for other kinds of counselors or therapists, such as mental health counselors or marriage, family, and child counselors. These counselors usually complete two years of graduate school leading to a master's degree. Prior to certification or licensing, they usually must complete two years of internship or postgraduate supervision. The content of these graduate programs varies considerably, but those that specifically train students to become marriage, family, and child counselors naturally include special training in couple counseling.

Choosing a Couple Therapist

Which of these mental health professionals is better at couple counseling? If we assume that those who have the most overall training are best, we would choose psychiatrists. Generally, they have spent a longer time getting their education and training than any of the other professions. Furthermore, if we assume that cost and quality are related, we would also choose psychiatrists, since they are generally the most expensive. However, much of the training of psychiatrists is completely irrelevant to couple therapy, particularly if the couple's problems are not tied to physical or mental health problems. In fact, most psychiatrists have had little or no formal training in couple counseling. One could pay out a lot for very little.

If we exclude medical training and look for the professional with the largest amount of psychological training, then we will naturally choose doctorate-level psychologists. During their training, they may spend more time and effort studying human behavior than the other mental health professions. However, unless they specialized in couple or family therapy, they may not have had much experience working with couples.

If we assume that it is not the overall amount of training that matters but rather the amount of specific training in couple counseling, we might choose marriage, family, and child counselors. Although less educated overall than the doctoral mental health professions, these counselors have had special training in marital and family therapy. Furthermore, they will be less expensive than the doctorate-level providers. However, the programs that train master's-level clinicians show great differences in quality. Admissions standards tend to be lower than for doctorate-level programs. Therefore, the therapist who has a counselor license or certification may not be a better couple counselor than one with another professional identification.

Furthermore, the qualities that make a good couple therapist may have less to do with professional training and experience than with the therapist's own personal qualities. There is considerable evidence for this point in individual therapy. We recently reviewed the large research literature on training and experience in individual psychotherapy and found that it has little to do with client success. Thus clients are as likely to have a successful result of psychotherapy with a less experienced and less trained therapist than with a more experienced and more trained therapist.

We believe that couple therapy is more challenging than individual therapy simply because there are two people in the room rather than one and these two people are often adversaries. Being a good listener can take one a long way in individual therapy. Much more is required in couple therapy. Therefore, training and experience in couple therapy may make much more of a difference than training and experience in individual therapy. Nevertheless, no good research exists at this time on how training and experience in couple therapy affects the success of that therapy. The research literature on individual therapy should give us pause and make us look at factors other than simple training and experience when we choose a couple therapist.

The best couple therapist is one who has been successful with other couples. Therefore, a good place to get a referral is from friends who have been helped by couple counseling. Another good place to get a referral is from professionals, such as therapists, physicians, and ministers, who have referred people for couple therapy and gotten reports of their success. Getting in touch with professionals who can provide such referrals might mean calling a university psychology clinic or a community mental health center or the intake counselor at your health care organization. But be sure to ask whether the referring person knows couples who have been satisfied with the therapist being suggested to you. Reports of satisfied clients are still the best way to find satisfactory therapy yourself.

In choosing a therapist, remember that costs can vary widely and are not necessarily an indication of quality. Psychiatrists may charge $150 or more a session, clinical psychologists $100 or more a session, and master's-level therapists $80 or more a session. If asked, these therapists will sometimes take clients for less than their normal fee. Furthermore, your health insurance may provide some coverage of your couple therapy, particularly if you use a therapist who is employed by or who has a contract with your health care company.

Evaluating Your Couple Therapist

Just because you have carefully chosen a therapist who has been successful with other couples does not mean that this therapist will be successful with you. Even if the therapist has had 100 percent success before, if he or she cannot help you, you have not found the right therapist. The process of being a discriminating consumer does not end with the selection of a therapist. You should evaluate how your therapist affects you and your partner.

First, both of you should feel comfortable with your therapist. Being in therapy means disclosing your personal feelings, some of which may be uncomfortable or embarrassing. You certainly don't want to feel that your therapist is judging you for your feelings and positions. But more than that, you want to feel that it is easy to talk in front of your therapist, that he or she encourages open communication.

Second, both of you should feel that your therapist is an understanding ally. He or she should be neutral about your particular issues, not taking sides with you or your partner. But neutrality does not preclude understanding. Both of you should feel that your therapist understands your point of view, that he or she can see why you feel the way you do.

Third, discussions about your problems should be more constructive in therapy sessions than they have been elsewhere. You came to therapy because you avoided talking about your problems or got into destructive arguments. Unless your therapist can keep you from interrupting each other or translate your messages so you can better understand each other or refocus the discussion so it is more productive, you are not gaining anything from therapy.

The ultimate measure of success, however, is not what happens in the therapy session but what happens at home. No matter what wonderful things happen in session, if tension between the two of you does not decrease at home and satisfaction between the two of you does not increase outside of session, then therapy is a failure. Furthermore, these positive effects of therapy should not take forever. Couple therapy is not psychoanalysis. It does not take years. Most of the research on couple therapy shows that couples can improve with a dozen or so sessions. In our research, which is more extensive than any research published to date, we provide couples with a maximum of twenty-six sessions.

Improvement in your relationship, like improvement in any other important endeavor in life, is not a straight line upward. There are setbacks. Sometimes couples experience an initial "honeymoon effect" of therapy followed by some setback, as they see the problems are deeper or more complex than they first thought. However, despite some ups and downs, by ten to fifteen sessions of therapy you should experience some genuine progress. The two of you are confronting issues directly. You are able to talk about them more constructively. Even if you have a way to go, you should have a sense of progress.

If therapy isn't helping, discuss your concerns with your therapist. Perhaps the three of you can chart a more productive path. If therapy still isn't helpful, try another therapist. Couple therapy is hardly a panacea, but in the right hands, it can definitely alter relationships for the better.

YOU NEED HELP!

When does a personal problem become an interpersonal problem? Almost invariably, when one partner in a relationship has a serious personal problem, that problem intrudes on their relationship, causing conflict and sometimes preventing effective resolution of conflict.

At first Justin complained of chest pains but attributed them to indigestion. He dismissed Selena's concerns that they might be something more serious. When he started perspiring and getting nauseous, he continued to insist that it must be something he ate, but Selena insisted that he go to the emergency room. "If you won't do it for yourself," she said, "at least do it for me."

At the hospital, their deepest fears were confirmed. Justin was having a heart attack. However, because Selena had insisted he go to the emergency room, the doctors were able to intervene early and minimize the damage to his heart. He later told her, "You may have saved my life."

Selena's efforts did not end with this dramatic event. When Justin returned from the hospital, both he and Selena decided to make some dramatic lifestyle changes. He quit smoking and cut back on his drinking. They both tried to eat less fat and more fruits and vegetables. They started an exercise program. At first, Selena's enthusiasm and support for these changes was a welcome aid for Justin. She cheered him on and was sympathetic to his suffering, particularly when he gave up cigarettes. She was even tolerant of his bad moods.

But gradually Selena took on a supervisory, parental role with Justin. She monitored his diet and looked on disapprovingly when he indulged in a steak or treated himself to ice cream or cookies. She served him vegetables even when he didn't want to eat them. She reminded him when he didn't do his exercises. Concerned about his stress level, she urged him not to stay up so late.

Justin's contact with Selena created its own stresses for him. He resisted her efforts to control him, no matter how well intentioned they were. He found himself sneaking cookies when she wasn't looking. He looked forward to eating without her because it was more relaxing for him. Occasionally he lied to her about going to the gym. He felt diminished by the whole process: somehow he had gone from a competent, respected husband to an errant child.

For her part, Selena felt increasingly frustrated at Justin's lame efforts on his own behalf. Didn't he realize how close to death he had come? Did he want to bring more stress on himself and the family? Why couldn't he do what everyone agreed was healthy for him? In a moment of insight, Selena realized that she cared more about Justin's problem than he did. She had gone from helping him with his problem to taking it on as her own.

In this example, Justin is clearly the one with the health problem. It is his heart that suffered the damage. It is he who must take medication and change his lifestyle. In a marriage, however, one can rarely have a problem in isolation. His heart attack affected Selena in dramatic ways—she was faced with the possible loss of her mate or with the potential of caring for an invalid. It was almost as if their marriage had suffered a heart attack as well.

As any loving mate would, Selena tried to help Justin with his problem. But over time her help turned into pressure and control. Maybe Justin needed some of that pressure, but it created its own stress for him. And Justin's difficulties making lifestyle changes created stress for Selena. A health problem became an interpersonal problem.

With a physical health problem, it is relatively easy to sort out who has the problem, what should be done about it, and how a mate can help out with the problem. When someone in a relationship has a psychological problem, it is more difficult to make these simple distinctions. Unless the problem is extreme, partners may not even agree on whether a problem exists. A husband who suggests that his wife has a problem with depression may be met with the response that any depression on her part is only the result of his bad treatment of her. Even if both partners agree that one has a psychological problem, they may differ about what should be done about it. The wife may suggest marital therapy while the husband proposes antidepressant medication. Furthermore, they may differ on the role the "well" partner should take. Our depressed wife may want active emotional support from her husband as she struggles with depression, while he may want to avoid contact with what he sees as her "downward spiral into misery." In each of these situations, whatever personal problem exists can rapidly become an interpersonal problem. Furthermore, the personal problem may have had its genesis, in part, in the relationship.

If your partner has a serious personal problem, how can you avoid rejecting your partner for having the problem and abandoning your partner to deal with it on his or her own without taking on the problem as your own? If you can navigate these difficult waters, you will not only help your partner with his or her problem, but you may increase the intimacy in your relationship. A joint struggle against an important problem can bring about greater closeness.

It is beyond the scope of this book to deal specifically with all the possible psychological problems that a partner can have, or even to deal specifically with the most common of these psychological problems, such as anxiety, depression, alcohol and drug problems, and sexual dysfunction. Each of these problems is complicated on its own and can impose specific challenges on an intimate relationship. What we can do here is offer some general guidelines, based on the principles of this book, for dealing with a partner who has a psychological disorder.

Think of Your Partner's Difficulties as a Psychological Problem or Disorder, Not as a Character Flaw

It is relatively easy to handle a partner's physical problems. If your husband is injured in an accident or has a bona fide illness, you feel genuine concern and sympathy for him. If your wife needs surgery, you gladly visit her in the hospital. You don't begrudge your partner time away from responsibilities but instead take on some of your partner's share of the load while he or she cannot handle it.

Emotional and behavioral difficulties are harder to handle. You may believe your partner brought an emotional problem on himself and thus is responsible. You may suspect your partner of malingering out of laziness. You may view emotional difficulties, such as anxiety or depression, as a personal weakness, an inadequacy in handling life's stresses. You may fear your partner is manipulating you emotionally.

Behavioral difficulties, even more than emotional difficulties, may suggest character flaws. People may not be responsible for their emotions, but they certainly are responsible for their behavior. An alcohol abuser makes a decision to drink; he or she is not forced to do so. Because behavioral problems such as alcohol and drug abuse involve such clearly voluntary behavior, it may seem inappropriate to dignify them by calling them psychological disorders. Doesn't that allow your partner to escape responsibility for his or her behavior?

Not at all. Viewing your partner as having a psychological disorder does not absolve your partner of responsibility or rob her of the choice to take care of or not to take care of this disorder. Just as cancer victims make the choice to seek treatment even when the treatment is painful and scary, people with alcohol or gambling problems can seek and cooperate in difficult treatment.

There are many good reasons for us to think of emotional and behavioral problems as psychological disorders rather than as character flaws. First, an abundance of evidence suggests a genetic vulnerability to almost all of the psychological disorders. Anxiety, depression, and alcoholism are not flaws in something as nebulous as character; they are complicated products of biological and environmental factors over which we may have little control.

Second, if emotional and behavioral problems are accepted as psychological problems, some of the shame and blame associated with them can be dispelled. Rather than propelling them toward change, the shame and guilt that many people feel over depression or alcohol abuse may sink them more deeply into their problems. When self-blame is echoed by blame from family and friends, a downward spiral can easily occur.

Third, people can admit that they have a disorder more easily than they can admit that they are bad, inadequate, or failures as people. Coming to the realization that they have a drinking or gambling problem or a problem with depression is often the first major step for people with a psychological disorder. This step, no matter how difficult, is usually easier if the admission doesn't destroy their dignity.

Finally, viewing emotional and behavioral problems as disorders makes it easier to seek help for them. There are specific treatments for psychological disorders. Concrete steps can be taken to seek those treatments: making an appointment, participating in an evaluation, going to a meeting. It is unclear how to treat character flaws, a failure of will, an inadequate personality, or failure as a person.

You may find it easier to think of your partner's problem as a psychological disorder if you learn more about the disorder. The Appendix lists resources for several common psychological disorders that may be a starting point in your search for more information about a particular disorder. However, disorders always occur in unique human beings. If you want to know more about your partner's problems, you will need to talk and listen to him or her.

Talk about the Problem

Sometimes psychological problems are the elephant in the room that no one discusses. A husband rarely discusses his wife's difficulty in leaving the house because of her anxiety; nor does she. A wife notices but doesn't mention the quantity of alcohol her husband consumes each day; neither does he. The spouse with the problem may deny the seriousness of the condition; the partner may be afraid to bring it up.

Other couples may discuss the problems of one partner frequently but unproductively. A husband complains of his wife's drug problems, but she dismisses or ignores his complaints. A wife complains about her husband's complete disinterest in sex, but he passively tunes out her concerns.

If you have a partner with a serious psychological disorder, you may suggest that your partner seek treatment, you may even apply pressure in that direction. Yet your recommendations, especially if they are based on some readings about the problem, may come across as domineering advice from self-designated "experts." Or your recommendations may carry an accusatory subtext: "You are so bad you need a psychiatrist." Your advice may come out of your own frustration and carry the message "You are impossible for me to deal with; maybe the professionals can deal with you." These recommendations reflect your own needs and not your partner's needs: "I don't want to have to deal with this anymore. Go to a professional." These recommendations are often personally rejecting: "Take your problems elsewhere."

It is hardly surprising when a partner reacts negatively to recommendations that contain these messages. Your partner may argue with you, reject your calls for treatment, or criticize you in return. He may resist your suggestions, simply because you made them. Your recommendations for treatment can then prevent your partner from seeking it or at least delay it.

It is best to talk to your partner about her problem when you are not frustrated by it. When you are not upset, you can approach your partner with concern; your message is less likely to have overtones of accusation. Also, it is usually better to talk about your partner's problem when she is not angry with you. For then she is less likely to anticipate accusation and more likely to hear your concern. Finally, it is usually best not to mention treatment right away. Your partner will need to admit to his problem before he will be willing to seek treatment for it. If he is defensive about his problems, it may take considerable constructive talk before he can face the possibility of treatment.

You Cannot Control Your Partner's Emotions or Behavior

A special kind of pain comes when we see those we love do damaging things to themselves. We watch an alcoholic partner take the first drink, knowing what will follow. We watch a depressed partner berate himself relentlessly. Usually these actions not only bring us vicarious pain but affect us directly as well. We are embarrassed by our partners' drinking binges and clean up after them. We fear that the downward spiral of depression may lead to a job loss. We want to stop this self-destructive emotion and behavior, for their sake as well as our own. We cannot sit by helplessly and watch. So we try to control their destructive behavior. We may pressure a depressed partner to get out of bed and try to enjoy the day. We may remind an alcoholic partner not to drink at a party. We may try to distract an anxious partner.

If the problem is serious, it is unlikely that these prompts and reminders will have much impact. We may become more of a nagging partner than a helpful one. As we see the failure of our efforts to control our partners, we can get angry. We complain about their destructive behavior. We criticize them for their problem.

In our foiled efforts to help our partners by controlling their behavior, we may inadvertently contribute to their difficulties. There is considerable research on how family members respond to a spouse or child with a serious emotional disorder. Criticism, hostility, and even overinvolvement in the patient's life and problems have consistently been shown to have negative effects on the patient. For example, Jill Hooley, a psychologist at Harvard University, examined relapse in depressed patients. She and her colleagues followed depressed patients after they were released from the hospital and looked at what predicts whether their depression would return. Those patients whose spouses had critical and hostile attitudes toward them were most likely to relapse. In fact, in one study, the response of depressed patients to the question "How critical is your spouse of you?" was the best predictor of relapse—better than the overall marital satisfaction of the couple and better than another variable previously shown to predict depression, and even better than these two variables combined!

It may be difficult to accept that you cannot control your partner's destructive emotions and behavior. You have, however, some power to control yourself. To give up some of your fruitless efforts to try to control your partner, you may need to take better care of yourself.

Take Care of Yourself

Some emotional and behavioral problems in your partner can present threats to your own safety and security as well as to your partner's. A focus on taking care of yourself, even if you can't take care of your partner, is essential. You may not be able to prevent your partner from driving under the influence of alcohol or drugs, but you can refuse to ride along. You may not be able to prevent your partner from gambling, but you can take steps to protect your money and perhaps the family money.

Even in less dramatic circumstances, you may need to take better care of yourself. Dealing with a partner who has a serious anxiety disorder or a serious depression can be demanding. Your life can become focused on his needs to the exclusion of your own. You take over his responsibilities because he has such difficulty with them. Your antennas are precisely tuned to his emotional state, so you detect his mood changes even before he does. As your life becomes restricted by his demands, you naturally feel resentful toward him and criticize him for depressed and anxious behavior. This criticism may then exacerbate your partner's own difficulties with anxiety or depression and create tension between the two of you. Furthermore, you may feel guilt along with your resentment, because you see your partner's struggle. This is another example of the effort to cope with an initial problem creating an additional, reactive problem.

By not losing yourself in your efforts to help your partner, by taking care of your own needs as well as hers, you may have to face some disappointment, possibly even anger, from your partner. However, you may limit your own resentment and guilt and be able to be more energetic and supportive toward your partner. By taking care of yourself, you may also be better able to take care of your partner.

Seek Professional Help

Psychological disorders usually require professional assistance. Once your partner has admitted to a serious psychological problem, you may be able to assist with obtaining treatment. In fact, it may be helpful if you participate in treatment. Sex therapy is best done with both partners. Some treatments for substance problems, such as alcoholism, involve both partners. Marital therapy is a useful treatment for depression when one partner suffers from depression and marital problems exist as well. Even if you don't participate in the treatment itself, you can support your partner's efforts in treatment.

Some of the suggestions we made about finding couple therapy are applicable to individual therapy. Contact friends and professionals to find a mental health professional who specializes in the disorder and who has successfully treated the disorder. Your partner needs to feel comfortable with the therapist and confident in him or her. The therapist should practice a treatment that has scientific evidence to support it. For example, of the psychological treatments, behavior therapy and cognitive behavior therapy have proven effective with both anxiety and depressive disorders. Interpersonal psychotherapy has also been proven effective for depression. There are also medications that are effective for depression and anxiety, particularly for depression. Don't be afraid to ask your therapist about the scientific evidence in support of the treatment he or she is to provide or to ask for readings about the treatment.

It Could Be Me

We have discussed individual psychological disorders that affect your partner. Of course, one of these disorders could affect you, not your partner. In that case, your openness and willingness to examine yourself will help not only you but also your relationship. It also may enable your partner to assist you more actively.

RECAP

Despite your best efforts, you may be faced with relationship problems that you are unable to resolve. You may need couple therapy to improve your relationship. Dozens of studies done throughout the world have shown that therapy can help couples improve their satisfaction with each other. Couple therapy is certainly no panacea for relationship problems: some couples are not helped, and others relapse after treatment. But therapy can help a majority of couples resolve their problems and improve their relationship.

A psychological disorder in your partner, such as depression or alcoholism, presents problems for both of you. In the worst of all cases, the relationship problems contribute to the individual psychological disorder and the disorder contributes to the relationship problems. In the best of all cases, the relationship can support and even heal the individual problems of your partner, contributing to a greater intimacy between you. If you both are able to discuss the problem constructively, you can join forces to face the problem together rather than letting it alienate you. You can seek professional help and use that help effectively.

Internet Resources

AUTHORS' WEB SITES

Andrew Christensen, PhD
   www.psych.ucla.edu/faculty/christen

Neil S. Jacobson, PhD
   http://depts.washington.edu/ccrstaff

PROFESSIONAL ORGANIZATIONS

The Web sites of the major professional organizations that deal with mental health issues provide information on the particular profession, provide assistance with getting a therapist, and provide information on mental health problems.

American Association for Marriage and Family Therapy
   www.aamft.org/

Association for Advancement of Behavior Therapy
   www.aabt.org/aabt

American Psychological Association
   www.apa.org/

American Psychiatric Association
   www.psych.org/

National Association of Social Workers
   www.naswdc.org/

RESOURCES FOR MENTAL DISORDERS

We have listed several sites where information on some of the most common mental disorders, which were mentioned briefly in Chapter 17, can be found.

National Institute of Mental Health
www.nimh.nih.gov/

National Institute on Alcoholism Abuse and Alcoholism
www.niaaa.nih.gov/

National Institute on Drug Abuse
www.nida.nih.gov/

Anxiety Disorder Association of America
www.adaa.org/

Bibliography

CHAPTER 2

Karney, B. R., & Bradbury, T. N. (1995). The longitudinal course of marital quality and stability: A review of theory, methods, and research. *Psychological Bulletin, 118,* 3–34.

Peterson, D. R. (1979). Assessing interpersonal relationships by means of interaction records. *Behavioral Assessment, 1,* 221–236.

CHAPTER 3

Huston, T. L., & Houts, R. M. (1998). The psychological infrastructure of courtship and marriage: The role of personality and compatibility in romantic relationships. In T. N. Bradbury (Ed.), *The developmental course of marital dysfunction* (pp. 114–151). New York: Cambridge.

Milgram, S. (1963). Behavioral study of obedience. *Journal of Abnormal and Social Psychology, 67*(4), 371–378.

McGue, M., & Lykken, D. T. (1992). Genetic influence on risk of divorce. *Psychological Science, 3,* 368–373.

Pope, H., & Mueller, C. W. (1976). The intergenerational transmission of marital instability: Comparisons by race and sex. *Journal of Social Issues, 32,* 49–66.

Widom, C. S. (1989). Does violence beget violence?: A critical examination of the literature. *Psychological Bulletin, 106,* 3–28.

CHAPTER 4

Biernat, M., & Wortman, C. B. (1991). Sharing of home responsibilities between professionally employed women and their husbands. *Journal of Personality and Social Psychology, 60,* 844–860.

CHAPTER 5

Levinger, G. (1983). Development and change. In H. Kelley, E. Berscheid, A. Christensen, J. Harvey, J. Huston, G. Levinger, E. McClintock, L. Peplau, & D. Peterson, *Close relationships* (pp. 397–448). San Francisco: Freeman.

CHAPTER 6

Kleck, R. E., & Strenta, A. (1980). Perceptions of the impact of negatively valued physical characteristics on social interaction. *Journal of Personality and Social Psychology, 39,* 861–873.

Langer, E. J., & Rodin, J. (1976). The effects of choice and enhanced personal responsibility for the aged: A field experiment in an institutional setting. Journal *of Personality and Social Psychology, 34,* 191–198.

CHAPTER 12

Christensen, A., Sullaway, M., & King, C. C. (1983). Systematic error in behavioral reports of dyadic interaction: Egocentric bias and content effects. *Behavioral Assessment, 5,* 129–140.

CHAPTER 15

Goodman, G., & Esterly, G. (1988). *The talk book: The intimate science of communication in close relationships.* Emmaus, PA: Rodale Press.

CHAPTER 16

Barling, J., O'Leary, K. D., Jouriles, E. N., Vivian, D., & MacEven, K. E. (1987). Factor similarity of the Conflict Tactics Scale across samples, spouses, and sites: Issues and implications. *Journal of Family Violence, 2,* 37–54.

Evans, P. (1992). *The verbally abusive relationship: How to recognize it and how to respond.* Holbrook, MA: Bob Adams.

Gagnon, J. H., Michael, R. T., Laumann, E. O., & Kolata, G. (1994). *Sex in America: A definitive survey.* Boston: Little, Brown.

Jacobson, N. S., & Gottman, J. (1998). *When men batter women: New insights into ending abusive relationships.* New York: Simon & Schuster.

Lawson, A. (1988). *Adultery.* New York: Basic Books.

NiCarthy, G. (1986). *Getting free: You can end abuse and take back your life.* Seattle: Seal Press.

O'Leary, K. D., Vivian, D., & Malone, J. (1992). Assessment of physical aggression against women in marriage: The need for multimodal assessment. *Behavioral Assessment 14,* 5–14.

Straus, M. A., & Gelles, R. J. (1986). Societal change and change in family violence from 1975 to 1985 as revealed in two national surveys. *Journal of Marriage and the Family, 48,* 465–479.

CHAPTER 17

Christensen, A., & Jacobson, N. S. (1994). Who (or what) can do psychotherapy: The status and challenge of nonprofessional therapies. *Psychological Science, 5,* 8–14.

Halford, W. K., & Bouma, R. (1997). Individual psychopathology and marital distress. In W. K. Halford & H. J. Markman (Eds.), *Clinical handbook of marriage and couple intervention* (pp. 291–321). New York: Wiley.

Hooley, J. M., & Teasdale, J. D. (1989). Predictors of relapse in unipolar depressives: Expressed emotion, marital distress, and perceived criticism. *Journal of Abnormal Psychology, 98,* 229–235.

Index

About the Authors

ANDREW CHRISTENSEN, PHD, is a professor in the Department of Psychology at the University of California, Los Angeles. He has published widely on couple conflict and couple therapy. He is coauthor of *Close Relationships* (1983). More recently, he coauthored *Acceptance and Change in Couple Therapy: A Therapist's Guide for Transforming Relationships* (1996) with Neil S. Jacobson. His therapy approach and research have been cited in *Newsweek, Time, U.S. News & World Report, USA Today,* and the *Los Angeles Times,* as well as other magazines and newspapers.

With Neil Jacobson, Dr. Christensen developed a treatment program for couples called integrative couple therapy. Currently he is directing (with Dr. Jacobson, until his recent death) a multisite study at UCLA and the University of Washington, sponsored by the National Institute of Mental Health, which compares integrative couple therapy with traditional behavioral couple therapy. This is the largest study to date of the effectiveness of marital therapy. The current book is a couples' guide to their approach.

NEIL S. JACOBSON, PHD, was a professor of psychology at the University of Washington until his death in 1999. One of the most widely cited family therapists in the world, he was author of 200 articles and 9 books. He received awards from both the American Family Therapy Academy and the American Association for Marriage and Family Therapy (AAMFT) for his cumulative, distinguished, and lifetime contributions to family therapy research. He also received MERIT and Research Scientist Awards from the National Institutes of Health for his seminal and prolific contributions to mental health research. Dr. Jacobson was a past president of the Association for Advancement of Behavior Therapy, and was designated Master Lecturer by the AAMFT.